AMBULANCE CARE

Clinical Skills

Printing History

This edition first published in 2022. Reprinted in 2023.

The authors and publishers welcome feedback from readers of this book. Please contact the publisher:

Class Professional Publishing

The Exchange, Express Park, Bristol Road, Bridgwater TA6 4RR

Telephone: 01278 427800

Email: info@class.co.uk

www.classprofessional.co.uk

Class Professional Publishing is an imprint of Class Publishing Ltd

A CIP catalogue record for this book is available from the British Library

Paperback ISBN: 9781801610346

ePub ISBN: 9781801610353

ePDF ISBN: 9781801610469

Cover design by Nicky Boroweic

Designed and typeset by S4Carlisle Publishing Services

Printed in the UK by Hobbs

This book is printed on disposable paper from responsible sources. Refer to local recycling guidance on disposal of this book.

FSC www.fsc.org MIX Paper from responsible sources FSC® C020438

WORLD LAND TRUST™ www.carbonbalancedprint.com CBP2250

AMBULANCE CARE
Clinical Skills

Richard Pilbery
and
Kris Lethbridge

CLASS
PROFESSIONAL
PUBLISHING

Contents

Disclaimer

The details in this book are presented for information purposes only. Some procedures included in the book may lie outside the reader's scope of practice and therefore anyone using the book must ensure they have the appropriate knowledge and skills to enable suitable interpretation. Paramedics and healthcare professionals should always follow local procedures and be aware of their own scope of practice.

Ambulance services may not adopt the exact same equipment shown within the text and therefore any equipment shown is for example purposes only. The information contained herein with regards to providers or equipment does not constitute endorsement or recommendation.

About the Authors

Richard Pilbery FCPara is a Research Paramedic employed by Yorkshire Ambulance Service NHS Trust and Associate Lecturer at Sheffield Hallam University. Richard is a co-author of *Ambulance Care Practice, Ambulance Care Essentials, First Responder Care Essentials*, and *Casualty Care for Fire and Rescue*, as well as *Paramedic Case Studies*.

Kris Lethbridge MCPara is a Critical Care Paramedic working for Cornwall Air Ambulance and as a practitioner in the critical care unit at Royal Cornwall Hospital. He is also co-author of *Ambulance Care Practice, Ambulance Care Essentials, First Responder Care Essentials,* and *Casualty Care for Fire and Rescue.*

Acknowledgements

Class Professional Publishing would like to thank the following for their co-operation in the production of *Ambulance Care Clinical Skills*:

- Paul Maskell, Vicky Pilbery, James Short, Peter Williams, the students at Coventry University and the University of Gloucester, and the teams at SWAST, WMS and YAS for modelling
- Charles L. Till and colleagues at Coventry University for the use of their facilities and equipment
- Martin Hilliard and colleagues at the University of Gloucestershire for the use of their facilities and equipment
- Cornwall Air Ambulance for the use of their facilities and equipment
- Tasnim Ali at YAS for sourcing volunteers for photoshoots
- Nigel Wilson for photography work
- Ferno, Reflex Medical, Safeguard Medical, SP Services, University of the West of England and Zoll for the loan of equipment

We would like to thank the following for their invaluable feedback on earlier drafts of the Ambulance Care series:

- The National Education Network of Ambulance Services (NENAS) for their contribution to the development of the text throughout
- Sinead Blanchette, West Midlands Ambulance Service
- John Ellison, West Midlands Ambulance Service
- Claire Gedge, South Central Ambulance Service
- Gary Heaps, North West Ambulance Service
- Clive James, St John Ambulance
- Stephen Jeffries, West Midlands Ambulance Service
- Steve Knowles, South West Ambulance Service
- Jim Lewis, St John Ambulance
- Sid Marshall, South Central Ambulance Service
- Clare McGonigle, South Central Ambulance Service
- Ken Morgan, North West Ambulance Service
- Carol Offer, North West Ambulance Service
- Julian Rhodes, Medicare EMS
- Lizzie Ryan, South West Ambulance Service Trust
- Rob Slee, University of Greenwich
- Allan Sunderland, East of England Ambulance Service
- Sam Taylor, University of Hertfordshire
- Ken Wheeler
- Trevor West, East Midlands Ambulance Service
- Mike Hoolihan, South Central Ambulance Service
- All anonymous reviewers for their insight and support.

We would like to thank the following for their kind permission to publish material contained herein:

- Chapter 8 Alcohol Handrub Procedure. Based on the 'How to Handrub' poster © World Health Organization 2009. All rights reserved
- Chapter 8 Handwashing Procedure. Based on the 'How to Handwash' poster © World Health Organization 2009. All rights reserved

The following images are the photography work of Kris Lethbridge:

- Chapter 3: Needle Thoracentesis, Step 2 (p. 135)
- Chapter 4: Intravenous Cannulation, Step 16 (p. 180)
- Chapter 5: Inhalers (pp. 135–211); Infusion (pp. 213–217); Drawing Up an Ampoule, Step 8 (p. 220); Nebuliser (pp. 226–228); Reconstituting Medications, Step 5 (p. 231); Intranasal (pp. 244–246)
- Chapter 6: Cervical Collar (pp. 296–298) and Figure 6.1 (p. 295)
- Chapter 7: LUCAS Chest Compression (pp. 376–381)
- Chapter 8: Donning PPE for Standard Infection Prevention Control (pp. 399–402); Donning PPE for AGPs (pp. 403–406); Doffing PPE for Standard Infection Prevention Control (pp. 407–411); Doffing PPE for AGPs (pp. 413–416).

Every effort has been made to secure permission to reproduce copyright images. If any have been inadvertently overlooked, the copyright holders are invited to contact Class Professional Publishing and the omission will be rectified in the next printing as well as all further editions.

Introduction

Clinical skills are a fundamental part of any clinician's practice, regardless of their seniority or role. Developing these skills can take time and significant experience before they are mastered. The highly variable nature of prehospital practice means there are a great number of skills that must be learnt and that, when required, need to be performed proficiently in potentially challenging and stressful situations. Being familiar with the steps required to complete a skill, as well as understanding the rationale for why procedures should be done a certain way, will help you optimally perform potentially life-saving interventions when the time comes, even if they may be infrequently required in practice (applying an arterial tourniquet, for example).

This text has been created to support the development and maintenance of skills required by prehospital practitioners in a wide variety of roles. Detailed steps for each procedure have been outlined to support the initial acquisition of the skill; for most steps, a rationale has also been provided, so not only can you learn **how** to perform a skill appropriately, but also understand **why** each step is undertaken. In our experience of prehospital education and training, the 'why' is often omitted from learning, but understanding the rationale is fundamental, not least of all so that when you encounter a situation where circumstances dictate a need to deviate from the normal procedure, you can understand the implications of doing so.

In writing this text, we have sought out evidence to support the rationale for why procedures should be performed in certain ways, although this has highlighted the lack of evidence for many procedures. Where evidence is lacking we have drawn on our own experience, as well as seeking expert feedback from others, to determine the current perceived 'best way' to perform that procedure. As evidence grows and evolves, it may become evident that there are better ways to undertake the skills included, and we will endeavour to keep pace with this evidence in future editions. We are also always open to feedback and advice from readers who can contribute to improving the procedures contained within.

A clinician's scope of practice will be determined by their role, experience, and the clinical governance arrangements put in place by their employer or governing agency supporting them to provide clinical care within the role they are currently deployed. We have not set out to create a definitive list of procedures within this text for any specific role or organisation; instead we have selected skills which we believe will benefit from detailed explanation to support practitioners who may be called upon to undertake such interventions.

We hope that both students and experienced practitioners alike will find this text a valuable resource for learning and maintaining the skills which are core to their role, and would encourage all practitioners to regularly refresh their knowledge, particularly for those skills which may not be carried out as frequently in practice. While we believe that the information contained within will be a valuable tool to support skill maintenance, this does not negate the need for regular hands-on practice. This book should be read in partnership with regular physical practice of skills so that you are ready when the day comes that they are needed.

Chapter

1 Patient Assessment

The key to every patient encounter is a good patient assessment. Management decisions hinge on them, so it is important that they are undertaken competently. Many of the skills in this chapter do not even require specialist equipment, but all can affect which treatment or management plan is implemented. If patient assessment is not undertaken properly, for example poor ECG electrode placement (1) or inaccurate estimation of respiratory rate (2), then patient harm can result (3).

References

1. Gregory P, Lodge S, Kilner T, et al. Accuracy of ECG chest electrode placements by paramedics: an observational study. *British Paramedic Journal*. 2019 Dec 1;4(3):51–52.
2. Rimbi M, Dunsmuir D, Ansermino JM, et al. Respiratory rates observed over 15 and 30 s compared with rates measured over 60s: practice-based evidence from an observational study of acutely ill adult medical patients during hospital admission. *QJM: An International Journal of Medicine*. 2019 Jul 1;112(7):513–517.
3. Johansson H, Lundgren K, Hagiwara MA. Reasons for bias in ambulance clinicians' assessments of non-conveyed patients: a mixed-methods study. *BMC Emergency Medicine*. 2022 May 6;22(1):79.

Respiratory Rate

Indications

- Any patient requiring a physiological assessment.
- Before and after the administration of medication that might alter respiratory function, for example beta-2 agonist drugs, opiates and benzodiazepines (1).

Contraindications

- Prior to correction of a life-threatening airway/breathing/circulation (ABC) problem, for example occluded airway, tension pneumothorax or exsanguinating haemorrhage.
- Suspected cardiac arrest.

Advantages

- Respiratory rate can provide an early warning of severe illness (1).
- A routine observation to assess patient physiology.

Disadvantages

- Does not provide indication of efficacy of either oxygenation or ventilation.

Procedure – Respiratory Rate Measurement

Take the following steps to record a respiratory rate:

Action		Rationale
1.	Do not inform the patient you are intending to record their respiratory rate.	While typically you should obtain consent from patients, if they know you are recording their respiration, it is likely that they will become aware of their own respiratory rate with the potential for altering it (2).
2.	Don appropriate personal protective equipment (PPE), if required.	This reduces the risk of cross-infection (3).
3.	If possible, position the patient so their chest is clearly visible and not obscured by baggy clothing.	In order to record respirations accurately, it is necessary to have a clear view of the chest (2). Note that this might not always be possible, particularly for patients in respiratory distress, who may adopt a position which aides their breathing but makes respiratory-rate calculation difficult. On the other hand, excessive chest wall movement due to increased work of breathing may actually make counting a respiratory rate easier.

Action		Rationale
4.	Using a watch or clock with a second hand, or a timer, count the respiratory rate for a full minute. This can be achieved by watching the rise and fall of the chest, or by using an alternative method such as capnography (4,5) or an oxygen mask with an integrated respiratory rate indicator (6).	Counting for 60 seconds is the safest time period to ensure accurate recording of respiratory rate, particularly when determining early warning scores (7).
5.	Document the respiratory rate.	You must keep full, clear and accurate records for everyone you care for, treat, or provide other services to (8).

References

1. Loughlin PC, Sebat F, Kellett JG. Respiratory rate: the forgotten vital sign – make it count! *Joint Commission Journal on Quality and Patient Safety*. 2018 Aug;44(8):494–499.
2. Hill A, Kelly E, Horswill MS, et al. The effects of awareness and count duration on adult respiratory rate measurements: an experimental study. *Journal of Clinical Nursing*. 2018;27(3–4):546–554.
3. NHS England, NHS Improvement. Standard infection control precautions: national hand hygiene and personal protective equipment policy [Internet]. 2019 [cited 2021 Nov 11]. Available from: https://www.england.nhs.uk/publication/standard-infection-control-precautionsnational-hand-hygiene-and-personal-protectiveequipment-policy/.
4. Gaucher A, Frasca D, Mimoz O, et al. Accuracy of respiratory rate monitoring by capnometry using the Capnomask® in extubated patients receiving supplemental oxygen after surgery. *British Journal of Anaesthesia*. 2012 Feb 1;108(2):316–320.
5. Galka S, Berrell J, Fezai R, et al. Accuracy of student paramedics when measuring adult respiratory rate: a pilot study. *Australasian Journal of Paramedicine* [Internet]. 2019 Apr 17 [cited 2020 Jun 10];16. Available from: https://ajp.paramedics.org/index.php/ajp/article/view/566.
6. Breakell A. The clinical evaluation of the Respi-check mask: a new oxygen mask incorporating a breathing indicator. *Emergency Medicine Journal*. 2001 Sep 1;18(5):366–369.
7. Rimbi M, Dunsmuir D, Ansermino JM, et al. Respiratory rates observed over 15 and 30 s compared with rates measured over 60s: practice-based evidence from an observational study of acutely ill adult medical patients during hospital admission. *QJM: An International Journal of Medicine*. 2019 Jul 1;112(7):513–517.
8. Health and Care Professions Council. Standards of conduct, performance and ethics [Internet]. 2018 [cited 2019 Dec 29]. Available from: https://www.hcpc-uk.org/standards/standards-of-conduct-performance-and-ethics/.

Peak Flow

Indications

- Assess severity of bronchospasm in conditions such as asthma.
- Assess patient response to treatment, for example bronchodilators.

Contraindications

- Pre-school-aged children or patients with severe learning difficulties who cannot correctly perform the procedure (1).

Caution

- Can aggravate symptoms during severe life-threatening asthma exacerbations.

Advantages

- Simple, objective measurement.
- Patients with asthma often have their own peak flow meter.

Disadvantages

- Normal values chart less useful in patients with severe disease.

Procedure – Record a Peak Flow

Take the following steps to record a peak flow (2):

Action		Rationale
1.	Explain the procedure and obtain consent if appropriate to do so.	You must make sure that you have valid consent from service users or other appropriate authority before you provide care, treatment or other services (3,4).
	Ask if they know what their normal or best peak flow value is.	You can use the predicted value chart (see **Figure 1.1**), but a comparison with the patient's normal value is better.
2.	Don appropriate personal protective equipment (PPE), and undertake appropriate hand hygiene.	This reduces the risk of cross-infection (5).
3.	Insert the mouthpiece into the meter (these are single-patient use). 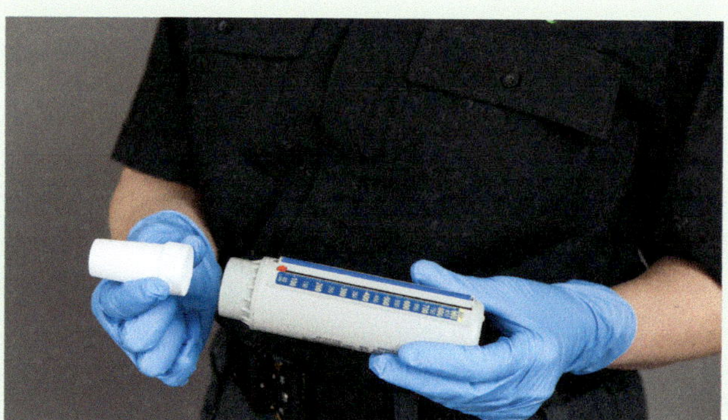	

Action		Rationale
4.	Ask the patient to hold the peak flow meter with their fingers clear of the scale and slot. Ensure that the holes at the end of the meter are not blocked. 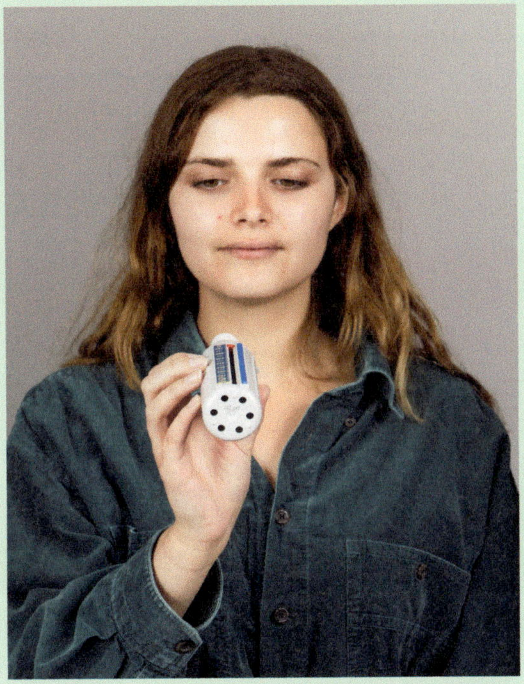	This helps to ensure an accurate peak flow reading.
5.	With the patient in a standing, or upright sitting, position, ask them to take a deep breath. Advise them not to flex their neck. 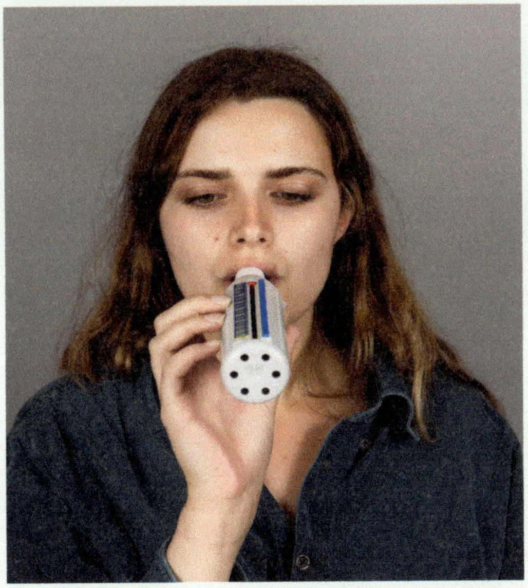	This position helps to maximise available lung volume. Flexing the neck will increase airflow resistance.

Action		Rationale
6.	Ask them to place the peak flow meter in their mouth and hold horizontally, closing their lips around the mouthpiece before blowing as hard and fast as they can. This should be a short, sharp 'huff'. 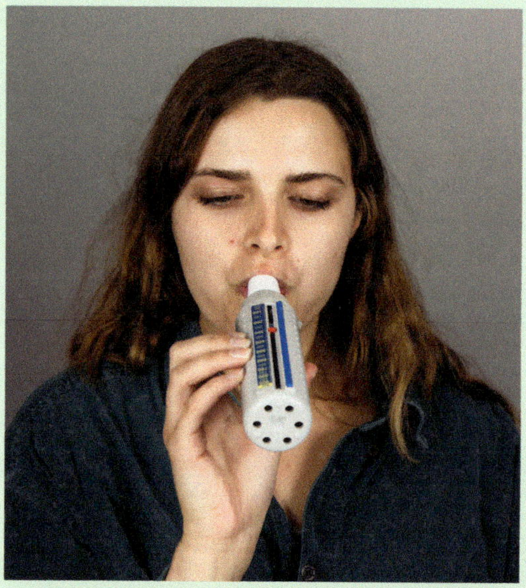	Patients should not hold their breath at maximum inspiration for more than a couple of seconds, so do not delay moving to this step from step 5. This is a forceful exhalation lasting about one second. This will ensure that it is the 'peak' flow being measured.
7.	Note the value on the scale indicated by the pointer. 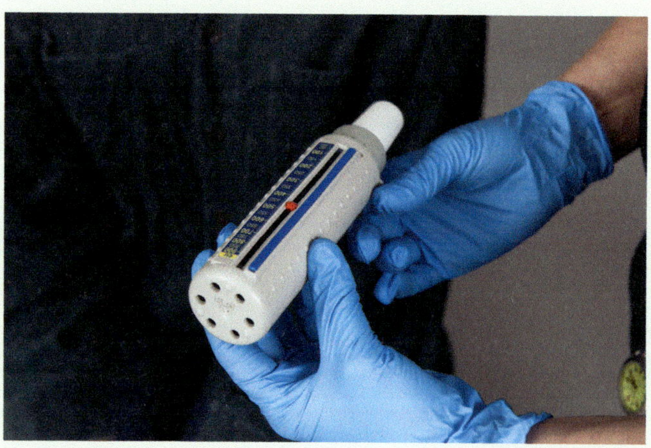	

	Action	Rationale
8.	Return the pointer to zero and repeat steps 4–7 twice to obtain three readings. The three values should be similar. 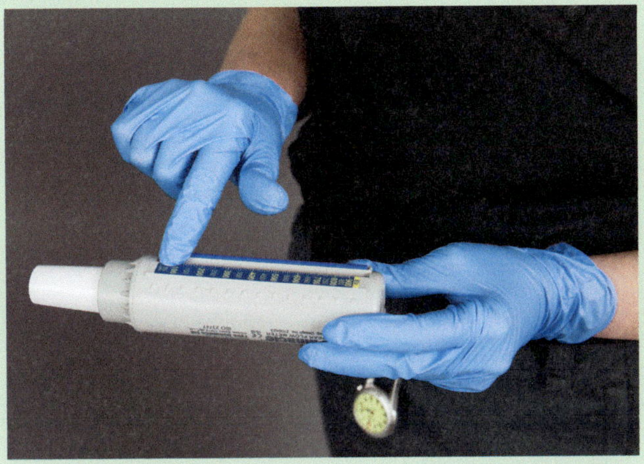	This will help mitigate incorrect readings due to poor technique or poor effort on one or more attempts (6).
9.	Document the highest value from the three readings. 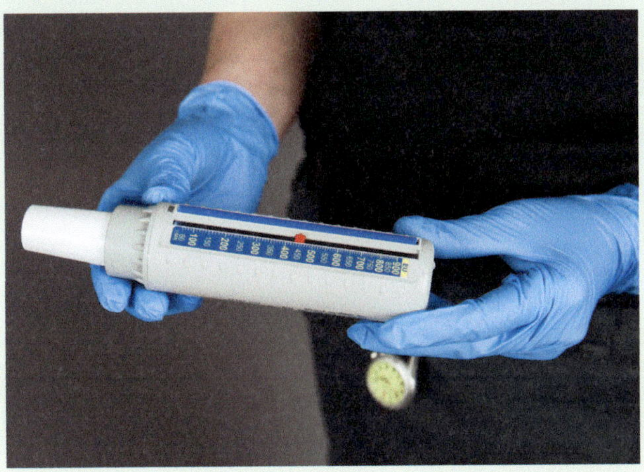	You must keep full, clear and accurate records for everyone you care for, treat, or provide other services to (4).

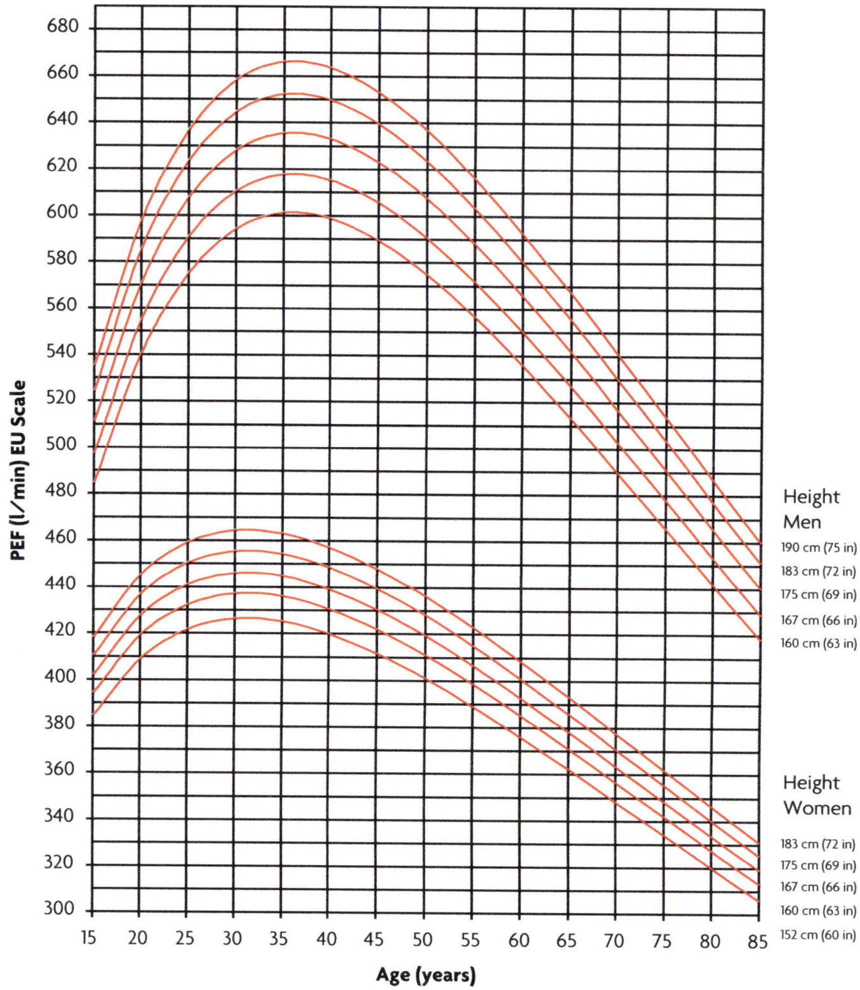

Figure 1.1 Normal peak flow values.

Source: Adapted by Clement Clarke for use with EN13826/EU scale peak flow meters from Nunn AJ and Gregg I. New regression equations for predicting peak expiratory flow in adults. *British Medical Journal*. 1989;298:1068–1070.

References

1. Joint Royal Colleges Ambulance Liaison Committee, Association of Ambulance Chief Executives. JRCALC Clinical Guidelines. Cited from JRCALC Plus (Version 1.2.13) [Mobile application software]. Bridgwater: Class Publishing Ltd; 2021.
2. Clement Clarke International. *Mini-Wright Peak Flow Meter Instructions for Use*. Edinburgh: Clement Clarke International; 2017.
3. British Medical Association. General information [Internet]. 2018 [cited 2019 Dec 29]. Available from: https://www.bma.org.uk/advice/employment/ethics/consent/consent-tool-kit/2-general-information.
4. Health and Care Professions Council. Standards of conduct, performance and ethics [Internet]. 2018 [cited 2019 Dec 29]. Available from: https://www.hcpc-uk.org/standards/.standards-of-conduct-performance-and-ethics/
5. NHS England, NHS Improvement. Standard infection control precautions: national hand hygiene and personal protective equipment policy [Internet]. 2019 [cited 2021 Nov 11]. Available from: https://www.england.nhs.uk/publication/standard-infection-control-precautions-national-hand-hygiene-and-personal-protective-equipment-policy/.
6. DeVrieze BW, Modi P, Giwa AO. Peak flow rate measurement [Internet]. StatPearls Publishing, Treasure Island (FL); 2020. Available from: http://europepmc.org/abstract/MED/29083754.

Pulse Oximetry

Indications

- As part of a cardiovascular or respiratory assessment of a patient.
- Titration of oxygen delivery.

Contraindications

- None.

Caution

- Pulse oximeters do not instantaneously reflect changes in blood oxygenation (1).
- Can give false values in the presence of carboxyhaemoglobin and methaemoglobinaemia.
- Using probes in different anatomical areas or age groups than specified can result in significant measurement errors.

Advantages

- Non-invasive and easy to measure.
- Can assist in accurate titration of oxygen.
- Provides an estimate of arterial oxygenation.

Disadvantages

- Not as accurate as invasive methods of measuring oxygenation.
- Does not provide sufficient information about adequacy of ventilation.
- Can give erroneous readings in cases of carbon monoxide poisoning (2) and methaemoglobinaemia (3), in the presence of poor peripheral perfusion, nail varnish, and during excessive motion (4,5).

Procedure – Record Oxygen Saturations with Pulse Oximetry

Take the following steps to record a patient's oxygen saturations with pulse oximetry (6):

Action		Rationale
1.	Explain the procedure and obtain consent if appropriate to do so.	You must make sure that you have valid consent from service users or other appropriate authority before you provide care, treatment or other services (7,8).
2.	Don appropriate personal protective equipment (PPE), and undertake appropriate hand hygiene.	This reduces the risk of cross-infection (9).
3.	Turn the pulse oximeter on. 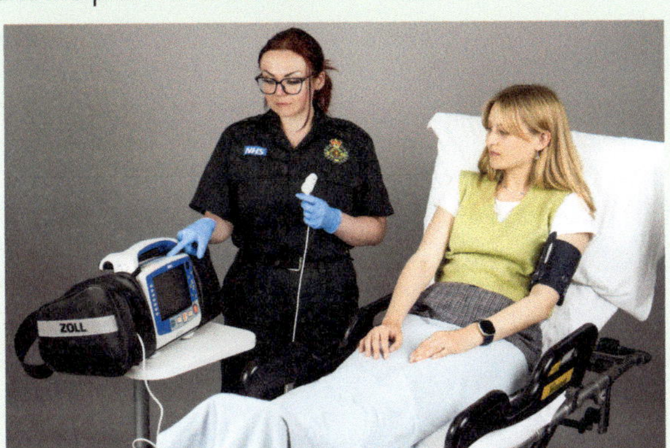	

Action		Rationale
4.	Select the appropriate probe with particular attention to correct sizing and where it will go (usually the finger, toe or ear). If used on a finger or toe, make sure the area is clean. Do not place probes designed for adults on babies or finger probes on ears, and vice versa.	Correct sizing and avoidance of excessive pressure will help obtain an accurate reading. Probes attached too tightly can lead to detection of venous pulsations and venous oxygen saturation presented as arterial blood oxygen saturation (SpO_2) (2). Using probes in different anatomical areas or age groups than specified can result in significant measurement errors (up to 50% lower or 30% higher) (10,11).
	If present, consider removing nail varnish or rotating the probe by 90°.	Some dark-coloured nail varnish can affect the accuracy of pulse oximeters. However, if a consistent reading is obtained throughout, then this is probably accurate (12,13). Rotating the probe can alleviate this.
5.	Connect the probe to the pulse oximeter.	
6.	Position the probe securely and, if possible, avoid the arm being used for blood pressure monitoring. 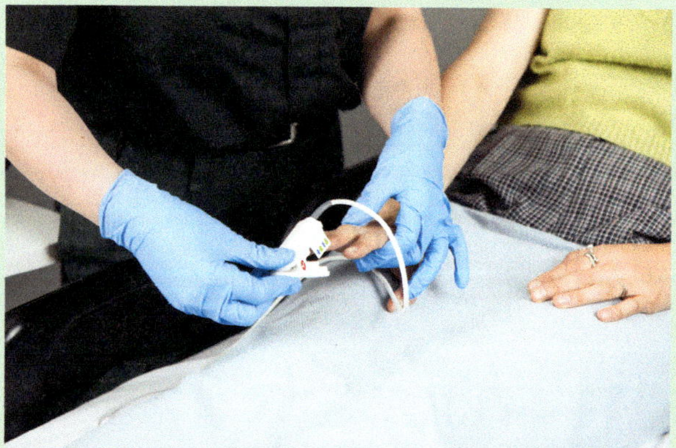	Cuff inflation will interrupt the pulse oximeter signal.

Action		Rationale
7.	Allow several seconds for the pulse oximeter to detect the pulse and calculate the oxygen saturation. Look for the displayed pulse indicator or waveform to indicate that the device has detected the pulse reliably. In addition, if your device can measure the perfusion index (PI), this should be above the manufacturer's minimum (1.0 for the X-Series (14)). If it is not, try another finger or limb. 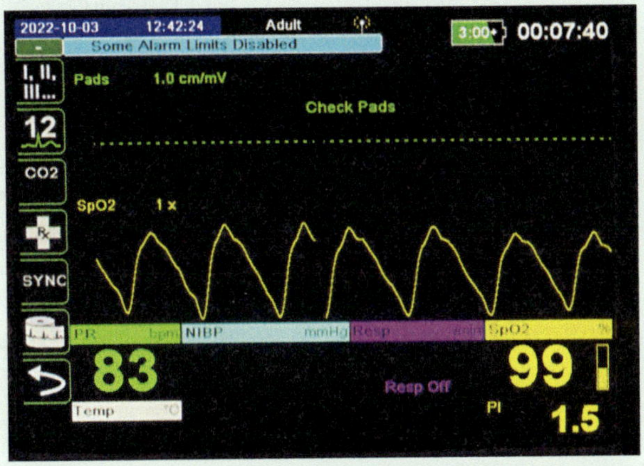	Without these signs, any readings may not be reliable (2,6).
8.	Once the unit has detected a good pulse, the oxygen saturation and pulse rate will be displayed. Like all machines, oximeters may occasionally give a false reading – if in doubt, rely on clinical judgement rather than the machine (15). You can check the pulse oximeter is working properly by placing it on your own finger (6).	
9.	Document your findings.	You must keep full, clear and accurate records for everyone you care for, treat, or provide other services to (8).

References

1. Aguilar SA, Davis DP. Latency of pulse oximetry signal with use of digital probes associated with inappropriate extubation during prehospital rapid sequence intubation in head injury patients: case examples. *Journal of Emergency Medicine*. 2012 Apr 1;42(4):424–428.
2. Chan ED, Chan MM, Chan MM. Pulse oximetry: understanding its basic principles facilitates appreciation of its limitations. *Respiratory Medicine*. 2013 Jun;107(6):789–799.
3. Barker SJ, Curry J, Redford D, et al. Measurement of carboxyhemoglobin and methemoglobin by pulse oximetry. *Anesthesiology*. 2006 Nov 1;105(5): 892–897.
4. Clarke GWJ, Chan ADC, Adler A. Effects of motion artifact on the blood oxygen saturation estimate in pulse oximetry. In: 2014 IEEE International Symposium on Medical Measurements and Applications (MeMeA). 2014. pp. 1–4.

5. O'Driscoll BR et al. BTS guideline for oxygen use in adults in healthcare and emergency settings. *Thorax*. 2017 Jun;72(Suppl 1):ii1–ii90.
6. World Health Organization. Pulse oximetry training manual [Internet]. 2011 [cited 2020 Jun 20]. Available from: https://cdn.who.int/media/docs/default-source/patient-safety/pulse-oximetry/who-ps-pulse-oxymetry-training-manual-en.pdf?sfvrsn=322cb7ae_6.
7. British Medical Association. General information [Internet]. 2018 [cited 2019 Dec 29]. Available from: https://www.bma.org.uk/advice/employment/ethics/consent/consent-tool-kit/2-general-information.
8. Health and Care Professions Council. Standards of conduct, performance and ethics [Internet]. 2018 [cited 2019 Dec 29]. Available from: https://www.hcpc-uk.org/standards/standards-of-conduct-performance-and-ethics/.
9. NHS England, NHS Improvement. Standard infection control precautions: national hand hygiene and personal protective equipment policy [Internet]. 2019 [cited 2021 Nov 11]. Available from: https://www.england.nhs.uk/publication/standard-infection-control-precautionsnational-hand-hygiene-and-personal-protectiveequipment-policy/.
10. NHS Improvement. Risk of harm from inappropriate placement of pulse oximeter probes [Internet]. 2018 [cited 2020 Jul 3]. Available from: https://improvement.nhs.uk/documents/3603/Patient_Safety_Alert_-_Placement_of_oximetry_probes_FINAL.pdf.
11. Johnson CL, Anderson MA, Hill PD. Comparison of pulse oximetry measures in a healthy population. *MEDSURG Nursing*. 2012 Apr;21(2):70–75; quiz 76.
12. Chan MM, Chan MM, Chan ED. What is the effect of fingernail polish on pulse oximetry? *Chest*. 2003 Jun;123(6):2163–2164.
13. Hinkelbein J et al. Effect of nail polish on oxygen saturation determined by pulse oximetry in critically ill patients. *Resuscitation*. 2007 Jan 1;72(1):82–91.
14. Zoll. X Series® Operator's guide. 2019 [cited 2022 Jun 9]. Available from: https://www.zoll.com/-/media/public-site/products/x-series/9650-003355/9650-003355-05-sf_c.ashx.
15. Yönt GH, Korhan EA, Khorshid L. Comparison of oxygen saturation values and measurement times by pulse oximetry in various parts of the body. *Applied Nursing Research*. 2011 Nov;24(4):e39–43.

Pulse Measurement

Indications
- As part of initial assessment to determine whether the patient is in cardiac arrest.
- Routine cardiovascular physiological assessment.

Contraindications
- None.

Advantages
- Gives early indication of the adequacy of cardiac output.
- Greater accuracy when estimating the rate of irregular heart rhythms than electronic devices (if count conducted over 60 seconds).

Disadvantages
- Requires physical contact with the patient and the use of one hand, making other simultaneous activities difficult.
- Can take up to 60 seconds to perform accurately.

Procedure – Record a Pulse

Take the following steps to record a pulse:

Action		Rationale
1.	Explain the procedure and obtain consent if appropriate to do so.	You must make sure that you have valid consent from service users or other appropriate authority before you provide care, treatment or other services (1,2).
2.	Don appropriate personal protective equipment (PPE), and undertake appropriate hand hygiene.	This reduces the risk of cross-infection (3).
3.	Place your index and middle fingers (and your ring finger, optionally) along the artery and press gently. As a general rule for adults, palpate the radial pulse first in conscious patients and the carotid pulse first in unconscious patients. 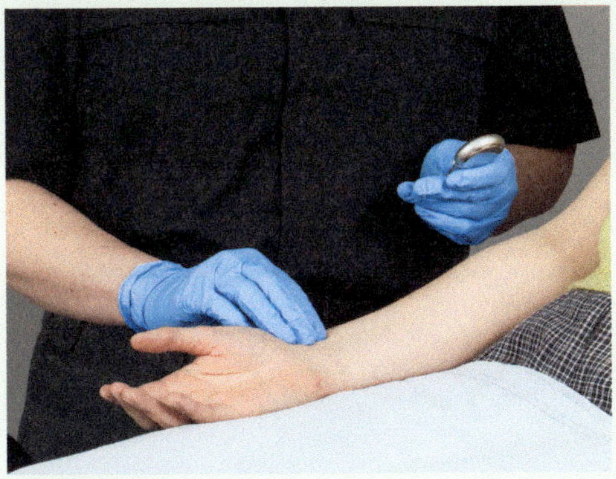	Avoid using your thumb as the arteries run along the palmar surface and may be palpable (4). Do not push too hard, or you will occlude the artery. Palpating a pulse at the wrist is less threatening than moving your hand towards the patient's neck! In unconscious patients, who may have a low BP, you will want to ascertain whether they have a pulse or not, and the carotid artery is generally the best place to determine this (although the femoral artery is also used).

Action		Rationale
	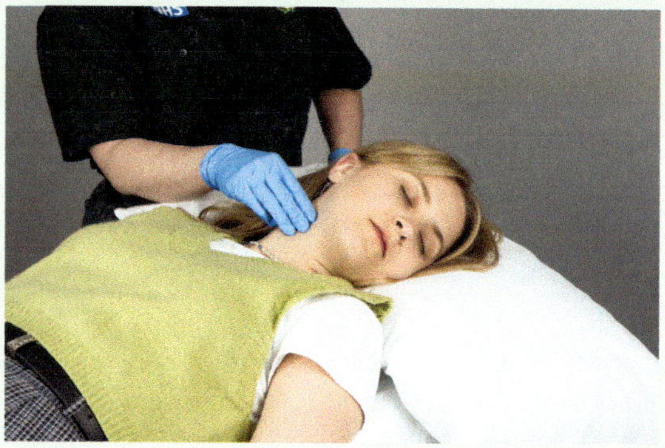	A patient who does not have a radial pulse but does have a carotid pulse is likely to have poor peripheral perfusion. However, it is not possible to accurately determine systolic blood pressure (BP) from the absence or presence of pulses (5,6).
4.	If the pulse has a regular rhythm, count for 15 seconds and then multiply by four. If the pulse is very fast or slow or irregular, then count for a full 60 seconds.	Counting for 60 seconds is most accurate but may not always be practical to achieve. Counting for 15 seconds will probably not result in a clinically important error, but expect an error of up to 5 beats per minute (bpm) in this case (7). Note: If you suspect a cardiac arrest, then pulse checks should be conducted for no more than 10 seconds (8).
5.	Document the procedure.	You must keep full, clear and accurate records for everyone you care for, treat, or provide other services to (2).

References

1. British Medical Association. General information [Internet]. 2018 [cited 2019 Dec 29]. Available from: https://www.bma.org.uk/advice/employment/ethics/consent/consent-tool-kit/2-general-information.
2. Health and Care Professions Council. Standards of conduct, performance and ethics [Internet]. 2018 [cited 2019 Dec 29]. Available from: https://www.hcpc-uk.org/standards/standards-of-conduct-performance-and-ethics/.
3. NHS England, NHS Improvement. Standard infection control precautions: national hand hygiene and personal protective equipment policy [Internet]. 2019 [cited 2021 Nov 11]. Available from: https://www.england.nhs.uk/publication/standard-infection-control-precautions-national-hand-hygiene-and-personal-protective-equipment-policy/.
4. Miletin J, Sukop A, Baca V, et al. Arterial supply of the thumb: systemic review: arterial supply of the thumb. *Clinical Anatomy*. 2017 Oct;30(7):963–973.
5. Naylor JF, Fisher AD, April MD, et al. An analysis of radial pulse strength to recorded blood pressure in the Department of Defense Trauma Registry. *Military Medicine*. 2020 Nov 1;185(11–12):e1903–1907.
6. Deakin CD, Low JL. Accuracy of the advanced trauma life support guidelines for predicting systolic blood pressure using carotid, femoral, and radial pulses: observational study. *BMJ*. 2000 Sep 16;321(7262):673–674.
7. Kobayashi H. Effect of measurement duration on accuracy of pulse-counting. *Ergonomics*. 2013 Dec;56(12):1940–1944.
8. Resuscitation Council (UK). *Advanced Life Support*. London: Resuscitation Council (UK); 2021.

Capillary Refill Time Measurement

Indications

- Part of the circulatory assessment of a patient.
- Suspicion of dehydration.
- Assessment of response to treatment.

Contraindications

- Very sick children where distress may lead to decline of current condition, for example life-threatening asthma.
- Low-ambient light makes accurate assessment diffcult (1).

Advantages

- Does not require equipment to perform.
- Provides some measure of circulatory adequacy when blood pressure measurement is not possible.

Disadvantages

- Sick infants or children can have a normal capillary refill time (CRT) (2).
- Does not predict mild-to-moderate hypotension in adults (3) and its usefulness in adults has been questioned (4).
- Accuracy affected by ambient temperature and light, the site and poor inter-observer agreement.

Procedure – Capillary Refill Time Measurement

Take the following steps to measure the CRT:

Action		Rationale
1.	Explain the procedure to the patient and the patient's caregiver (depending on age) and obtain consent if appropriate to do so.	You must make sure that you have valid consent from service users or other appropriate authority before you provide care, treatment or other services (5,6).
2.	Don appropriate personal protective equipment (PPE), and undertake appropriate hand hygiene.	This reduces the risk of cross-infection (7).
3.	Ensure the environment is warm and well lit. Choose one person to record all CRT measurements.	Cool or cold skin and poor lighting affect the accuracy of CRT measurement, as does having multiple clinicians recording CRT (1).

	Action	Rationale
4.	Select either the upper part of the sternum (manubrium) or the fingertip pulp as the site for measurement. Site-specific advice: • Sternum: Place your index finger on the patient's manubrium. • Fingertip: Place the fingertip pulp between your thumb and index finger and hold the hand at the level of the patient's heart (8). 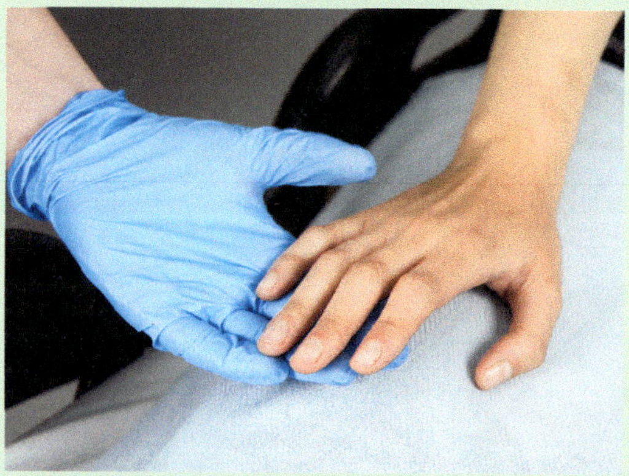	The sternum is generally a convenient site for children, and recording a CRT in small fingers can be a challenge. However, sternal CRT is difficult to assess in patients with darker skin tone (9). There is poor correlation between sternal and fingertip CRT, so do not use them interchangeably (9).
5.	Provide sufficient pressure to make the tip of your nail blanch (turn pale) (10). Press for 5 seconds. 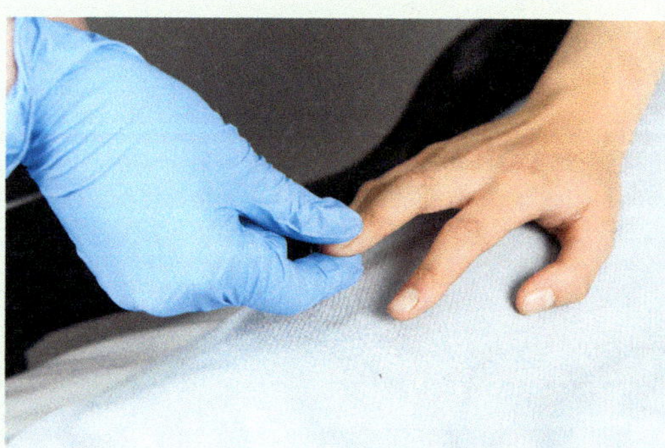	There is no universal agreement about the time pressure should be applied for, but 5 seconds is commonly reported (8–12).

Action		Rationale
6.	Remove the pressure and immediately count aloud how long it takes for the skin to return back to the pre-test colour. 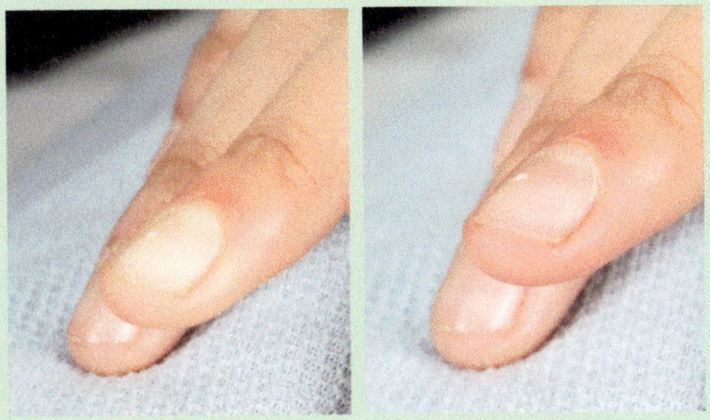	The time in seconds will be the patient's CRT.
7.	Consider repeating steps 4–5 and then average the results.	This may improve the accuracy of the result (10).
8.	Document the procedure. A normal CRT is 2–3 seconds. A CRT of more than 3 seconds in a child is clinically important (2).	You must keep full, clear and accurate records for everyone you care for, treat, or provide other services to (6).

References

1. Resuscitation Council UK. *European Paediatric Advanced Life Support*. 5th edition. London: RC(UK); 2021.
2. Fleming S, Gill P, Jones C, et al. The diagnostic value of capillary refill time for detecting serious illness in children: a systematic review and meta-analysis. *PLoS ONE* [Internet]. 2015 Sep 16 [cited 2020 May 3];10(9). Available from: https://www.ncbi.nlm.nih.gov/pmc/articles/PMC4573516/.
3. Pickard A, Karlen W, Ansermino JM. Capillary Refill time: is it still a useful clinical sign? *Anesthesia & Analgesia*. 2011 Jul;113(1):120–123.
4. Lewin J, Maconochie I. Capillary refill time in adults. *Emergency Medical Journal*. 2008 Jan 6;25(6): 325–326.
5. British Medical Association. General information [Internet]. 2018 [cited 2019 Dec 29]. Available from: https://www.bma.org.uk/advice/employment/ethics/consent/consent-tool-kit/2-general-information.
6. Health and Care Professions Council. Standards of conduct, performance and ethics [Internet]. 2018 [cited 2019 Dec 29]. Available from: https://www.hcpc-uk.org/standards/standards-of-conduct-performance-and-ethics/.
7. NHS England, NHS Improvement. Standard infection control precautions: national hand hygiene and personal protective equipment policy [Internet]. 2019 [cited 2021 Nov 11]. Available from: https://www.england.nhs.uk/publication/standard-infection-control-precautions-nationalhand-hygiene-and-personal-protective-equipmentpolicy/.
8. Alsma J, van Saase JLCM, Nanayakkara PWB, et al. The power of flash mob research. *Chest*. 2017 May;151(5):1106–1113.
9. Crook J, Taylor RM. The agreement of fingertip and sternum capillary refill time in children. *Archives of Disease in Childhood*. 2013 Jan 4;98(4):265–268.
10. Ait-Oufella H, Bige N, Boelle PY, et al. Capillary refill time exploration during septic shock. *Intensive Care Medicine*. 2014 May 9;1–7.
11. Anderson B, Kelly A-M, Kerr D, et al. Impact of patient and environmental factors on capillary refill time in adults. *American Journal of Emergency Medicine*. 2008 Jan;26(1):62–65.
12. Skellett S, Hampshire S, Bingham R, et al. *European Paediatric Advanced Life Support*. 4th edition. London: RC(UK); 2016.

Blood Pressure

Blood pressure (BP) is the measurement of the pressure by the blood on the walls of a blood vessel. It is highest in the aorta and large systemic arteries (1).

The BP that you record consists of two measurements:

- **Systolic BP:** The BP during the systole phase of the cardiac cycle, when the ventricles contract and blood is forced out of the heart. This is the higher reading of BP.
- **Diastolic BP:** The BP during the diastole phase of the cardiac cycle, when the ventricles are relaxed. This is the lower reading of BP.

It is usually measured in millimetres of mercury (mmHg) and recorded as the systolic value over the diastolic, for example 120/80 mmHg.

Measurement of BP

BP can be measured directly, by inserting a sensor into a patient's artery (invasive), or indirectly using a cuff (non-invasive), which is applied to a patient's arm. The advantage of direct measurement is that it is accurate and continuous; it is typically used in hospital intensive care units. This method is not routinely available outside of hospital and so non-invasive methods are used.

Non-invasive BP (NIBP) Measurement

There are two methods of NIBP measurement used by the ambulance service:

- **Auscultatory:** This method uses a stethoscope and an aneroid sphygmomanometer, a device consisting of an inflatable cuff and an aneroid manometer to measure the pressure on a dial (**Figure 1.2**).
- **Automated:** This consists of an inflatable cuff connected to a sensor that detects the oscillations generated by turbulent blood flow and calculates systolic and diastolic values using an algorithm.

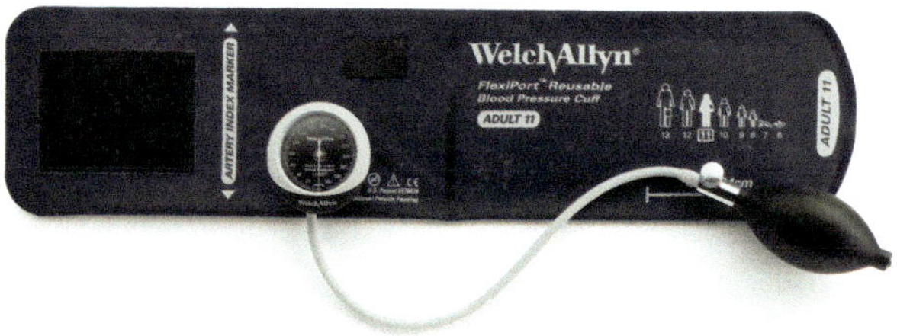

Figure 1.2 An aneroid sphygmomanometer.
Image reproduced by the kind permission of Welch Allyn.

Korotkoff Sounds

When using the auscultatory method of measuring BP, you will place a stethoscope over the patient's brachial artery and listen for turbulent blood flow, known as the Korotkoff sounds after a Russian surgeon, Nikolai Korotkoff, who first described them in 1905 (2).

The sounds are split into five phases (3):

1. The first appearance of faint, repetitive, clear tapping sounds that gradually increase in intensity for at least two consecutive beats is the systolic BP. This corresponds to the restoration of blood flow and is confirmed by the presence of a palpable pulse. This is the systolic pressure.
2. A brief period may follow during which the sounds soften and acquire a swishing quality. In some patients, sounds may disappear altogether for a short time.
3. The return of sharper sounds, which become crisper, to match or even exceed the intensity of phase 1 sounds.
4. The distinct abrupt muffling of sounds, which become soft and blowing in quality.
5. The point at which all sounds finally disappear completely is the diastolic pressure.

Note that in some groups of patients, the phase 4 sounds may be heard until the BP measurement reaches 0 mmHg. In these cases, the onset of phase 4 is taken to be the diastolic BP measurement (3).

References

1. Tortora GJ, Derrickson BH. *Principles of Anatomy and Physiology*. Hoboken: John Wiley Inc; 2017.
2. Talley NJ, O'Connor S. *Clinical Examination: A Systematic Guide to Physical Diagnosis*. 5th edition. London: Elsevier; 2006.
3. O'Brien E, Asmar R, Beilin L, et al. European Society of Hypertension recommendations for conventional, ambulatory and home blood pressure measurement. *Journal of Hypertension*. 2003;21(5):821–848.

Manual Blood Pressure Measurement

Indications
- Need to undertake a cardiovascular assessment of a patient.
- Patient showing signs of shock.
- Assessment of response to treatment.

Contraindications
- Patients who have an arteriovenous shunt should not have a BP recorded in the ipsilateral (same side of the body) arm.

Caution
- Korotkoff sounds are not reliably audible in infants under six months and in some older infants and children (1). Automated blood pressure (BP) measurement is preferable in these age groups (2).

Advantages
- Provides reliable assessment of BP in the presence of slow or irregular heart rhythms such as atrial fibrillation.
- Mechanical process (no need for electrical power).

Disadvantages
- Not as accurate as invasive BP monitoring.
- Takes time to perform with no opportunity for conducting other clinical care at the same time.

Procedure – Manual Blood Pressure Measurement

Take the following steps to manually record a BP (2,3):

Action		Rationale
1.	Explain the procedure and obtain consent if appropriate to do so.	You must make sure that you have valid consent from service users or other appropriate authority before you provide care, treatment or other services (4,5).
2.	Don appropriate personal protective equipment (PPE), and undertake appropriate hand hygiene.	This reduces the risk of cross-infection (6).

Action		Rationale
3.	If possible, allow the patient to sit for 3–5 minutes before measuring their BP, with feet flat on the floor and legs uncrossed. Ideally, the patient should have an empty bladder and have not experienced acute exposure to cold temperatures. The patient should have their back and arm supported, with the arm at the level of their heart (level with the mid-sternum). 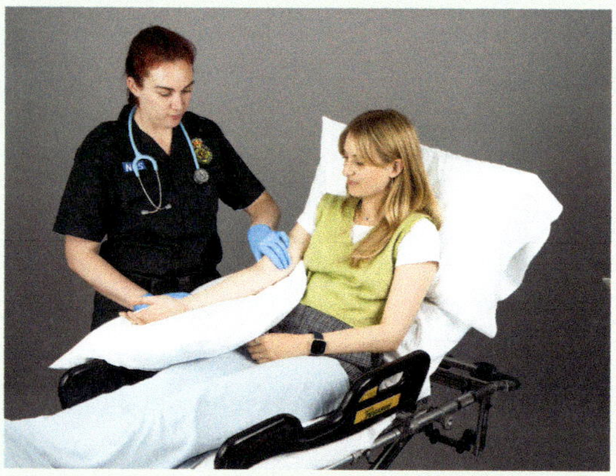	All are patient-related factors that can lead to erroneously raised BP (7). An unsupported arm, or an arm that is not level with the heart, can lead to inaccuracies of measurement (3).
4.	Ask about any medical conditions that might prevent a BP being recorded on a particular arm, such as paretic limbs, for example due to stroke, or arteriovenous shunts in dialysis patients.	Measurement in a paretic arm can lead to small but significant increases in BP readings (8). There is a risk of trauma or thrombosis as a result of checking BP in a limb with an arteriovenous shunt (9). There is no evidence that patients with, or at risk of, lymphoedema should not have their BP taken on the affected side (10,11). However, in the absence of high-quality evidence, use of the unaffected side, if possible, is advocated.
5.	Ensure the arm is free of restrictive clothing. Do not apply a cuff over clothes, if possible.	Restrictive clothing can create a tourniquet effect (12). Current guidelines advocate measurement with the cuff placed on bare skin. However, this is not supported by existing studies. Measurement over thin clothing is unlikely to result in clinically important errors (8).

Action		Rationale
6.	Palpate the brachial artery. This can be found by placing the pads of the index and middle fingers of one hand on the biceps tendon and then moving medially and pressing deeply. 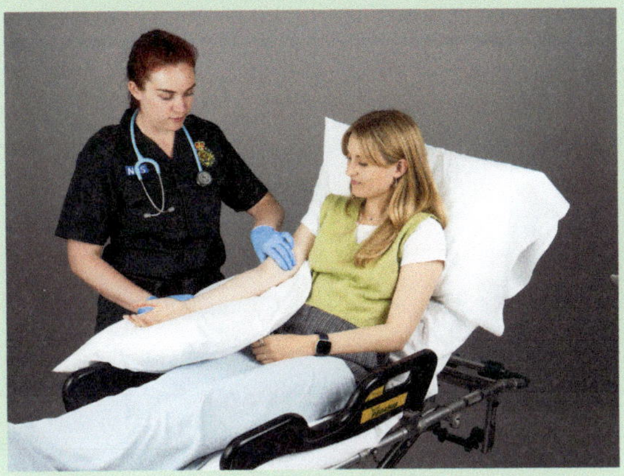	This ensures that the stethoscope will be placed in the correct position for an accurate reading (13).
7.	Select the appropriate cuff size. A standard bladder is 12–13 cm wide and 35 cm long, but ensure you have smaller and larger sizes available. 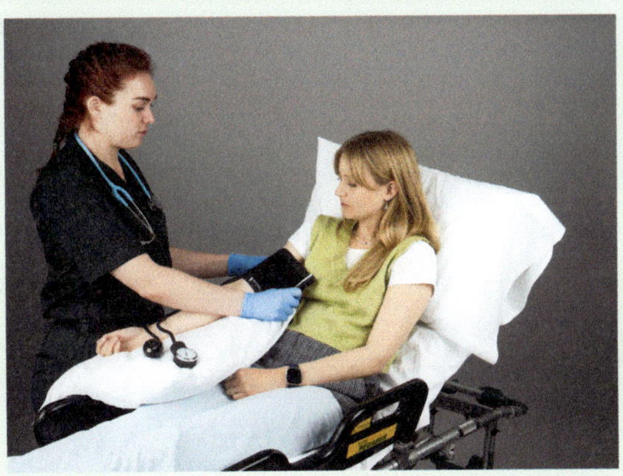	Using a cuff that is too small will result in an artificially elevated BP reading, and using a cuff that is too large will result in a reading that is artificially low (8).

	Action	Rationale
8.	Place the artery marker on the cuff over the patient's brachial artery. The artery marker should be located within the sizing markers on the cuff. 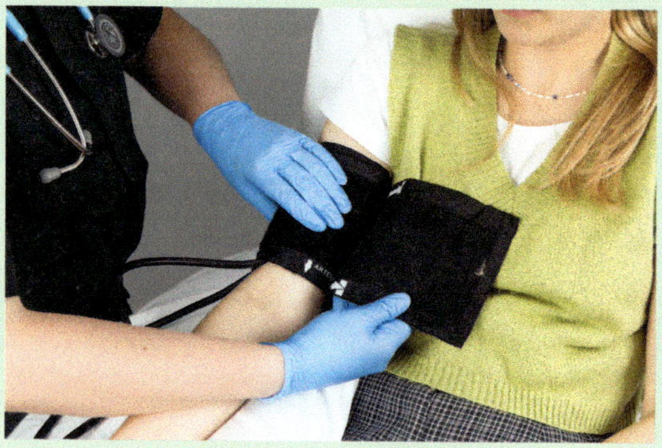	This will ensure the cuff bladder is centred over the brachial artery, providing a more accurate reading (13).
9.	Wrap the cuff snugly around the patient's upper arm, with the lower edge of the cuff 2–3 cm above the palpated brachial artery. Ensure it is clear of the antecubital fossa and does not touch the stethoscope. 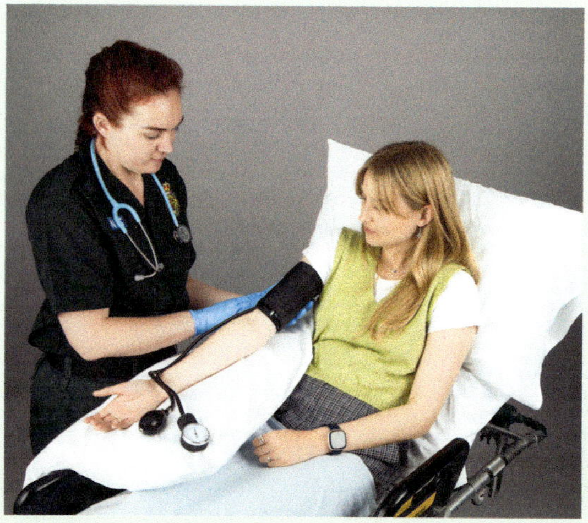	If the stethoscope is under the cuff, raised systolic and lowered diastolic BP readings will be obtained (8).
10.	Ask the patient to remain still and not talk during the BP measurement.	Talking and movement can artificially increase BP (7).

	Action	Rationale
11.	Palpate the brachial artery and inflate the cuff until the pulse disappears. Continue to inflate to 20–30 mmHg above this point. 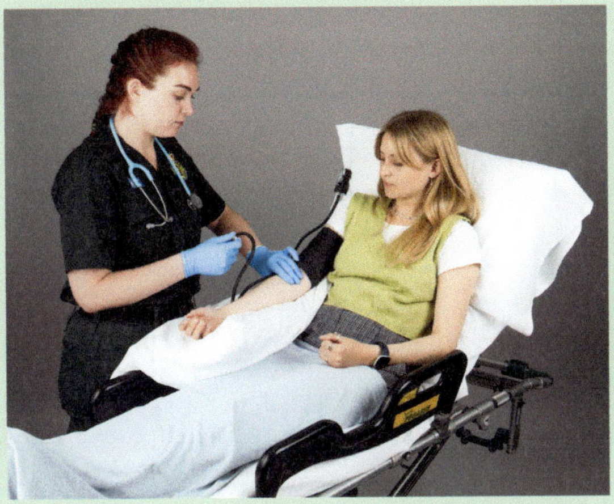	This avoids undue discomfort to the patient from excessive cuff pressure while ensuring that patients with an auscultatory gap have an accurate systolic BP reading recorded (12,14).
12.	Slowly deflate the cuff and note when the pulse returns. This gives an estimation of the systolic BP.	
13.	Wait for 30 seconds. Then put the diaphragm of the stethoscope in position. Place it firmly, but not with too much pressure, over the brachial artery. 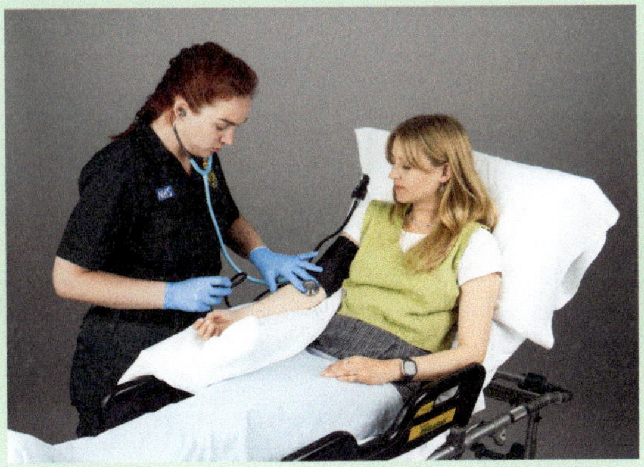	This will prevent venous congestion of the arm (2). While the bell may make the Korotkoff sounds easier to hear, the diaphragm is easier to hold in place (2). Excessive force may partially occlude the brachial artery (8).
14.	Rapidly inflate the cuff to 20–30 mmHg above your estimation of the systolic BP.	As for step 11.
15.	Deflate at a rate of 2–3 mmHg per pulse beat.	This prevents inaccurate measurement of BP (8).

Action		Rationale
16.	Note the pressure at which you first hear the Korotkoff sounds (phase 1, the systolic BP), the point at which they become muffled (phase 4) and then disappear (phase 5). The disappearance of sounds is usually taken to be the diastolic BP. If phase 5 does not occur until 0 mmHg, then the onset of phase 4 measurement should be taken as the diastolic value. 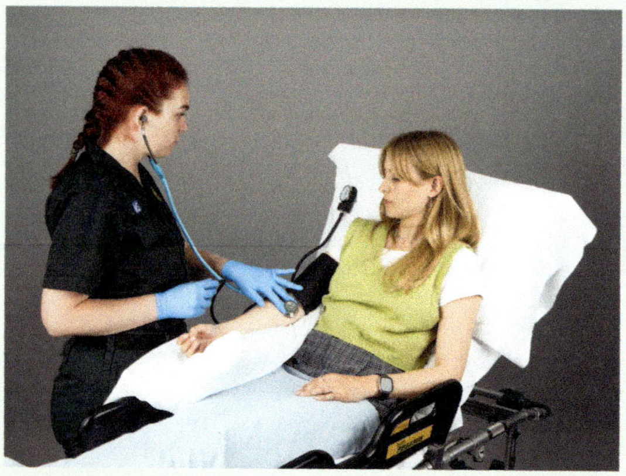	This ensures an accurate BP measurement (12).
17.	Document the BP as soon as possible, including the position of the patient and which arm the measurement was taken from, since these can affect the BP result.	Measurements may be forgotten if not documented promptly (2). You must keep full, clear and accurate records for everyone you care for, treat, or provide other services to (5).

References

1. Knecht KR, Seller JD, Alpert BS. Korotkoff sounds in neonates, infants, and toddlers. *American Journal of Cardiology*. 2009 Apr 15;103(8):1165–1167.
2. O'Brien E, Asmar R, Beilin L, et al. European Society of Hypertension recommendations for conventional, ambulatory and home blood pressure measurement. *Journal of Hypertension*. 2003;21(5):821–848.
3. Williams B, Mancia G, Spiering W, et al. 2018 ESC/ESH guidelines for the management of arterial hypertension: the Task Force for the management of arterial hypertension of the European Society of Cardiology (ESC) and the European Society of Hypertension (ESH). *European Heart Journal*. 2018 Sep 1;39(33):3021–3104.
4. British Medical Association. General information [Internet]. 2018 [cited 2019 Dec 29]. Available from: https://www.bma.org.uk/advice/employment/ethics/consent/consent-tool-kit/2-general-information.
5. Health and Care Professions Council. Standards of conduct, performance and ethics [Internet]. 2018 [cited 2019 Dec 29]. Available from: https://www.hcpc-uk.org/standards/standards-of-conduct-performance-and-ethics/.
6. NHS England, NHS Improvement. Standard infection control precautions: national hand hygiene and personal protective equipment policy [Internet]. 2019 [cited 2021 Nov 11]. Available from: https://www.england.nhs.uk/publication/standard-infection-control-precautions-nationalhand-hygiene-and-personal-protective-equipmentpolicy/.
7. Nerenberg KA, Zarnke KB, Leung AA, et al. Hypertension Canada's 2018 guidelines for diagnosis, risk assessment, prevention, and treatment of hypertension in adults and children. *Canadian Journal of Cardiology*. 2018 May 1;34(5):506–525.
8. Kallioinen N, Hill A, Horswill MS, et al. Sources of inaccuracy in the measurement of adult patients' resting

blood pressure in clinical settings: a systematic review. *Journal of Hypertension*. 2017;35(3):421–441.
9. Frese EM, Fick A, Sadowsky HS. Blood pressure measurement guidelines for physical therapists. *Cardiopulmonary Physical Therapy Journal*. 2011 Jun;22(2):5–12.
10. Asdourian MS, Swaroop MN, Sayegh HE, et al. Association between precautionary behaviors and breast cancer-related lymphedema in patients undergoing bilateral surgery. *Journal of Clinical Oncology*. 2017 Dec 10;35(35):3934–3941.
11. Cheng C-T, Deitch JM, Haines IE, et al. Do medical procedures in the arm increase the risk of lymphoedema after axillary surgery? A review. *ANZ Journal of Surgery*. 2014;84(7–8):510–514.
12. Muntner Paul, Shimbo D, Carey RM, et al. Measurement of blood pressure in humans: a scientific statement from the American Heart Association. *Hypertension*. 2019 May 1;73(5):e35–66.
13. Dougherty L, Lister S, West-Oram A. *Royal Marsden Manual of Clinical Nursing Procedures*. 9th edition. Hoboken: John Wiley & Sons Inc; 2015.
14. Reeves RA. Does This Patient Have Hypertension?: How to measure blood pressure. *Journal of American Medical Association*. 1995 Apr 19;273(15):1211.

Automated Blood Pressure Measurement

Indications

- Need for general physiological assessment of a patient.
- Patient showing signs of shock.
- To assess response to treatment.

Contraindications

- Patients who have an arteriovenous shunt should not have blood pressure (BP) recorded in the ipsilateral (same side of the body) arm.

Caution

- Some automated BP devices (for example, LifePak15 and Corpuls3) will not give an accurate reading when the patient has an irregular pulse (arrythmia) (1,2).

Advantages

- Provides reliable assessment of BP in infants under six months and in some older infants and children (3).
- Allows the clinician to undertake other tasks simultaneously.
- Unaffected by environments where there is excessive noise or lack of light.

Disadvantages

- Not as accurate as invasive BP monitoring.
- Requires batteries or external power source to function.

Procedure – Automated Blood Pressure Measurement

Generic steps to obtain an accurate automated BP are presented here. However, you should follow the manufacturer's instructions for device-specific guidance (1,2,4):

Action		Rationale
1.	Explain the procedure and obtain consent if appropriate to do so.	You must make sure that you have valid consent from service users or other appropriate authority before you provide care, treatment or other services (5,6).
2.	Don appropriate personal protective equipment (PPE), and undertake appropriate hand hygiene.	This reduces the risk of cross-infection (7).
3.	If possible, allow the patient to sit for 3–5 minutes before measuring their BP, with feet flat on the floor and legs uncrossed. Ideally, the patient should have an empty bladder and have not experienced acute exposure to cold temperatures.	All are patient-related factors that can lead to erroneously raised BP (8).
	The patient should have their back and arm supported, with the arm at the level of their heart (level with the mid-sternum).	An unsupported arm, or an arm that is not level with the heart, can lead to inaccuracies of measurement (9).

Action		Rationale
4.	Ask about any medical conditions that might prevent a BP being recorded on a particular arm, for example paretic limbs or arteriovenous shunts in dialysis patients.	Measurement in a paretic arm can lead to small but significant increases in BP readings (10). There is a risk of trauma or thrombosis as a result of checking BP in a limb with an arteriovenous shunt (11). There is no evidence that patients with, or at risk of, lymphoedema should not have their BP taken on the affected side (12,13). However, in the absence of high-quality evidence, use of the unaffected side, if possible, is advocated.
5.	Ensure the arm is free of restrictive clothing. Do not apply a cuff over clothes, if possible.	Restrictive clothing can create a tourniquet effect (14). Current guidelines advocate measurement with the cuff placed on bare skin. However, this is not supported by existing studies. Measurement over thin clothing is unlikely to result in clinically important errors (10).
6.	Select the appropriate cuff size. If the cuff has sizing range markers or lines, ensure that cuff ends between the range markings. If it doesn't, select a larger or smaller cuff. If the cuff is not fully deflated, squeeze any remaining air out of the cuff. 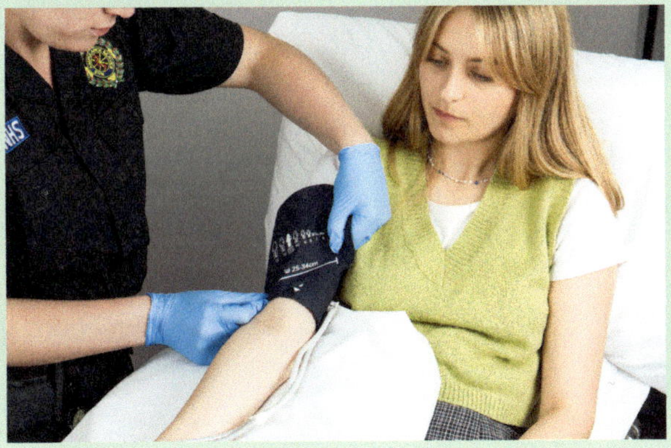	Using a cuff that is too small will result in an artificially elevated BP reading, and using a cuff that is too large will result in a reading that is artificially low (10).

Action		Rationale
7.	Connect the inflation tubing hose to the cuff and monitor. 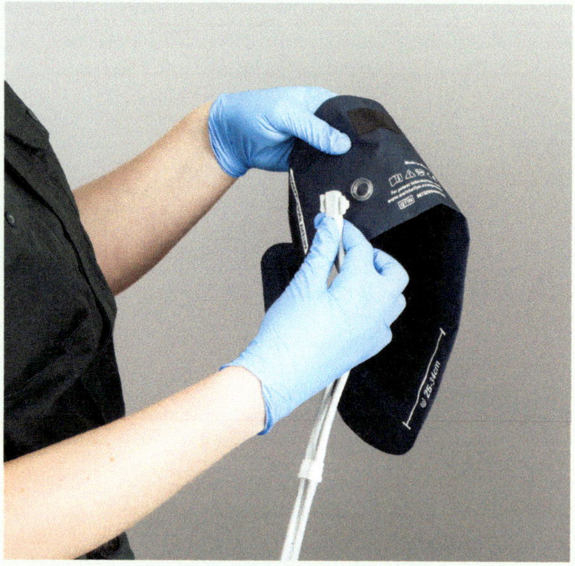	
8.	Wrap the cuff snugly around the patient's upper arm, with the lower edge of the cuff 2–3 cm above the elbow crease. If the cuff has an artery marker, this should be placed over the brachial artery with the arrow pointing towards the hand. 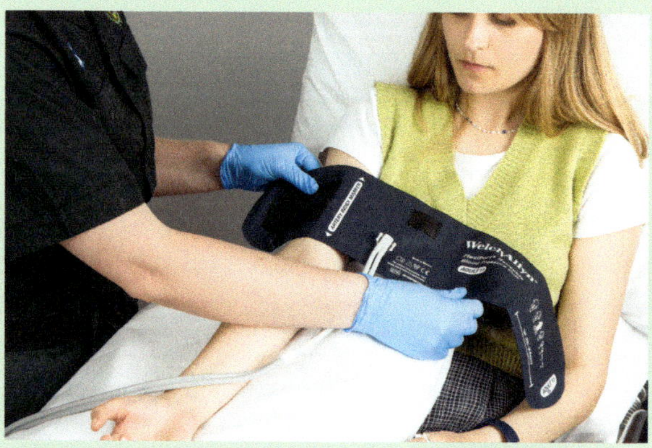	Cuffs that are too loose can result in artificially high BP readings (4).

Action		Rationale
9.	Check that the correct inflation setting has been selected. 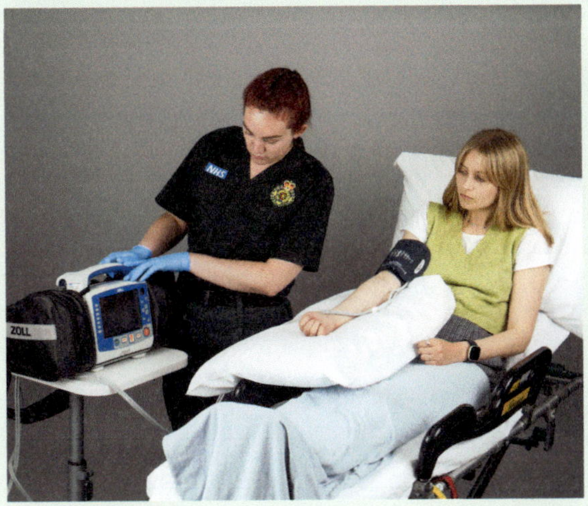	The inflation setting needs to be high enough to accurately capture the systolic BP, but not so high that it causes the patient unnecessary discomfort.
10.	Ask the patient to remain still and not talk during the BP measurement.	Talking and movement can artificially increase BP (8).
11.	Press the appropriate button on the monitor to measure the BP. 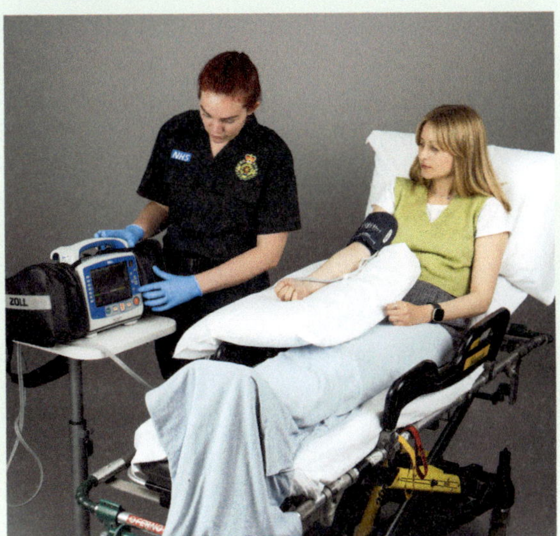	

Action		Rationale
12.	Document the BP as soon as possible, including the position of the patient, and which arm the measurement was taken from, since these can affect the BP result. 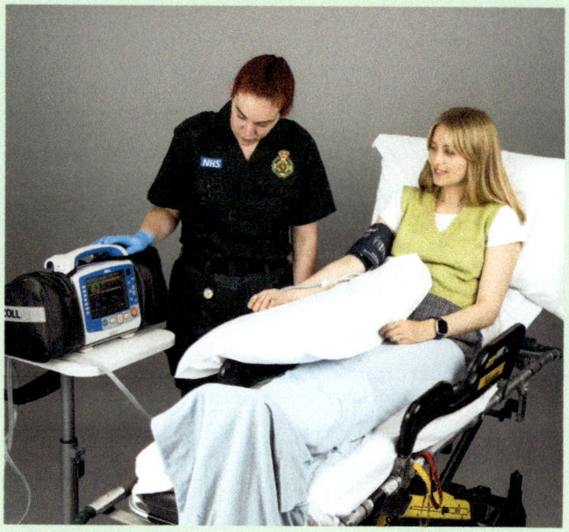	Measurements may be forgotten if not documented promptly (15). You must keep full, clear and accurate records for everyone you care for, treat, or provide other services to (6).

References

1. Physio-Control. LifePak 15 monitor/defibrillator operating instructions [Internet]. 2009 [cited 2013 Dec 20]. Available from: http://www.physio-control.com/uploadedFiles/Physio85/Contents/Emergency_Medical_Care/Products/Operating_Instructions/LIFEPAK15_OperatingInstructions_3306222-002.pdf.
2. GS Elektromedizinische Geräte. User Manual corpuls3. G. Stemple GmbH; 2013.
3. Knecht KR, Seller JD, Alpert BS. Korotkoff sounds in neonates, infants, and toddlers. *American Journal of Cardiology*. 2009 Apr 15;103(8):1165–1167.
4. Zoll. X Series® Operator's Guide. 2013 [cited 2020 May 20]; Available from: https://www.zoll.com/uk/medical-products/product-manuals.
5. British Medical Association. General information [Internet]. 2018 [cited 2019 Dec 29]. Available from: https://www.bma.org.uk/advice/employment/ethics/consent/consent-tool-kit/2-general-information.
6. Health and Care Professions Council. Standards of conduct, performance and ethics [Internet]. 2018 [cited 2019 Dec 29]. Available from: https://www.hcpc-uk.org/standards/.standards-of-conduct-performance-and-ethics/.
7. NHS England, NHS Improvement. Standard infection control precautions: national hand hygiene and personal protective equipment policy [Internet]. 2019 [cited 2021 Nov 11]. Available from: https://www.england.nhs.uk/publication/standard-infection-control-precautions-nationalhand-hygiene-and-personal-protective-equipmentpolicy/.
8. Nerenberg KA, Zarnke KB, Leung AA, et al. Hypertension Canada's 2018 guidelines for diagnosis, risk assessment, prevention, and treatment of hypertension in adults and children. *Canadian Journal of Cardiology*. 2018 May 1;34(5):506–525.
9. Williams B, Mancia G, Spiering W, et al. 2018 ESC/ESH Guidelines for the management of arterial hypertension: the Task Force for the management of arterial hypertension of the European Society of Cardiology (ESC) and the European Society of Hypertension (ESH). *European Heart Journal*. 2018 Sep 1;39(33):3021–3104.
10. Kallioinen N, Hill A, Horswill MS, et al. Sources of inaccuracy in the measurement of adult patients' resting blood pressure in clinical settings: a systematic review. *Journal of Hypertension*. 2017;35(3):421–441.

11. Frese EM, Fick A, Sadowsky HS. Blood pressure measurement guidelines for physical therapists. *Cardiopulmonary Physical Therapy Journal*. 2011 Jun;22(2):5–12.
12. Asdourian MS, Swaroop MN, Sayegh HE, et al. Association between precautionary behaviors and breast cancer-related lymphedema in patients undergoing bilateral surgery. *Journal of Clinical Oncology*. 2017 Dec 10;35(35):3934–3941.
13. Cheng C-T, Deitch JM, Haines IE, et al. Do medical procedures in the arm increase the risk of lymphoedema after axillary surgery? A review. *ANZ Journal of Surgery*. 2014;84(7–8):510–514.
14. Muntner P, Shimbo D, Carey RM, et al. Measurement of blood pressure in humans: a scientific statement from the American Heart Association. *Hypertension*. 2019 May 1;73(5):e35–66.
15. O'Brien E, Asmar R, Beilin L, et al. European Society of Hypertension recommendations for conventional, ambulatory and home blood pressure measurement. *Journal of Hypertension*. 2003;21(5):821–848.

Electrocardiograms

Indications

- 3-lead electrocardiogram (ECG):
  - Any seriously unwell or unstable patient.
  - Patients with arrhythmias.
- 12-lead ECG:
  - Patients presenting with a cardiovascular or respiratory complaint.

Contraindications

- Do not perform if the patient is in cardiac arrest. Assess the rhythm via the defibrillator pads instead.

Advantages

- Can aid patient management decisions, such as transporting appropriate patients directly for primary percutaneous coronary intervention (pPCI).
- Continuous ECG monitoring can provide instant feedback when arrythmias occur.

Disadvantages

- An ECG cannot rule out an acute coronary syndrome.
- 12-lead ECGs require the patient to be exposed and take time to perform.

Procedure – Record a 3- and 12-lead ECG

Take the following steps to record a 3- and 12-lead ECG:

Action		Rationale
1.	Explain the procedure and obtain consent if appropriate to do so.	You must make sure that you have valid consent from service users or other appropriate authority before you provide care, treatment or other services (1,2).
2.	Don appropriate personal protective equipment (PPE), and undertake appropriate hand hygiene.	This reduces the risk of cross-infection (3).

	Action	Rationale
3.	Place the patient in a semi-recumbent position (at 45°). Appropriately expose the patient, being mindful of maintaining their dignity and preventing heat loss. 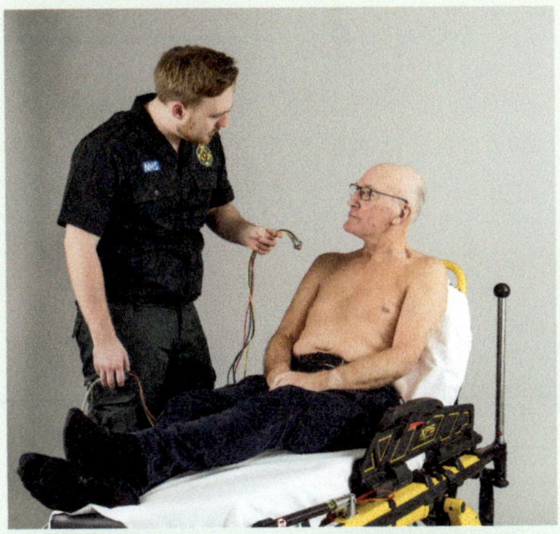	Patient position will affect the ECG appearance. Significant variations have been reported between patients lying supine and sitting up more than 60° (4–6). There is no evidence of significant ECG variation between the supine and 45° semi-recumbent positions (7).
4.	Prepare the skin. This will include shaving any hair at the electrode sites, cleaning oily skin with an alcohol wipe, and gently scraping the skin to remove the surface layer of dead skin cells. Patients who are sweating profusely can be a problem, but an alcohol wipe or gauze swabs should help. All of these will improve electrical conduction. 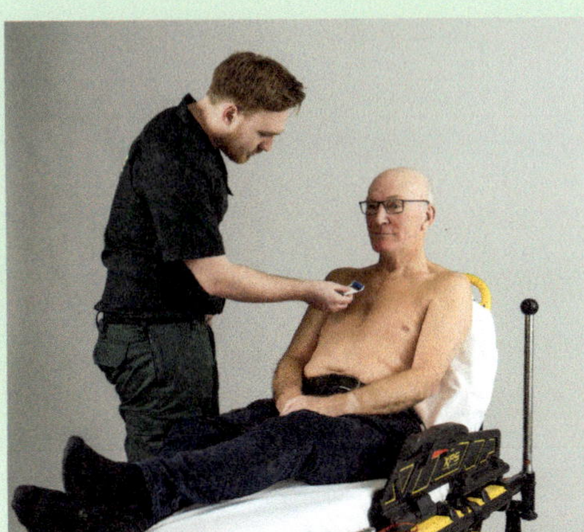	These steps will help reduce artefact on the ECG (7).

	Action	Rationale
5.	Check your electrodes are in date and then attach them to the leads prior to applying them to the patient's skin. Apply the electrodes flat to the skin, smoothing the tape outward and not pressing the centre of the electrode. Avoid placing electrodes over tendons and major muscle masses. 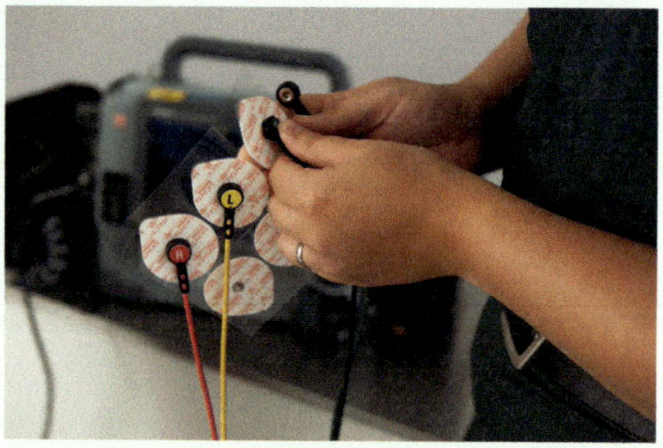	Good contact with the skin will help reduce arteact, as will avoiding large muscle masses and tendons.
6.	Apply the limb leads to the wrists and ankles where possible. However, in cases of patient or vehicular movement, a more proximal location may reduce artefact. Place the leads as follows: • **Red:** right wrist or arm • **Yellow:** left wrist or arm • **Green:** left ankle or leg • **Black:** right ankle or leg. 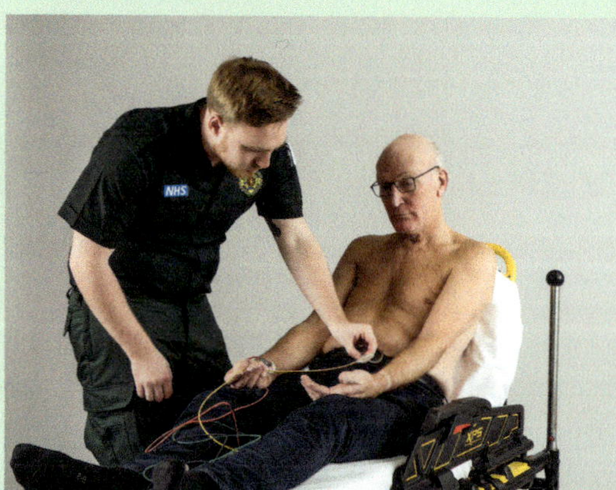	A more proximal location may alter the appearance of the ECG (7). Limb electrodes should not be placed on the torso as it can lead to significant changes in ECG wave height (amplitude) (8–10).
7.	Turn on the monitor and record a 3-lead ECG. Label it with the patient's name and date of birth.	The ECG forms part of the patient's care record and so needs to be identifiable.

Action		Rationale
The instructions below relate to a 12-lead ECG only.		
8.	Prepare the chest skin as in step 4 and attach electrodes to the chest leads.	
9.	Move your finger downwards crossing the manubrium until you feel a small horizontal ridge. This is the sternal angle or angle of Louis, where the manubrium and body of the sternum join. 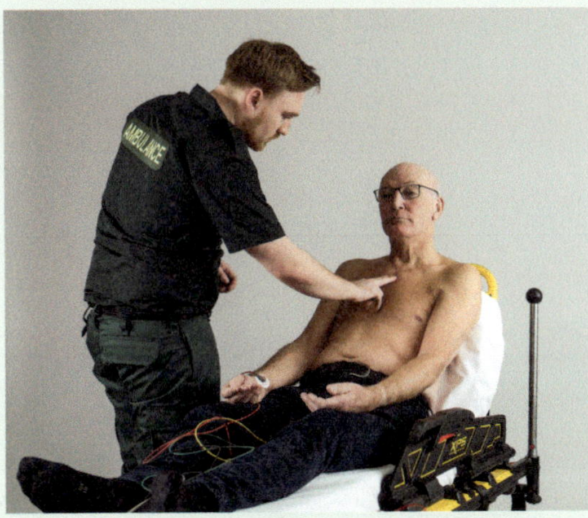	Standardised chest lead positioning is important to ensure that any changes seen on a patient's ECG are due to electrophysiological changes and not due to erroneous lead placement (11). One study involving paramedics found less than 6% could place all chest leads in the correct position (12).
10.	Slide your finger laterally and slightly downwards into the second intercostal space and move down two more intercostal spaces to locate the fourth intercostal space. Place lead V1 just to the left of the sternal border, and V2 just to the right. 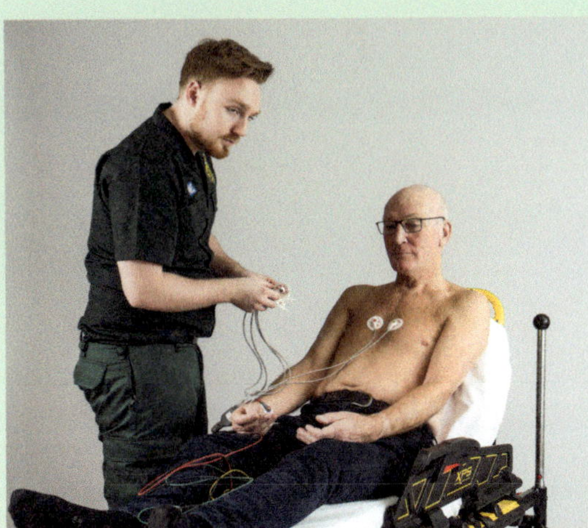	V1 and V2 electrodes are frequently placed too high (13,14).

Action		Rationale
11.	Move into the fifth intercostal space and laterally to the mid-clavicular line. This is the location of V4. 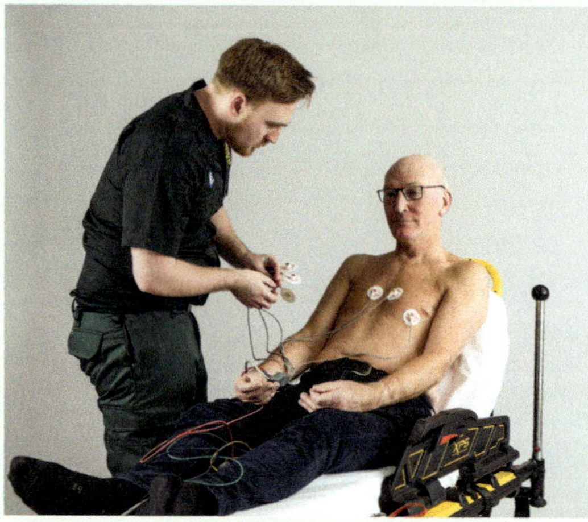	Leads V4, V5 and V6 are frequently placed too low (13,14).
12.	Place V3 midway between V2 and V4. 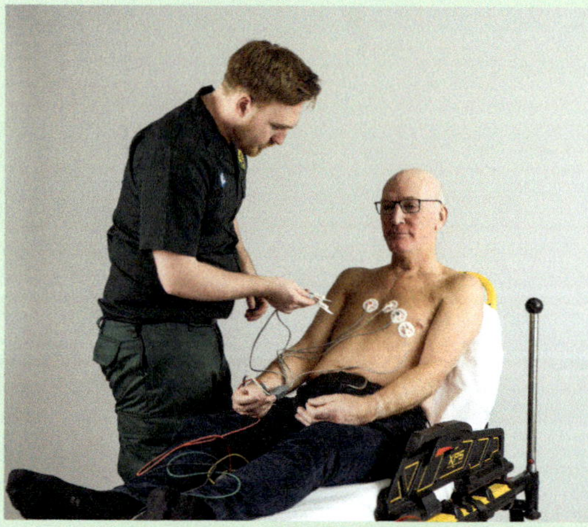	

Action		Rationale
13.	Place lead V6 level with V4, and in the mid-axillary line. 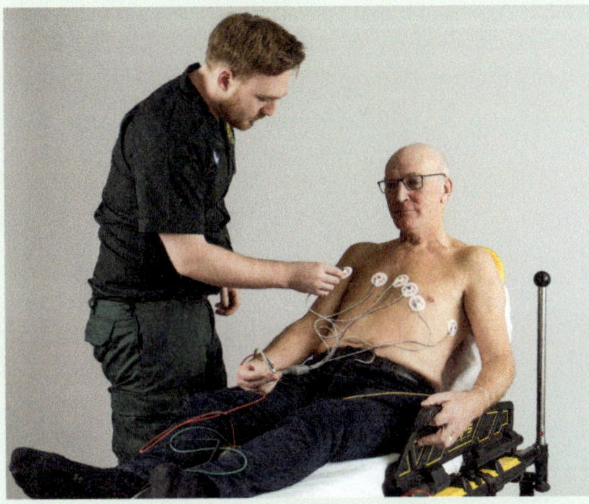	
14.	Place V5 level with, and midway between, V4 and V6 in the anterior axillary line. 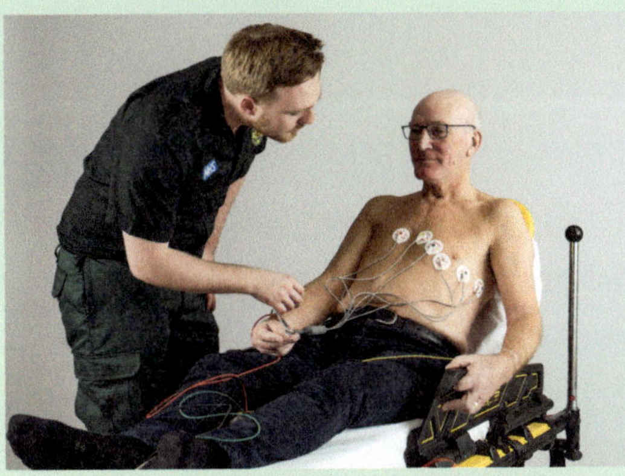	

	Action	Rationale
15.	Connect the cables to the monitor. 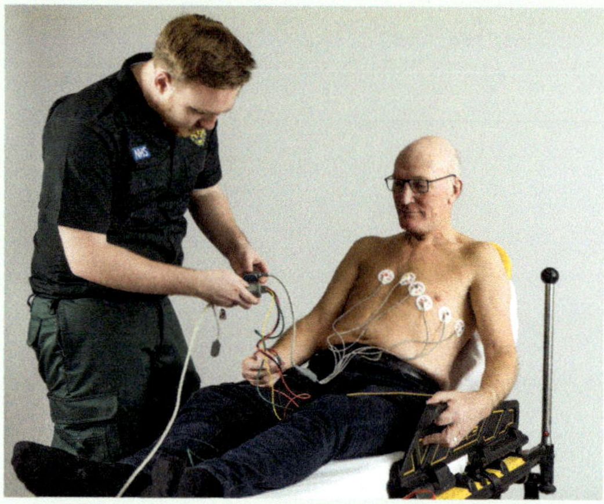	
16.	Press the 12-lead ECG Analyse button and record a 12-lead ECG. Review the 12-lead ECG to check it is of sufficient quality for diagnostic purposes. 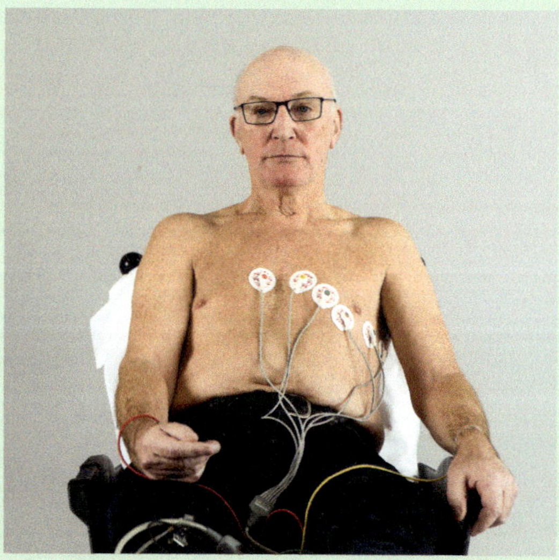	Important decisions (such as the need to transport the patient directly to a pPCI centre) may be made on the basis of the ECG you have recorded (7).
17.	Document the procedure and write the patient's name and date of birth on the ECG.	You must keep full, clear and accurate records for everyone you care for, treat, or provide other services to (2).

Additional ECG Lead Views

There are two important variations to the standard ECG lead placement: right-sided chest, and posterior. Both placements involve modifying the placement of V1–V6 which occur in steps 10–14 of the 12-lead ECG procedure (11).

To record a right-sided ECG, position V1–V6 in the same anatomical locations as for a standard ECG, but on the right-side of the chest (**Figure 1.3**).

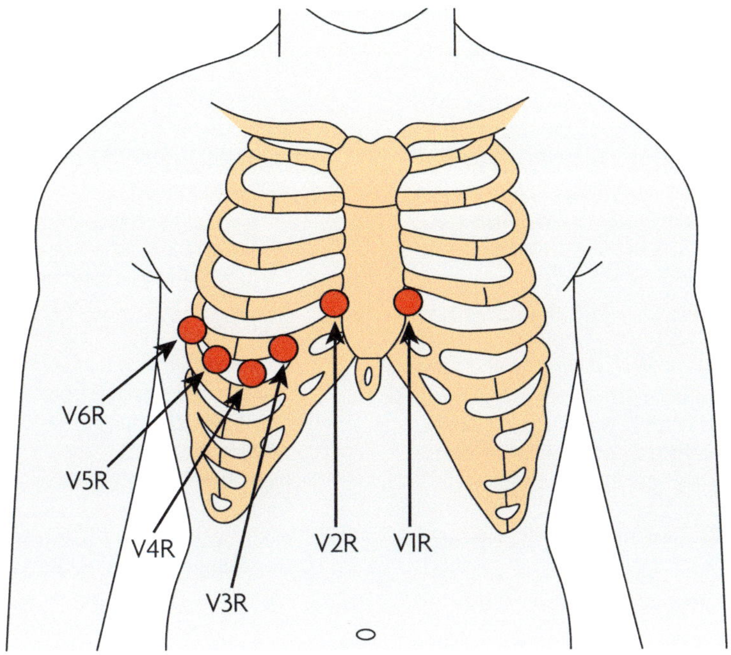

Figure 1.3 Right-sided chest lead placement.

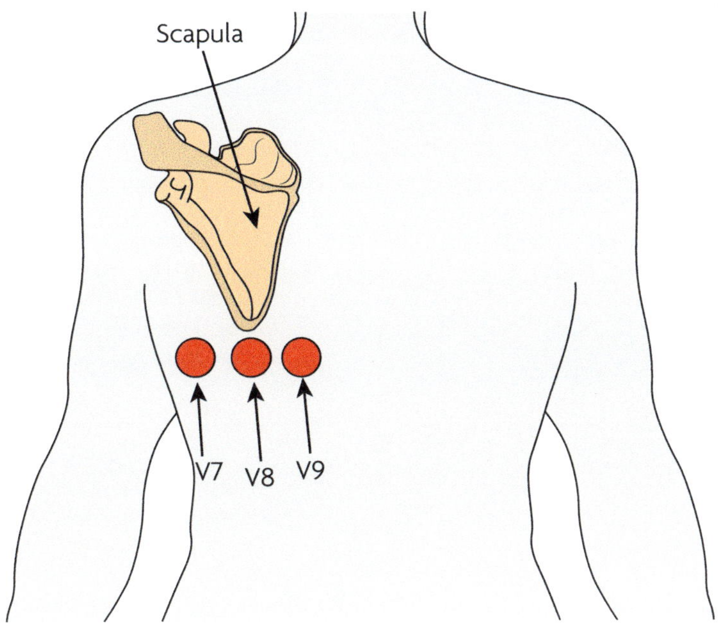

Figure 1.4 Posterior lead placement.

To record a posterior ECG, reposition V4, V5 and V6 in the same horizontal plane, but place V4 level with the posterior axillary line, V5 at the mid-scapular line, and V6 just to the left of the spine (**Figure 1.4**).

Don't forget to re-label the ECG so it is clear that alternative lead placements have been used. For right-sided leads, a small 'R' is added to V1–V6. For a posterior lead ECG, re-label V4, V5 and V6 as V7, V8 and V9, respectively.

References

1. British Medical Association. General information [Internet]. 2018 [cited 2019 Dec 29]. Available from: https://www.bma.org.uk/advice/employment/ethics/consent/consent-tool-kit/2-general-information.
2. Health and Care Professions Council. Standards of conduct, performance and ethics [Internet]. 2018 [cited 2019 Dec 29]. Available from: https://www.hcpc-uk.org/standards/standards-of-conduct-performance-and-ethics/.
3. NHS England, NHS Improvement. Standard infection control precautions: national hand hygiene and personal protective equipment policy [Internet]. 2019 [cited 2021 Nov 11]. Available from: https://www.england.nhs.uk/publication/standard-infection-control-precautions-nationalhand-hygiene-and-personal-protective-equipmentpolicy/.
4. Bergman KS, Stevenson WG, Tillisch JH, et al. Effect of body position on the diagnostic accuracy of the electrocardiogram. *American Heart Journal*. 1989 Jan;117(1):204–206.
5. Khare S, Chawala A. Effect of change in body position on resting electrocardiogram in young healthy adults. *Nigerian Journal of Cardiology*. 2016;13:125–129.
6. Baevsky RH, Haber MD, Blank FS, et al. Supine vs semirecumbent and upright 12-lead electrocardiogram: does change in body position alter the electrocardiographic interpretation for ischemia? *American Journal of Emergency Medicine*. 2007 Sep 1;25(7):753–756.
7. Society for Cardiological Science & Technology. Recording a standard 12-lead electrocardiogram [Internet]. 2017 [cited 2020 Jan 29]. Available from: http://www.scst.org.uk/resources/SCST_ECG_Recording_Guidelines_20171.pdf.
8. Arya A, Huo Y, Frogner F, et al. Effect of limb lead electrodes location on ECG and localization of idiopathic outflow tract tachycardia: a prospective study. *Journal of Cardiovascular Electrophysiology*. 2011;22(8):886–891.
9. Sevilla DC, Dohrmann ML, Somelofski CA, et al. Invalidation of the resting electrocardiogram obtained via exercise electrode sites as a standard 12-lead recording. *American Journal of Cardiology*. 1989 Jan 1;63(1):35–39.
10. Pahlm O, Haisty WK, Edenbrandt L, et al. Evaluation of changes in standard electrocardiographic QRS waveforms recorded from activity-compatible proximal limb lead positions. *American Journal of Cardiology*. 1992 Jan 15;69(3):253–257.
11. Kligfield P, Gettes LS, Bailey JJ, et al. Recommendations for the standardization and interpretation of the electrocardiogram part i: the electrocardiogram and its technology: a scientific statement from the American Heart Association Electrocardiography and Arrhythmias Committee, Council on Clinical Cardiology; the American College of Cardiology Foundation; and the Heart Rhythm Society Endorsed by the International Society for Computerized Electrocardiology. *Journal of the American College of Cardiology*. 2007 Mar 13;49(10):1109–1127.
12. Gregory P, Lodge S, Kilner T, et al. Accuracy of ECG chest electrode placements by paramedics: an observational study. *British Paramedic Journal*. 2019 Dec 1;4(3):51–52.
13. Bickerton M, Pooler A. Misplaced ECG electrodes and the need for continuing training. *British Journal of Cardiac Nursing*. 2019 Mar 2;14(3):123–132.
14. Medani SA, Hensey M, Caples N, et al. Accuracy in precordial ECG lead placement: improving performance through a peer-led educational intervention. *Journal of Electrocardiology*. 2018 Jan 1;51(1):50–54.

The AVPU Scale

Indications

- Any patient requiring a physiological assessment.
- Patients with illnesses that may rapidly affect the patient's level of consciousness (LOC).

Contraindications

- None.

Advantages

- Useful to determine a patient's LOC.
- Quick and easy to perform.

Disadvantages

- Not as comprehensive as the Glasgow Coma Scale score.
- The origins of the AVPU scale can be traced back to a 1966 paper on the assessment of barbiturate poisoning. There is no definitive guidance on each of the components and how they should be scored (1,2).

Procedure – Assessing Level of Consciousness with the AVPU Scale

Take the following steps to record the patient's LOC using the AVPU scale (3):

Action		Rationale
1.	Explain the procedure and obtain consent if appropriate to do so.	You must make sure that you have valid consent from service users or other appropriate authority before you provide care, treatment or other services (4,5).
2.	Don appropriate personal protective equipment (PPE), and undertake appropriate hand hygiene.	This reduces the risk of cross-infection (6).
3.	Observe the patient, noting any spontaneous eye, motor and verbal behaviours. If the patient has their eyes open or their eyes open spontaneously as you approach, they obey commands and can tell you their name, where they are and what month it is, record 'A'.	
4a.	If assessing LOC for a NEWS2 score and the patient cannot tell you their name, where they are and what month it is, and this is thought to be a new onset of confusion (this can be difficult to determine and others, such as family or caregivers, may be required to help), record 'C'. Otherwise, record 'V'.	NEWS2 includes an additional component: a new onset of confusion (7).

Action		Rationale
4b.	If the patient cannot tell you their name, where they are and what month it is, and either this is not a new onset of confusion or the assessment is not being conducted as part of the NEWS2 score, record 'V'.	
5.	If the patient does not respond to voice or from being shaken but responds to a trapezius pinch by moving their limbs (normally or abnormally), record 'P'. Note that the patient may have their eyes open but have a fixed gaze and may respond to pain with a single word, yet is still classed as being severely impaired and so their response should be recorded as a 'P', since the responses are abnormal and only occurred as a result of a pain stimulus.	
6.	If the patient's eyes remain closed and there is no limb movement, despite a painful stimulus such as a trapezius pinch, record 'U'.	
7.	Document the procedure.	You must keep full, clear and accurate records for everyone you care for, treat, or provide other services to (5).

References

1. Teasdale GM. National early warning score (NEWS) is not suitable for all patients. *BMJ*. 2012 Sep 4;345:e5875.
2. Matthew H, Lawson A. Acute barbiturate poisoning – A review of two years experience. *QJM: An International Journal of Medicine* [Internet]. 1966 Oct [cited 2021 Dec 14]; Available from: https://academic.oup.com/qjmed/article/35/4/539/1601974/ACUTE-BARBITURATE-POISONINGA-REVIEW-OF-TWO-YEARS.
3. Brunker C, Harris R. How accurate is the AVPU scale in detecting neurological impairment when used by general ward nurses? An evaluation study using simulation and a questionnaire. *Intensive Critical Care Nursing*. 2015 Apr;31(2):69–75.
4. British Medical Association. General information [Internet]. 2018 [cited 2019 Dec 29]. Available from: https://www.bma.org.uk/advice/employment/ethics/consent/consent-tool-kit/2-general-information.
5. Health and Care Professions Council. Standards of conduct, performance and ethics [Internet]. 2018 [cited 2019 Dec 29]. Available from: https://www.hcpc-uk.org/standards/standards-of-conduct-performance-and-ethics/.
6. Royal College of Physicians. National Early Warning Score (NEWS) 2 [Internet]. RCP London. 2017 [cited 2021 Dec 18]. Available from: https://www.rcplondon.ac.uk/projects/outputs/national-early-warning-score-news-2.
7. NHS England, NHS Improvement. Standard infection control precautions: national hand hygiene and personal protective equipment policy [Internet]. 2019 [cited 2021 Nov 11]. Available from: https://www.england.nhs.uk/publication/standard-infection-control-precautions-national-hand-hygiene-and-personal-protective-equipment-policy/.

Glasgow Coma Scale Score

Indications

- Any patient requiring a physiological assessment.
- Patients with illnesses that may rapidly affect the patient's level of consciousness (LOC).

Contraindications

- Patients who need immediate correction of an airway, breathing or circulation problem – use AVPU scale instead.

Advantages

- Helpful for monitoring changes in LOC.
- Provides an objective method to record and communicate the patient's LOC between healthcare professionals.

Disadvantages

- Takes time to perform compared to an AVPU assessment.
- Poor inter-rater reliability (different clinicians score the same patient presentation differently), especially in the emergency setting.

Procedure – Glasgow Coma Scale Score Measurement

Take the following steps to record a Glasgow Coma Scale (GCS) score (1):

Action		Rationale
1.	Explain the procedure to the patient (even if they are unconscious) and obtain consent if appropriate to do so.	You must make sure that you have valid consent from service users or other appropriate authority before you provide care, treatment or other services (2,3).
2.	Don appropriate personal protective equipment (PPE), and undertake appropriate hand hygiene.	This reduces the risk of cross-infection (4).
3.	Check for factors that may affect your assessment. This might include the patient not speaking your language, having a hearing impairment or eye-swelling, for example.	These will affect the ability of the patient to respond appropriately to any commands you provide as part of the assessment.
4.	Observe the patient, noting any spontaneous eye, motor and verbal behaviours. If the patient has their eyes open or their eyes open spontaneously as you approach, record a score of 4 and a rating of 'spontaneous'.	
5.	If eye-opening is not spontaneous, use a verbal stimulus. Introduce yourself and instruct the patient to open their eyes. Shouting may be necessary in some circumstances. If the patient opens their eyes, record a score of 3 and a rating of 'to sound'.	Raising your voice may be necessary if the patient is hard of hearing.

Action		Rationale
6.	If there is no response to sound, apply a painful stimulus centrally for up to 10 seconds. If the patient opens their eyes, record a score of 2 and a rating of 'to pressure'.	Ten seconds is sufficient time to provoke a maximal pain stimulus without causing any tissue damage.
7.	If there is no response to painful stimulus, score a 1 for eye-opening and a rating of 'none'. If there are local factors such as eye-swelling which prevent the patient from opening their eyes, record eyes as 'not testable' (NT).	
8.	To assess verbal response, ask the patient to tell you their name, where they are and what month it is. If they answer correctly, record a score of 5 and a rating of 'orientated'.	This will help ensure the patient is orientated to time, place and person.
9.	If the patient is unable to answer the questions in step 8 but is otherwise able to hold a conversation with you, record a score of 4 and a rating of 'confused'. If they cannot talk in sentences, but utter single words (unless there is another physiological reason why they cannot speak in full sentences, for example shortness of breath), record a score of 3 and a rating of 'words'. If the patient moans and groans but makes no recognisable speech, record a score of 2 and a rating of 'sounds'. If the patient makes no sound at all, score verbal response as 1 and a rating of 'none'. Note that inability to speak can be caused by other conditions and not just LOC – for example if the patient has a tracheostomy and no speech valve. In these cases, record as NT.	
10.	To test the motor response, ask the patient to perform a two-step action – for example ask them to grasp and release your fingers with their hand, or open their mouth and stick out their tongue. If they do this, record a score of 6 and a rating of 'obey commands'. Be mindful of conditions, such as spinal injury, which may prevent the patient from moving their arms.	Patients can reflexively grasp something placed in their hand, which is why it is important to undertake a two-step action (1).

	Action	Rationale
11.	If the patient does not obey commands, apply a trapezius squeeze for up to 10 seconds. If the patient moves their hand above their clavicle to move the stimulus away, record a score of 5 and a rating of 'localising'. If their arm does not reach above the clavicle but does flex, then they are either normally, or abnormally, flexing. In normal flexion, the elbow bends and the arm moves rapidly away from the body and the stimulus. In abnormal flexion, the elbow bends slowly (**Figure 1.5.1**). If in doubt, record a score of 4 and a rating of 'normal flexion'. If you are confident that the patient is exhibiting abnormal flexion, record a score of 3 and a rating of 'abnormal flexion'. If the patient extends their elbows rather than flexes, record a score of 2 and a rating of 'extension' (**Figure 1.5.2**). If there is no response, record a score of 1 and a rating of 'none'. In cases where the patient has been paralysed by drugs, record as NT. 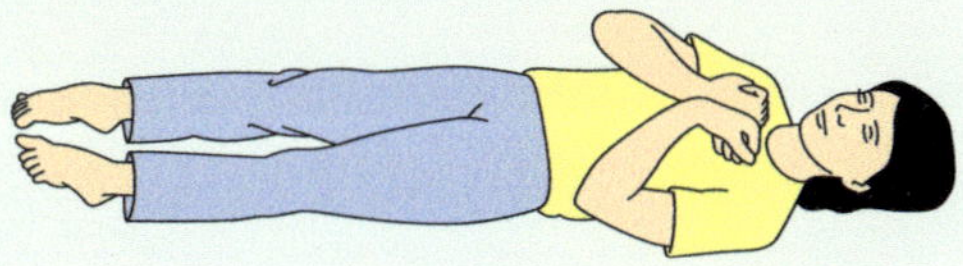 ***Figure 1.5.1*** Abnormal flexion response. 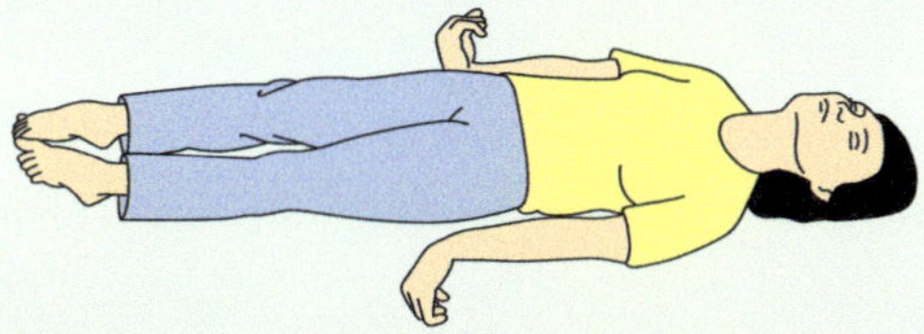 ***Figure 1.5.2*** Abnormal extension response.	Reducing scores suggest injury at different levels of the central nervous system. For example, abnormal flexion suggests injury within the cerebral hemisphere or internal capsule, whereas extension may indicate midbrain or upper pontine injury (5).
12.	If there are different responses on the right and left sides, record the 'best' response (the response with the higher score).	The response of the worst side may reflect focal brain damage or local injury.
13.	Document each component and the total score clearly. Ideally, both the descriptor and score should be recorded, for example E4V5M6 eyes opening, confused, obeys commands.	The total score does not communicate more detailed description of each response. You must keep full, clear and accurate records for everyone you care for, treat, or provide other services to (3).

References

1. Teasdale G, Allen D, Brennan P, et al. The Glasgow Coma Scale: an update after 40 years. *Nursing Times*. 2014;110:12–16.
2. British Medical Association. General information [Internet]. 2018 [cited 2019 Dec 29]. Available from: https://www.bma.org.uk/advice/employment/ethics/consent/consent-tool-kit/2-general-information.
3. Health and Care Professions Council. Standards of conduct, performance and ethics [Internet]. 2018 [cited 2019 Dec 29]. Available from: https://www.hcpc-uk.org/standards/standards-of-conduct-performance-and-ethics/.
4. Middleton PM. Practical use of the Glasgow Coma Scale: a comprehensive narrative review of GCS methodology. *Australasian Emergency Nursing Journal* [Internet]. 2012 [cited 2012 Aug 31]; Available from: http://www.sciencedirect.com/science/article/pii/S1574626712000651.
5. NHS England, NHS Improvement. Standard infection control precautions: national hand hygiene and personal protective equipment policy [Internet]. 2019 [cited 2021 Nov 11]. Available from: https://www.england.nhs.uk/publication/standard-infection-control-precautions-national-hand-hygiene-and-personal-protective-equipment-policy/.

Face, Arm, Speech Test

Indications

- Patient with suspected stroke or transient ischaemic attack.

Contraindications

- None.

Advantages

- Quick and straightforward to undertake.
- Can facilitate direct referral to hyper-acute stroke pathways in eligible patients.

Disadvantages

- Does not detect symptoms such as unilateral leg weakness or vision loss (1,2).
- Requires the patient to be able to understand and follow commands.

Procedure – Face, Arm, Speech Test

Take the following steps to undertake a Face, Arm, Speech Test (FAST) (3):

Action		Rationale
1.	Explain the procedure to the patient and obtain consent. 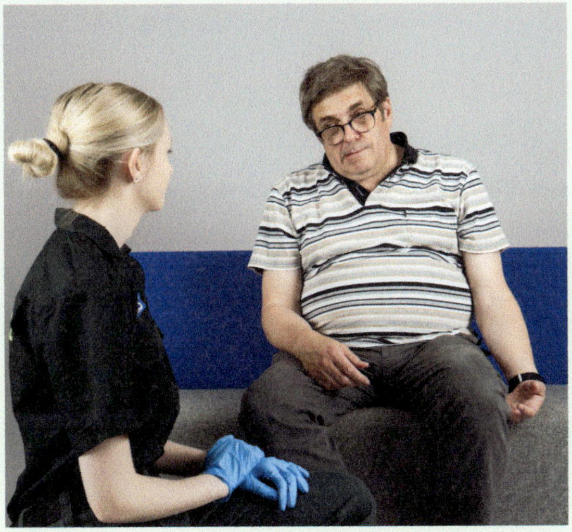	You must make sure that you have valid consent from service users or other appropriate authority before you provide care, treatment or other services (4,5).
2.	Don appropriate personal protective equipment (PPE), and undertake appropriate hand hygiene.	This reduces the risk of cross-infection (6).

<table>
<tr><th colspan="2">Action</th><th>Rationale</th></tr>
<tr><td>3.</td><td>Ask the patient to smile or show their teeth. Look for a new lack of symmetry. This is positive if there is an unequal smile, grimace or obvious facial asymmetry.
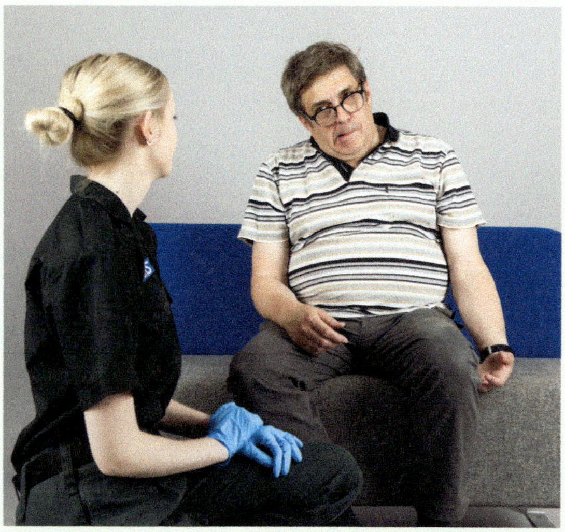</td><td>The tests in steps 3, 4 and 5 are designed to detect the most commonly involved artery (middle cerebral) in strokes (7).</td></tr>
<tr><td>4.</td><td>Lift the patient's arms together to 90° (45° if they are lying on their back) with palms uppermost. Ask them to hold that position for 5 seconds. Look for one arm drifting or falling rapidly.
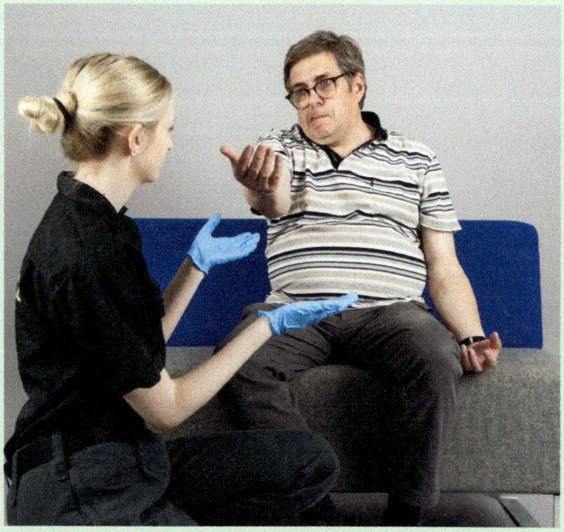</td><td>Note that this step does not instruct the patient to close their eyes, although it may be common practice to do so (3).</td></tr>
</table>

Action		Rationale
5.	During conversation (if the patient can speak), look for new speech disturbance. This may require asking someone who knows the patient. Specifically, look for slurred speech and word-finding difficulties. Ask the patient to identify common objects (such as keys, a cup, a chair or a pen). If the patient has a severe visual disturbance, place the object in the patient's hand and ask them to name it. 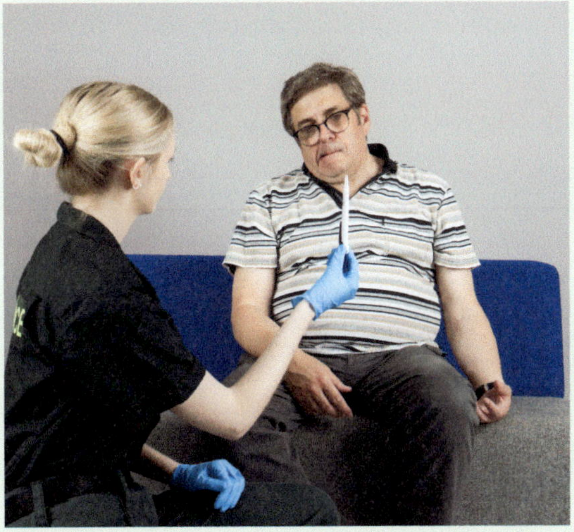	The assessment of dysphasia (a disorder of language production) requires assessment of the patient's comprehension and ability to produce spontaneous speech and name objects (8).
6.	Document the procedure; the presence of one or more of the signs above constitutes a positive test.	You must keep full, clear and accurate records for everyone you care for, treat, or provide other services to (5).

References

1. Intercollegiate Stroke Working Party. National clinical guideline for stroke [Internet]. 2016 [cited 2018 Nov 22]. Available from: https://www.strokeaudit.org/SupportFiles/Documents/Guidelines/2016-National-Clinical-Guideline-for-Stroke-5t-(1).aspx.
2. McClelland G. Paramedic identification of stroke mimic presentations: development and preliminary evaluation of a pre-hospital clinical assessment tool. Newcastle; 2018.
3. Harbison J, Hossain O, Jenkinson D, et al. Diagnostic accuracy of stroke referrals from primary care, emergency room physicians, and ambulance staff using the Face Arm Speech Test. *Stroke*. 2003 Jan 1;34(1):71–76.
4. British Medical Association. General information [Internet]. 2018 [cited 2019 Dec 29]. Available from: https://www.bma.org.uk/advice/employment/ethics/consent/consent-tool-kit/2-general-information.
5. Health and Care Professions Council. Standards of conduct, performance and ethics [Internet]. 2018 [cited 2019 Dec 29]. Available from: https://www.hcpc-uk.org/standards/standards-of-conduct-performance-and-ethics/.
6. NHS England, NHS Improvement. Standard infection control precautions: national hand hygiene and personal protective equipment policy [Internet]. 2019 [cited 2021 Nov 11]. Available from: https://www.england.nhs.uk/publication/standard-infection-control-precautions-national-hand-hygiene-and-personal-protective-equipment-policy/.
7. Marieb E, Hoehn K. *Human Anatomy & Physiology*. 11th edition. Harlow: Pearson; 2019.
8. Ross J, Horton-Szar D. *Crash Course Nervous System*. 4th edition. Smith C, Ed. London: Mosby; 2015.

Blood Sugar Measurement

Indications
- Patients with acute illness.
- Patients suspected of having hypo- or hyper-glycaemia.
- As part of reassessment following treatment for hypoglycaemia.
- Any patient with confusion or reduced level of consciousness.

Contraindications
- None in the emergency setting, but see cautions.

Cautions
The following conditions can adversely affect the accuracy of capillary blood glucose measurement. A laboratory-analysed venous sample is preferable in the following presentations (1):
- Patients on home dialysis.
- Peripheral circulatory failure, for example shock (venous sample from a cannula probably suitable).
- Severe dehydration.
- Extremes of haematocrit (can be seen in neonates and pregnant patients).
- Hyperlipidaemia.

Advantages
- Can be performed at the patient's side.
- Easy to perform.

Disadvantages
- Not as accurate as a laboratory-analysed blood sample.
- Painful.
- Invasive; infection prevention and control measures must be in place.

Procedure – Blood Sugar Measurement

Take the following steps to measure a patient's blood sugar (2):

Note: The SD Codefree monitor is used here, but the steps are likely to be the same for most other devices. However, make sure you are familiar with the blood glucose meters you will be using.

Action		Rationale
1.	Explain the procedure to the patient and obtain consent if appropriate to do so.	You must make sure that you have valid consent from service users or other appropriate authority before you provide care, treatment or other services (3,4).

Action		Rationale
2.	Don appropriate personal protective equipment (PPE), and undertake appropriate hand hygiene.	This reduces the risk of cross-infection (5).
3.	Select an appropriate site, which is typically the side of a finger in an adult or older child (the non-dominant hand, if possible) and the heel of the foot in a younger child or infant. Clean the area with water or water-soaked gauze and dry thoroughly. 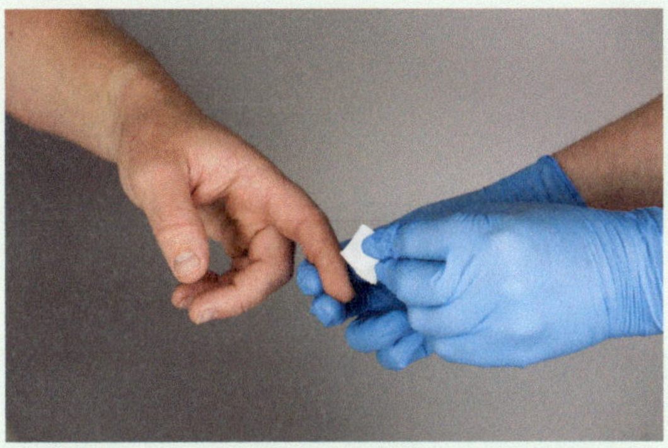	The side of a finger and heel are less painful than other areas, for example the pads of the fingers, due to lower density of nerve fibres (6). Contamination of the test finger with glucose-rich foods or dilutional error due to inadequate hand drying or the patient licking their finger clean, will result in artificially high or low results (7). Alcohol swabs do not remove traces of glucose as effectively as water so should not be used (8,9). There is little evidence to suggest that alcohol itself leads to errors in blood sugar results, but you should consult the manufacturer's guidelines for the device you use (9,10).
4.	Check the use-by date on the test strip container. Do not use test strips past their use-by date. 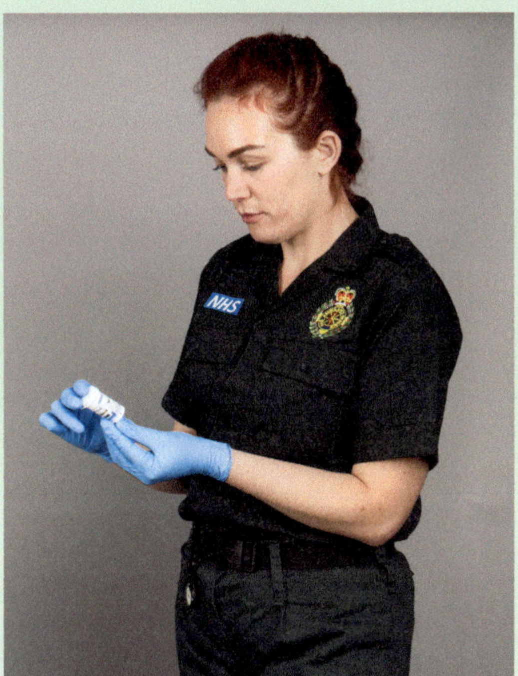	Out-of-date strips could lead to incorrect results.

Action		Rationale
5.	Insert a test strip into the bottom of the meter. This will turn it on (some models will beep too). 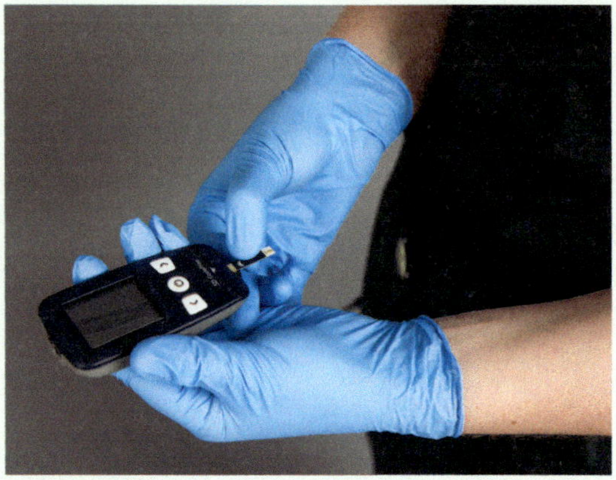	
6.	On the screen, an icon showing the test strip and a flashing blood drop will appear. Ask the patient to dangle their arm down at their side to encourage blood flow to their fingertips. 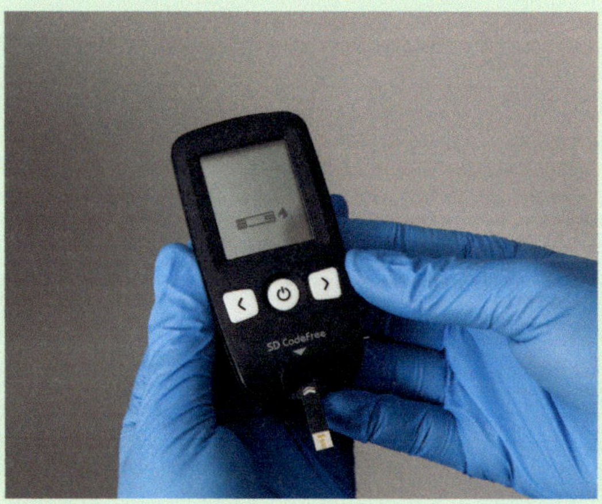	

Action		Rationale
7.	Prick the target area with a lancet, disposing of it in a sharps bin after use. 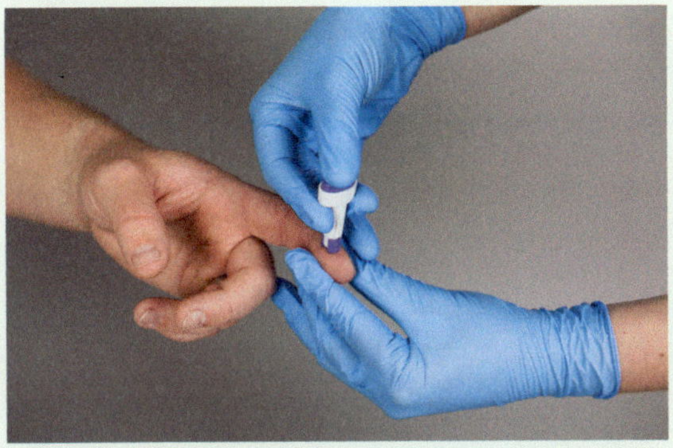	While most lancets will automatically withdraw the needle back inside the outer container, it should be treated as a contaminated sharp and disposed of appropriately.
8.	Wait a couple of seconds and then, with the patient's hand facing downwards, gently squeeze their finger to assist the flow of blood. 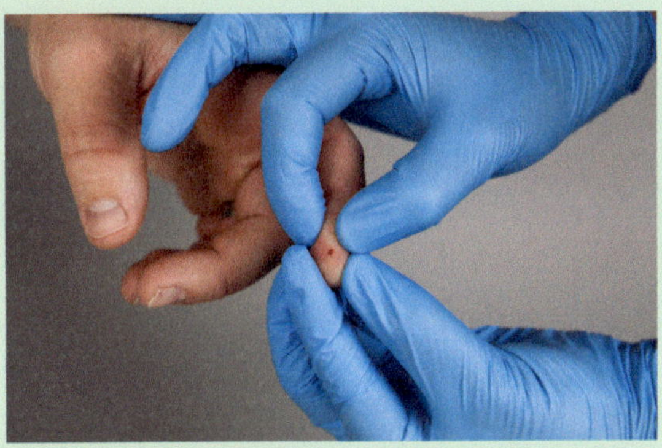	This will help ensure enough blood for a sample is available.
9.	Touch the blood drop to the front edge of the yellow window of the test strip. When you have enough blood, you will see a countdown timer. 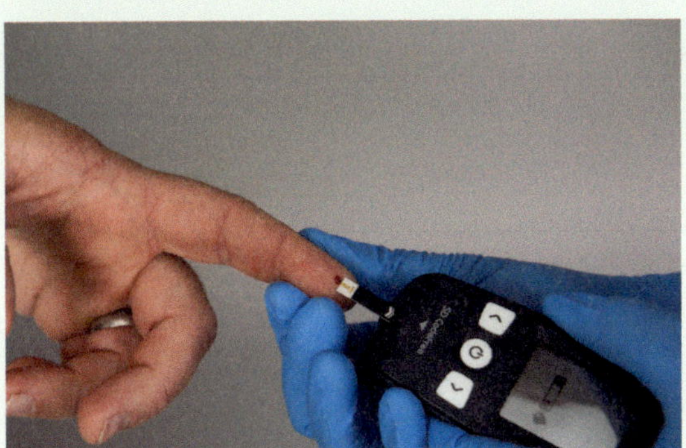	Blood is drawn up from the tip of the test strip; this will not happen if you place blood on top of the strip (11).

Action		Rationale
10.	Ask the patient to apply pressure to the puncture site with gauze until bleeding has stopped. 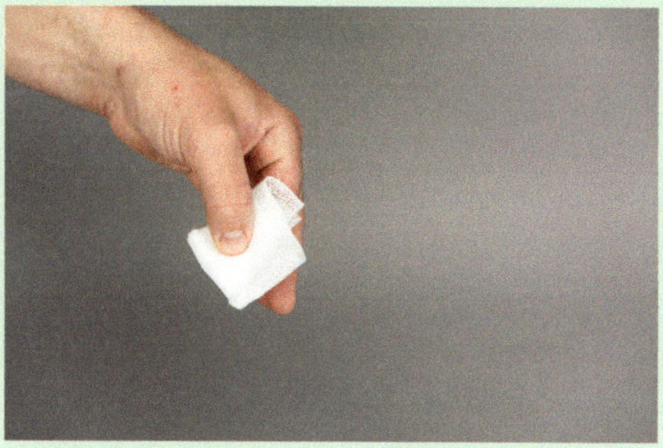	
11.	The blood sugar result will appear on the display. Check that the unit of measure is mmol/l and not mg/dL. Document the procedure and the result. 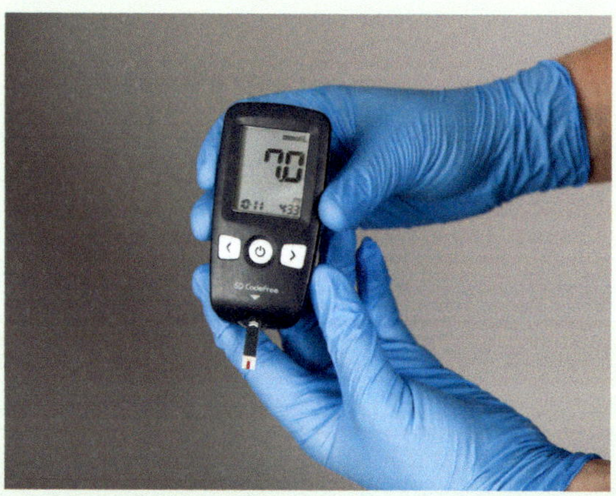	Using mg/dL could result in the blood sugar being interpreted as a higher value than it actually is (1). You must keep full, clear and accurate records for everyone you care for, treat or provide other services to (4).
12.	Document the procedure.	You must keep full, clear and accurate records for everyone you care for, treat, or provide other services to (5).

References

1. Medicines and Healthcare Regulatory Agency. Point of care testing with blood glucose meters: leaflet [Internet]. GOV.UK. 2013 [cited 2021 Nov 4]. Available from: https://www.gov.uk/government/publications/point-of-care-testing-with-blood-glucose-meters-leaflet.
2. Roche. ACCU-CHEK Aviva user's manual [Internet]. 2019 [cited 2021 Nov 6]. Available from: https://www.accu-chek.co.uk/download/file/fid/27771.
3. British Medical Association. General information [Internet]. 2018 [cited 2019 Dec 29]. Available from: https://www.bma.org.uk/advice/employment/ethics/consent/consent-tool-kit/2-general-information.
4. Health and Care Professions Council. Standards of conduct, performance and ethics [Internet]. 2018 [cited 2019 Dec 29]. Available from: https://www.hcpc-uk.org/standards/standards-of-conduct-performance-and-ethics/.
5. NHS England, NHS Improvement. Standard infection control precautions: national hand hygiene and personal protective equipment policy [Internet]. 2019 [cited 2021 Nov 11]. Available from: https://www.england.nhs.uk/publication/standard-infection-control-precautions-national-hand-hygiene-and-personal-protective-equipment-policy/.
6. Marieb E, Hoehn K. *Human Anatomy & Physiology*. 11th edition. Harlow: Pearson; 2019.
7. Lunt H, Florkowski C, Bignall M, et al. Capillary glucose meter accuracy and sources of error in the ambulatory setting. *New Zealand Medical Journal*. 2010;123(1310):74–85.
8. Kotwal N, Pandit A. Variability of capillary blood glucose monitoring measured on home glucose monitoring devices. *Indian Journal of Endocrinology Metabolism*. 2012 Dec;16(Suppl 2):S248–251.
9. Palese A, Chiandetti R, Mansutti I. The effect of 2% chlorhexidine and cleansing wipes on capillary blood glucose sampling accuracy of a fingertip soiled with apple: a case crossover study design. *Journal of Clinical Nursing*. 2014 Sep 1;23(17–18):2672–2675.
10. Sagkal Midilli T, Ergın E, Baysal E, et al. Comparison of glucose values of blood samples taken in three different ways. *Clinical Nursing Research*. 2019 May 1;28(4):436–455.
11. Roche. ACCU-CHEK Aviva User's Manual [Internet]. 2019 [cited 2021 Nov 6]. Available from: https://www.accuchek.co.uk/download/fi le/fi d/27771.

Axillary Temperature Measurement

Indications

- Routine physiological assessment.
- Aids recognition of local and systemic infection.
- Guides treatment in cases of hypothermia and hyperthermia.

Contraindications

- None.

Advantages

- Minimally invasive.
- Can be performed even on very small infants.

Disadvantages

- Underestimates core body temperature (1).
- Left and right axilla temperatures may be different (2).
- Can take up to 90 seconds to return a reading (3).

Procedure – Axillary Temperature Measurement

Take the following steps to record an axillary temperature:

Action		Rationale
1.	Explain the procedure and obtain consent if appropriate to do so.	You must make sure that you have valid consent from service users or other appropriate authority before you provide care, treatment or other services (4,5).
2.	Don appropriate personal protective equipment (PPE), and undertake appropriate hand hygiene.	This reduces the risk of cross-infection (6).
3.	Turn on the thermometer, check it is clean and functional, and apply a fresh cover to the probe. Once you have turned it on, the thermometer will be able to perform any self-checks.	This reduces the risk of cross-infection (6).
4.	Place the tip of the thermometer high in the axilla, in the fold where the arm meets the chest. Adduct the patient's arm so it is flush with the side of the chest and ensure the thermometer is covered.	The armpit is not a closed cavity and so cool ambient air can affect readings (3).
5.	Leave in place until the thermometer has finished measuring. Usually there will be a visual or audible indication that this has happened.	Removing the thermometer early may lead to an underestimate of temperature (3).

Action		Rationale
6.	Remove from the axilla and read the temperature. Check the temperature is recorded in degrees Celsius (°C).	Temperature readings in degrees Fahrenheit (°F) will be higher.
7.	Document the procedure.	You must keep full, clear and accurate records for everyone you care for, treat, or provide other services to (5).

References

1. Oguz F, Yildiz I, Varkal M, et al. Axillary and tympanic temperature measurement in children and normal values for ages. *Pediatric Emergency Care*. 2016 Apr 5;34(3):169–173.
2. Vardasca R et al. Bilateral assessment of body core temperature through axillar, tympanic and inner canthi thermometers in a young population. *Physiological Measurement*. 2019 Sep 30;40(9):094001.
3. Braun. PRT1000 instruction manual. Kaz Europe Sarl; 2015.
4. British Medical Association. General information [Internet]. 2018 [cited 2019 Dec 29]. Available from: https://www.bma.org.uk/advice/employment/ethics/consent/consent-tool-kit/2-general-information.
5. Health and Care Professions Council. Standards of conduct, performance and ethics [Internet]. 2018 [cited 2019 Dec 29]. Available from: https://www.hcpc-uk.org/standards/standards-of-conduct-performance-and-ethics/.
6. NHS England, NHS Improvement. Standard infection control precautions: national hand hygiene and personal protective equipment policy [Internet]. 2019 [cited 2021 Nov 11]. Available from: https://www.england.nhs.uk/publication/standard-infection-control-precautions-national-hand-hygiene-and-personal-protective-equipment-policy/.

Tympanic Temperature Measurement

Indications

- Routine physiological assessment.
- Aids recognition of local and systemic infection.
- Guides treatment in cases of hypothermia and hyperthermia.

Contraindications

- Infants under 4 weeks of age (use electronic axilla thermometer instead) (1).

Advantages

- Quick.
- Minimally invasive.

Disadvantages

- Can give inaccurate results in cases of: excessive ear wax; if the ears have been covered for any period of time, for example wearing of ear muffs or lying on one side; and where the patient is susceptible to environmental conditions, for example if they have been outside for a prolonged period of time (2).
- Temperatures may be different between ears (3).

Procedure – Record a Temperature with a Tympanic Thermometer

Take the following steps to record a temperature with a tympanic thermometer (4):

Action		Rationale
1.	Explain the procedure and obtain consent if appropriate to do so.	You must make sure that you have valid consent from service users or other appropriate authority before you provide care, treatment or other services (5,6).
2.	Don appropriate personal protective equipment (PPE), and undertake appropriate hand hygiene.	This reduces the risk of cross-infection (7).
3.	Turn on the thermometer, check it is clean and functional, and apply a fresh cover to the probe. Once you have turned it on, the thermometer will perform a self-check. 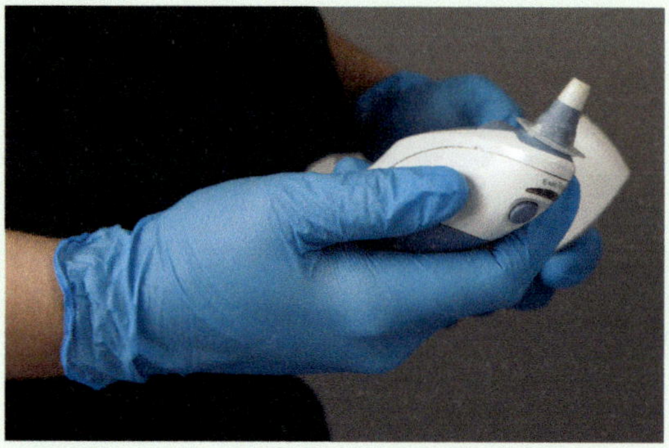	This reduces the risk of cross-infection (7).

Action		Rationale
4.	If your model of thermometer has an age setting, select the correct age group.	
5.	Place the probe into the ear and gently advance until the probe seals the opening. It should be placed straight down the ear canal, so the tip of the device is facing the tympanic membrane. Some thermometers will report if you do not have the thermometer in the correct position. 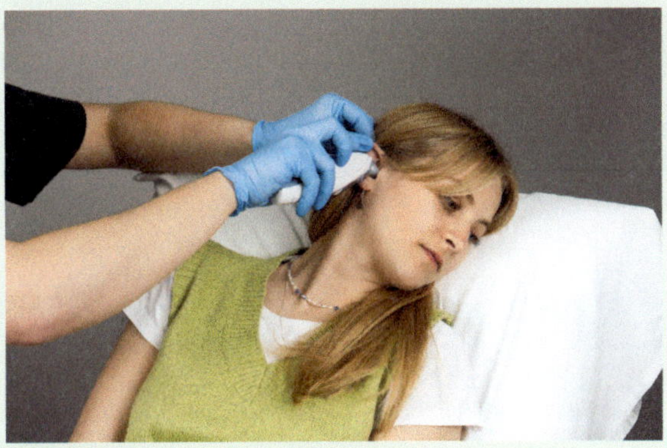	If external air can enter the ear canal, an inaccurate temperature reading may be obtained (8). The thermometer works by taking an infra-red reading of temperature directly from the tympanic membrane. In adults, the probe will probably work its way into the correct position (9). In children, there have been several suggested techniques. Most include gently pulling backwards on the pinna and then either pulling the ear slightly downwards or turning the probe towards the patient's eye (10,11). Follow local guidance.
6.	Push the button that measures temperature and hold the probe still until it has completed; this can take a few seconds.	
7.	Remove from the ear and read the temperature. Check the temperature is recorded in degrees Celsius (°C). 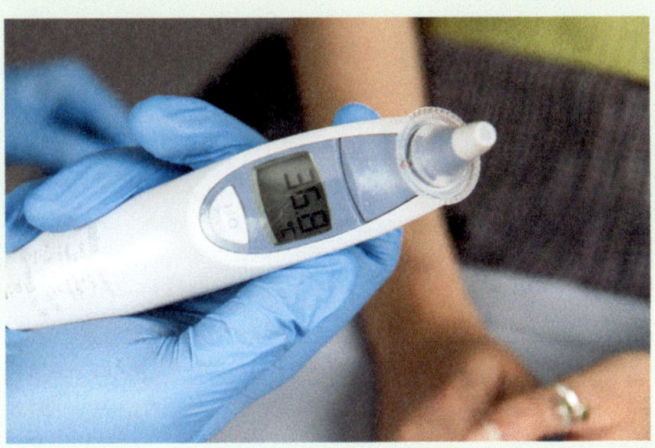	Temperature readings in degrees Fahrenheit (°F) will be higher.
8.	Document the procedure.	You must keep full, clear and accurate records for everyone you care for, treat, or provide other services to (6).

References

1. National Institute for Health and Care Excellence. Fever in under 5s: assessment and initial management [Internet]. NICE; 2019 [cited 2021 May 31]. Available from: https://www.nice.org.uk/guidance/ng143.
2. Arslan GG, Eser I, Khorshid L. Analysis of the effect of lying on the ear on body temperature measurement using a tympanic thermometer. *Journal of Pakistan Medical Association*. 2011 Nov;61(11):1065–1068.
3. Vardasca R, Magalhaes C, Marques D, et al. Bilateral assessment of body core temperature through axillar, tympanic and inner canthi thermometers in a young population. *Physiological Measurement*. 2019 Sep 30;40(9):094001.
4. Braun. Braun ThermoScan Ear Thermometer. Kaz Europe Sarl; 2014.
5. British Medical Association. General information [Internet]. 2018 [cited 2019 Dec 29]. Available from: https://www.bma.org.uk/advice/employment/ethics/consent/consent-tool-kit/2-general-information.
6. Health and Care Professions Council. Standards of conduct, performance and ethics [Internet]. 2018 [cited 2019 Dec 29]. Available from: https://www.hcpc-uk.org/standards/standards-of-conduct-performance-and-ethics/.
7. NHS England, NHS Improvement. Standard infection control precautions: national hand hygiene and personal protective equipment policy [Internet]. 2019 [cited 2021 Nov 11]. Available from: https://www.england.nhs.uk/publication/standard-infection-control-precautions-national-hand-hygiene-and-personal-protective-equipment-policy/.
8. Weiss ME, Sitzer V, Clarke M, et al. A comparison of temperature measurements using three ear thermometers. *Applied Nursing Research*. 1998 Nov;11(4):158–166.
9. Graveling R, MacCalman L, Cowie H. The use of infra-red (tympanic) temperature as a guide to signs of heat stress in industry [Internet]. 2013 [cited 2021 Nov 18]. Available from: https://www.hse.gov.uk/research/rrpdf/rr989.pdf.
10. Childs C, Harrison R, Hodkinson C. Tympanic membrane temperature as a measure of core temperature. *Archives of Disease in Childhood*. 1999 Mar 1;80(3):262–266.
11. Orkun N, Eşer I. The effect of pinna position on body temperature measurements made with a tympanic membrane thermometer in pediatric patients. *Journal of Pediatric Research*. 2020 May 14;7(2):132–138.

Chapter

2 Airway

More often than not, your patient will have a patent airway. However, some patients will need assistance with opening and maintaining their airway. Our experience suggests that when intervention is required, most patients will be successfully managed with simple techniques and adjuncts. Being familiar with how to perform these skills appropriately is essential. Many techniques that are considered basic, such as bag-valve-mask ventilation, can actually be very challenging and require experience and deliberate practice in order for clinicians to be able to master them in all situations. The same is true for inserting and successfully ventilating with supraglottic airway devices.

We would encourage all clinicians who may be called upon to do so, to deliberately practise airway management on a regular basis, including the 'basic' techniques. Being faced with the challenge of managing a difficult airway at a cardiac arrest and trying to remember some tips you last heard during mandatory training a year ago, is not sufficient.

We would like to draw your attention to a few items in this chapter. First, we have deliberately not included cricoid pressure. While we accept that it is still used in practice, there is evidence that it can worsen laryngeal view and may not result in occlusion of the oesophagus, even if applied correctly (1,2).

Second, the BURP manoeuvre (which stands for backward, upward, rightward pressure) and bimanual laryngoscopy with external laryngeal manipulation (ELM) are not the same thing. While they share similarities inasmuch that they both involve moving the larynx to improve the glottic view, bimanual laryngoscopy with ELM is probably the better technique since it enables the clinician with the best view (the intubator), to manoeuvre the larynx into the best position, with the assisting clinician then maintaining that position (3–5).

Finally, we believe that paramedics should, on the rare occasion it is required as part of airway management in cardiac arrest, be able to intubate. However, to do this safely, this needs to be undertaken within a service or system that has robust clinical governance in addition to opportunities for continual training, education, maintenance of competency and provision of the appropriate equipment (6).

References

1. Naik K, Frerk C. Cricoid force: time to put it to one side. *Anaesthesia* [Internet]. 2018 [cited 2018 Oct 31];74(1). Available from: https://onlinelibrary.wiley.com/doi/abs/10.1111/anae.14470.
2. Gautier N, Danklou J, Brichant JF, et al. The effect of force applied to the left paratracheal oesophagus on air entry into the gastric antrum during positive-pressure ventilation using a facemask. *Anaesthesia*. 2019;74(1):22–28.
3. Brown CA, Sakles JC, Mick NW, editors. *The Walls Manual of Emergency Airway Management*. 5th edition. Philadelphia, PA: Wolters Kluwer; 2018.
4. Kovacs G, Law JA. *Airway Management in Emergencies*. 2nd edition. Shelton: McGraw-Hill Medical; 2011.
5. Hwang J, Park S, Huh J, et al. Optimal external laryngeal manipulation: modified bimanual laryngoscopy. *American Journal of Emergency Medicine*. 2013 Jan;31(1):32–36.
6. Gowens P, Aitken-Fell P, Broughton W, et al. Consensus statement: a framework for safe and effective intubation by paramedics. *British Paramedic Journal*. 2018;3(1):23–27.

Recovery Position

Indications

- A spontaneously breathing but unconscious patient who does not have a spinal injury.

Contraindications

- Patients with spinal injuries.
- Patients who require assisted ventilation or insertion of an advanced airway.

Advantages

- Simple and quick to perform, even for a single rescuer.
- Does not require equipment.
- Encourages postural drainage of secretions or vomit from the patient's mouth.

Disadvantages

- Not a definitive airway (does not guarantee that the patient will not aspirate).
- Sometimes difficult to assess patient's breathing and undertake other examinations or monitoring.

Procedure – Recovery Position

Take the following steps to place a patient in the recovery position (1):

Action		Rationale
1.	Don appropriate personal protective equipment (PPE), and undertake appropriate hand hygiene.	This reduces the risk of cross-infection (2).
2.	With the patient lying supine, kneel beside the patient and straighten both of their legs. Quickly check if they have any items in their pockets that should be removed before rolling the patient. 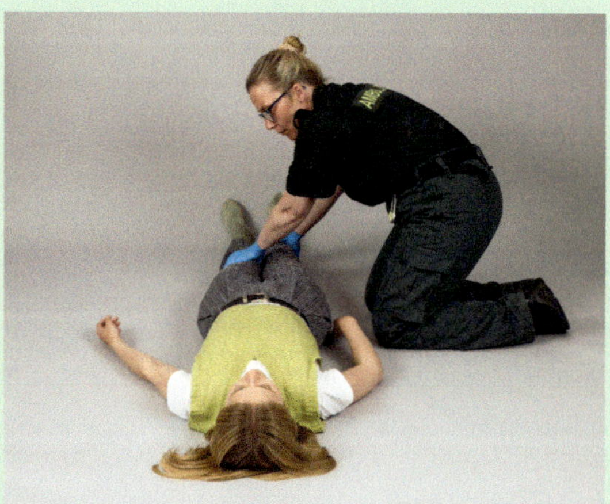	Sharp items such as keys could cause soft-tissue injury.

Action		Rationale
3.	Place the arm nearer to you at right angles to their body, with the arm bent at the elbow and palm of the hand facing upwards. 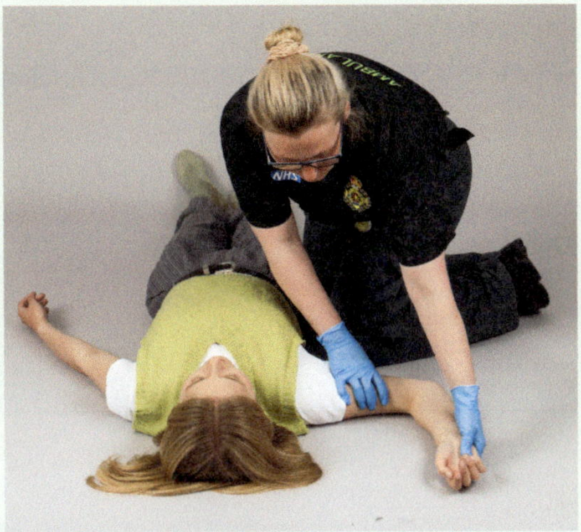	This will keep it clear of the torso when you roll the patient.
4.	Bring the other arm across the chest and hold the back of their hand against the cheek that is nearer to you. Don't let go. 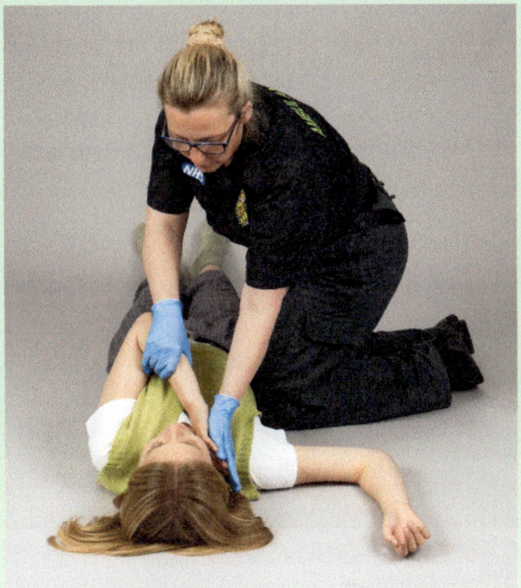	This will provide support for the head during the rolling manoeuvre.

Action		Rationale
5.	With your other hand, grasp the leg furthest away from you just above the knee and lift upwards so the leg flexes. Keep the foot on the ground. 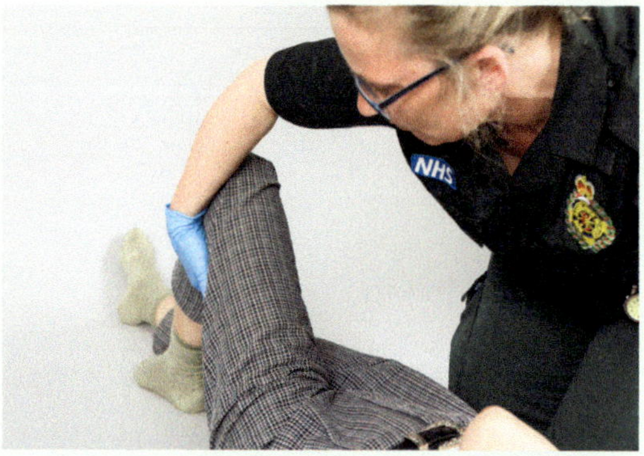 	The bent knee will act as a fulcrum, making it easier to roll the patient, even if they are much larger than the clinician.
6.	While supporting the head, pull the leg towards you, so that the patient rolls to face you. 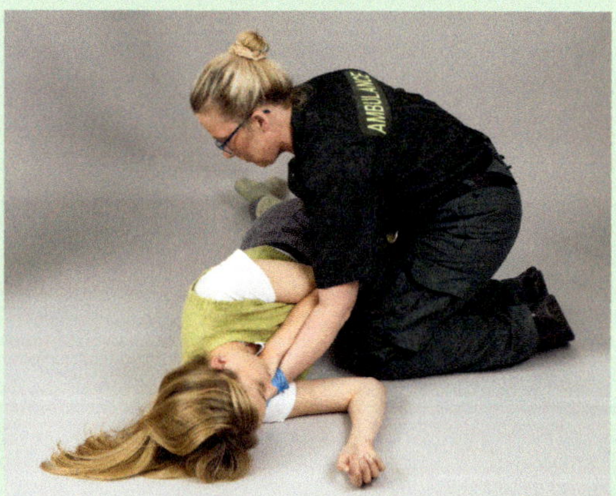 	
7.	Adjust the upper leg so that the patient's hip and knee are bent at right angles. 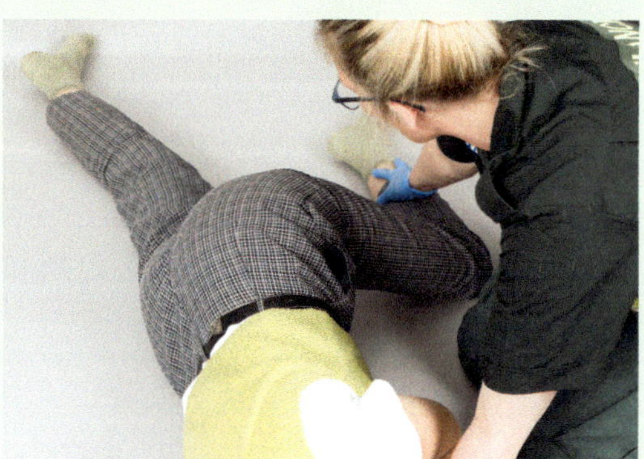	This will prevent the patient from rolling fully prone.

	Action	Rationale
8.	Tilt the head back to ensure the airway remains open. Adjust the patient's hand that is under their cheek if required, to maintain head tilt and keep the patient facing slightly downwards. Reassess frequently. 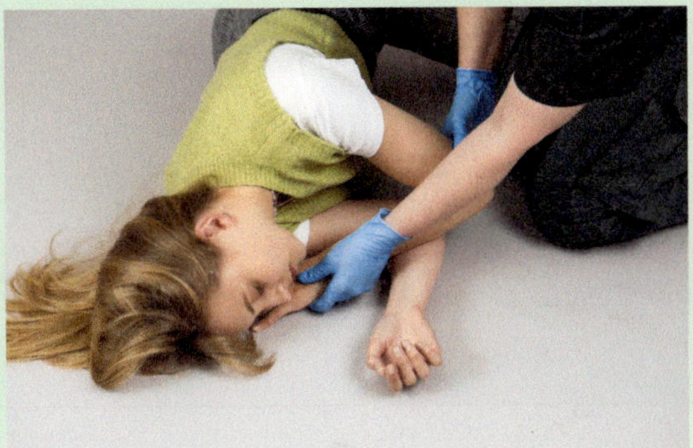	This helps keep the airway patent and allows free drainage of secretions from the mouth.
9.	Document the procedure.	You must keep full, clear and accurate records for everyone you care for, treat, or provide other services to (3).

References

1. Zideman DA, Singletary EM, Borra V, et al. European Resuscitation Council Guidelines 2021: first aid. *Resuscitation*. 2021 Apr;161:270–290.
2. NHS England, NHS Improvement. Standard infection control precautions: national hand hygiene and personal protective equipment policy [Internet]. 2019 [cited 2021 Nov 11]. Available from: https://www.england.nhs.uk/publication/standard-infection-control-precautions-national-hand-hygiene-and-personal-protective-equipment-policy/.
3. Health and Care Professions Council. Standards of conduct, performance and ethics [Internet]. 2018 [cited 2019 Dec 29]. Available from: https://www.hcpc-uk.org/standards/standards-of-conduct-performance-and-ethics/.

Head Tilt–Chin Lift

Indications

- Unresponsive patients who have an airway obstruction caused by loss of pharyngeal muscle tone.

Contraindications

- Suspected cervical spinal injury.

Advantages

- No equipment is required.
- Technique is simple and non-invasive.

Disadvantages

- Does not protect the airway from aspiration.
- Not suitable for patients with a suspected cervical spinal injury.
- Requires practice and experience to perform effectively, especially with more challenging airways, for example in obese patients.

Procedure – Head Tilt–Chin Lift

Take the following steps to perform a head tilt–chin lift (1):

Action		Rationale
1.	Don appropriate personal protective equipment (PPE), and undertake appropriate hand hygiene.	This reduces the risk of cross-infection (2).
2.	With your patient lying on their back (supine), position yourself at the patient's side. Place the hand closer to the patient's head on their forehead and gently tilt the head backwards. 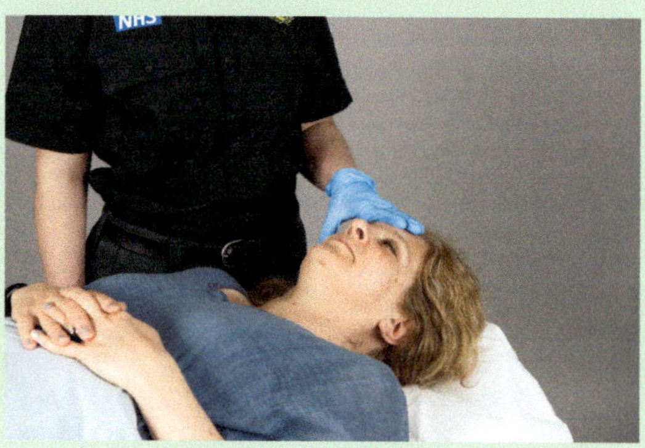	This elevates the tongue and epiglottis away from the posterior pharyngeal wall (3).

Action		Rationale
3.	Place two fingers on the bony part of the chin and gently lift upwards. Take care not to overextend the neck. 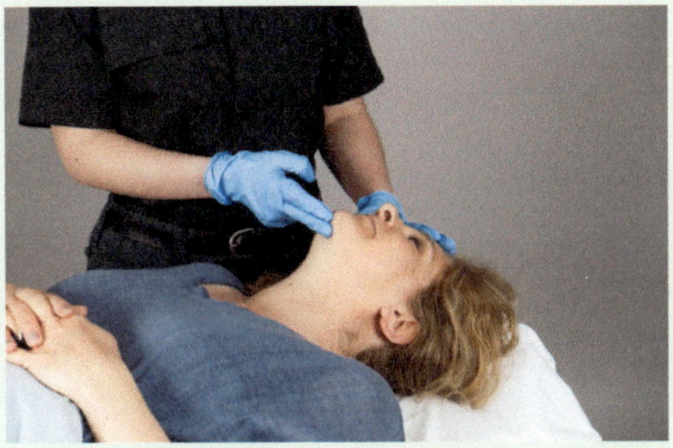	This moves the tongue away from the palate. Together with head extension, this should result in a patent airway (3). Hyperextending the airway can reduce the airway diameter.
4.	Check for procedure success by adopting a look, listen, feel approach (1). 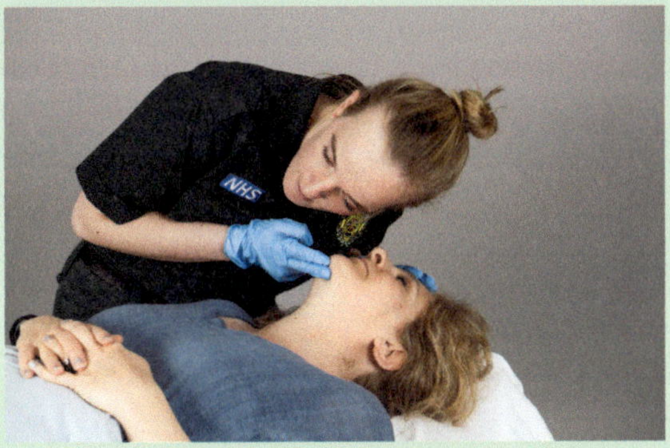	
5.	Document the procedure.	You must keep full, clear and accurate records for everyone you care for, treat, or provide other services to (4).

References

1. Resuscitation Council (UK). *Advanced Life Support*. London: Resuscitation Council (UK); 2021.
2. NHS England, NHS Improvement. Standard infection control precautions: national hand hygiene and personal protective equipment policy [Internet]. 2019 [cited 2021 Nov 11]. Available from: https://www.england.nhs.uk/publication/standard-infection-control-precautions-national-hand-hygiene-and-personal-protective-equipment-policy/.
3. Kovacs G, Law JA. *Airway Management in Emergencies*. 2nd edition. Shelton: McGraw-Hill Medical; 2011.
4. Health and Care Professions Council. Standards of conduct, performance and ethics [Internet]. 2018 [cited 2019 Dec 29]. Available from: https://www.hcpc-uk.org/standards/standards-of-conduct-performance-and-ethics/.

Jaw Thrust

Indications

- Unresponsive patients who have an airway obstruction caused by loss of pharyngeal muscle tone.
- Alternative technique when head tilt–chin lift has been unsuccessful.

Contraindications

- Responsive patients.

Advantages

- No equipment is required.
- Technique is simple and non-invasive.
- Maintains neutral alignment of the head when cervical spine injury is suspected.

Disadvantages

- Does not protect the airway from aspiration.
- Difficult to maintain for long periods.
- Requires an assistant to provide ventilations, if required.

Procedure – Jaw Thrust

Take the following steps to perform a jaw thrust (1):

Action		Rationale
1.	Don appropriate personal protective equipment (PPE), and undertake appropriate hand hygiene.	This reduces the risk of cross-infection (2).
2.	With your patient lying on their back (supine), identify the angle of the mandible. 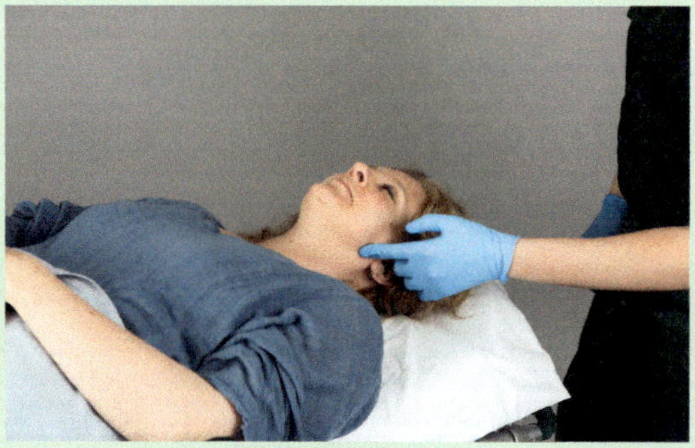	Identification of anatomical structures will ensure correct hand placement in step 3.

3.	Place your fingers behind the mandible and lift in an upwards and forwards direction. 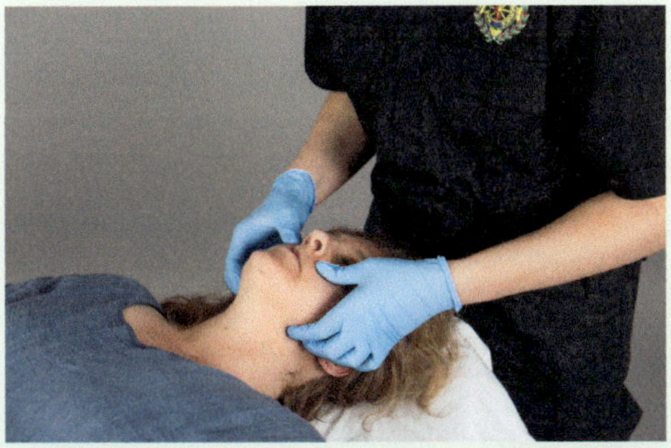	This moves the tongue away from the palate and posterior pharyngeal wall, resulting in a patent airway (3).
4.	Using your thumbs, open the patient's mouth. 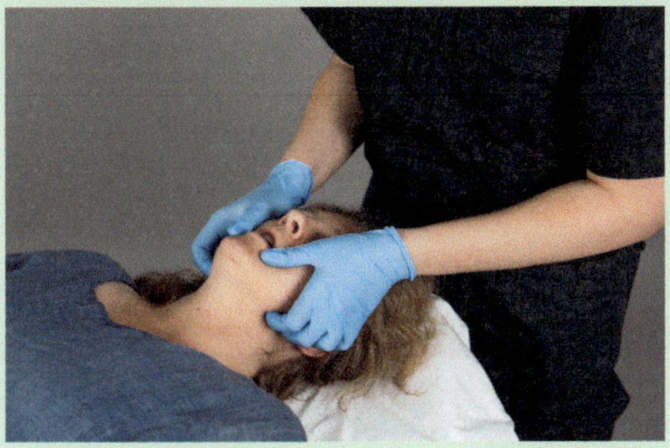	This improves the likelihood that the technique will be effective in obtaining a patent airway (1).
5.	Document the procedure.	You must keep full, clear and accurate records for everyone you care for, treat, or provide other services to (4).

References

1. Resuscitation Council (UK). *Advanced Life Support*. London: Resuscitation Council (UK); 2021.
2. NHS England, NHS Improvement. Standard infection control precautions: national hand hygiene and personal protective equipment policy [Internet]. 2019 [cited 2021 Nov 11]. Available from: https://www.england.nhs.uk/publication/standard-infection-control-precautions-national-hand-hygiene-and-personal-protective-equipment-policy/.
3. Kovacs G, Law JA. *Airway Management in Emergencies*. 2nd edition. Shelton: McGraw-Hill Medical; 2011.
4. Health and Care Professions Council. Standards of conduct, performance and ethics [Internet]. 2018 [cited 2019 Dec 29]. Available from: https://www.hcpc-uk.org/standards/standards-of-conduct-performance-and-ethics/.

Triple Airway Manoeuvre

Indications

- Unresponsive patients who have an airway obstruction caused by loss of pharyngeal muscle tone.
- Head tilt–chin lift and jaw thrust have been unsuccessful.

Contraindications

- Responsive patients.
- Suspected spinal injury.

Advantages

- No equipment is required.
- Technique is simple and non-invasive.

Disadvantages

- Does not protect the airway from aspiration.
- Not suitable for patients with a suspected cervical spinal injury.
- Difficult to maintain for long periods.
- Requires an assistant to provide ventilations, if required.

Procedure – Triple Airway Manoeuvre

Take the following steps to perform the triple airway manoeuvre (1):

Action		Rationale
1.	Don appropriate personal protective equipment (PPE), and undertake appropriate hand hygiene.	This reduces the risk of cross-infection (2).
2.	With your patient lying on their back (supine), identify the angle of the mandible. 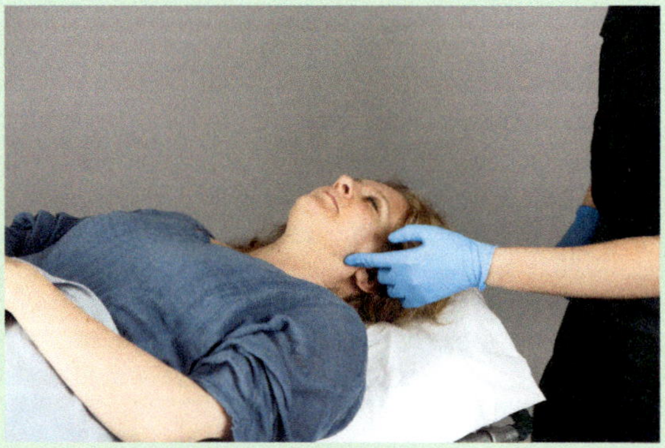	Identification of anatomical structures will ensure correct hand placement in step 3.

Action		Rationale
3.	Place your fingers behind the mandible and lift in an upwards and forwards direction. 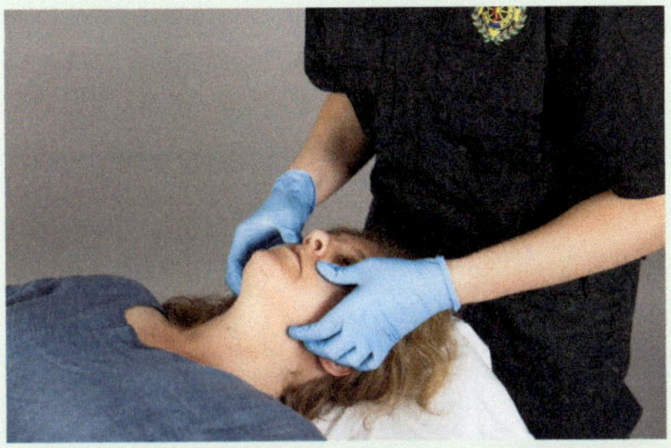	This moves the tongue away from the palate and posterior pharyngeal wall, resulting in a patent airway (3).
4.	Using your thumbs, open the patient's mouth. 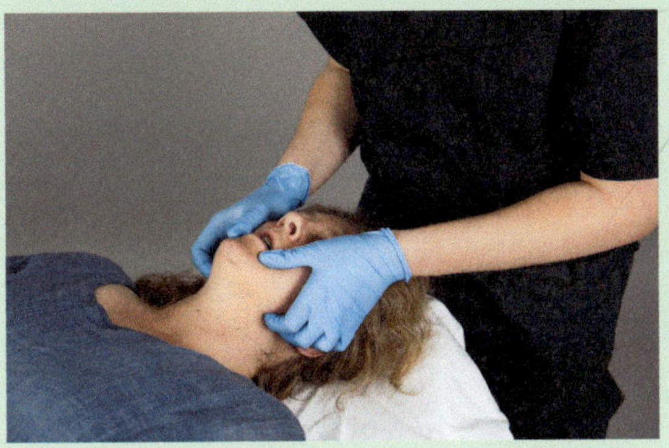	Improves the likelihood that the technique will be effective in obtaining a patent airway (4).
5.	Tilt the head backwards. 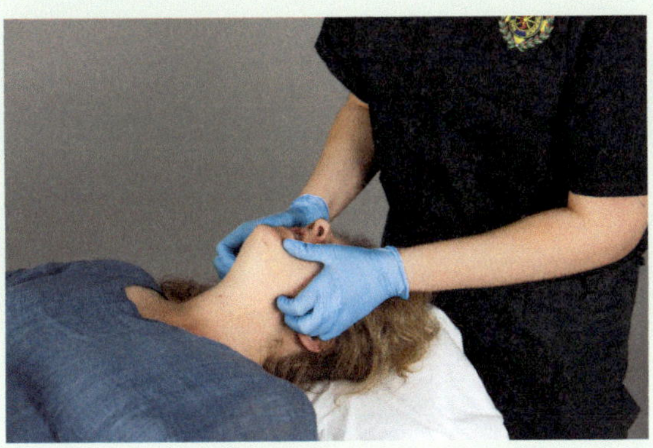	This further improves airway patency and, together with steps 3 and 4, may lead to increased supraglottic airway insertion success and reduced time to successful insertion (5,6).
6.	Document the procedure.	You must keep full, clear and accurate records for everyone you care for, treat, or provide other services to (7).

References

1. Queensland Ambulance Service. Clinical Practice Manual [Internet]. 2021 [cited 2022 Jan 2]. Available from: https://ambulance.qld.gov.au/clinical.html.
2. NHS England, NHS Improvement. Standard infection control precautions: national hand hygiene and personal protective equipment policy [Internet]. 2019 [cited 2021 Nov 11]. Available from: https://www.england.nhs.uk/publication/standard-infection-control-precautions-national-hand-hygiene-and-personal-protective-equipment-policy/.
3. Kovacs G, Law JA. *Airway Management in Emergencies*. 2nd edition. Shelton: McGraw-Hill Medical; 2011.
4. Resuscitation Council (UK). *Advanced Life Support*. London: Resuscitation Council (UK); 2021.
5. Aoyama K, Takenaka I, Sata T, et al. The triple airway manoeuvre for insertion of the laryngeal mask airway in paralyzed patients. *Canadian Journal of Anaesthesia*. 1995 Nov;42(11):1010–1016.
6. Baran Akkuş i, Kavak Akelma F, Emlek M, et al. Comparison of the standard and triple airway maneuvering techniques for i-gel™ placement in patients undergoing elective surgery: a randomized controlled study. *Journal of Anesthesia*. 2020 Aug 1;34(4):512–518.
7. Health and Care Professions Council. Standards of conduct, performance and ethics [Internet]. 2018 [cited 2019 Dec 29]. Available from: https://www.hcpc-uk.org/standards/standards-of-conduct-performance-and-ethics/.

BURP Manoeuvre

Indications

- To improve view of laryngeal inlet during intubation attempt.

Contraindications

- None.

Advantages

- May improve the view by as much as one full Cormack-Lahane grade (1).

Disadvantages

- Not as effective as external laryngeal manipulation.

Procedure – BURP Manoeuvre

Take the following steps to perform the BURP (backward, upward, rightward pressure) manoeuvre (1,2):

Action		Rationale
1.	Don appropriate personal protective equipment (PPE), and undertake appropriate hand hygiene.	This reduces the risk of cross-infection (3).
2.	When instructed to do so by the intubating clinician, place your thumb, index and middle fingers on the patient's thyroid cartilage. 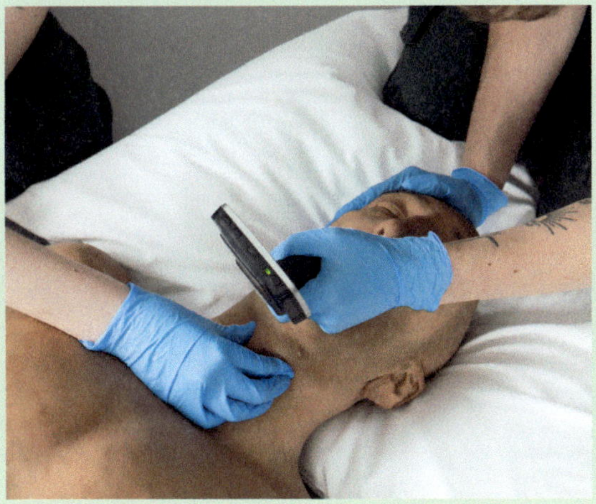	Clear communication with the intubating clinician will ensure the manoeuvre is choreographed.
3.	Provide backward, upward, rightward pressure, stopping when instructed to do so by the intubating clinician when a clear view is obtained. Note that the airway operator may choose to use their dominant hand to guide this movement and let go once they have an optimal view.	The whole manoeuvre may not need to be completed to obtain an optimal view.

Action		Rationale
4.	Maintain the position and steady pressure until instructed to remove it by the intubating clinician. If a video laryngoscope is being used, monitor the view to ensure that the correct pressure continues to be maintained.	Premature release may result in loss of view and abandonment of the intubation attempt.
5.	Document the procedure.	You must keep full, clear and accurate records for everyone you care for, treat, or provide other services to (4).

References

1. Brown CA, Sakles JC, Mick NW, editors. *The Walls Manual of Emergency Airway Management*. 5th edition. Philadelphia, PA: Wolters Kluwer; 2018.
2. Kovacs G, Law JA. *Airway Management in Emergencies*. 2nd edition. Shelton: McGraw-Hill Medical; 2011.
3. NHS England, NHS Improvement. Standard infection control precautions: national hand hygiene and personal protective equipment policy [Internet]. 2019 [cited 2021 Nov 11]. Available from: https://www.england.nhs.uk/publication/standard-infection-control-precautionsnational-hand-hygiene-and-personal-protectiveequipment-policy/.
4. Health and Care Professions Council. Standards of conduct, performance and ethics [Internet]. 2018 [cited 2019 Dec 29]. Available from: https://www.hcpc-uk.org/standards/standards-of-conduct-performance-and-ethics/.

Bimanual Laryngoscopy with External Laryngeal Manipulation

Indications
- To improve view of laryngeal inlet during intubation attempt.

Contraindications
- None.

Advantages
- More effective than BURP (backward, upward, rightward pressure) manoeuvre at improving glottic view (1,2).

Disadvantages
- None.

Procedure – Bimanual Laryngoscopy with External Laryngeal Manipulation

Take the following steps to perform bimanual laryngoscopy with external laryngeal manipulation (ELM) (2–4):

Action		Rationale
1.	Don appropriate personal protective equipment (PPE), and undertake appropriate hand hygiene.	This reduces the risk of cross-infection (5).
2.	The non-intubating clinician should place their thumb, index and middle fingers on the patient's thyroid cartilage. 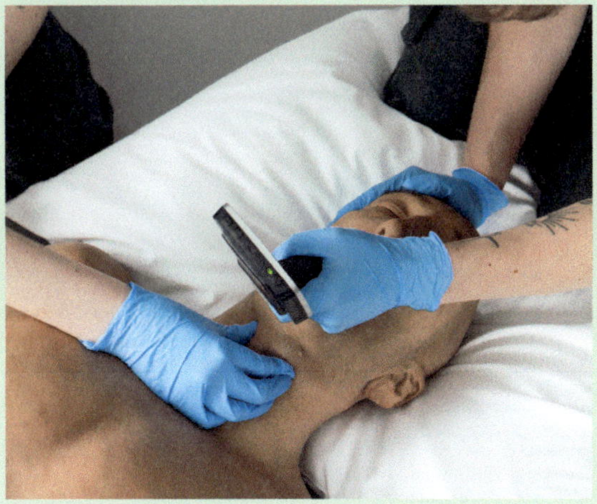	

Action		Rationale
3.	Once the laryngoscope has been placed into the vallecula, the intubating clinician places their right hand over the non-intubating clinician's hand and guides it into the optimal position which provides the best view of the glottic opening. 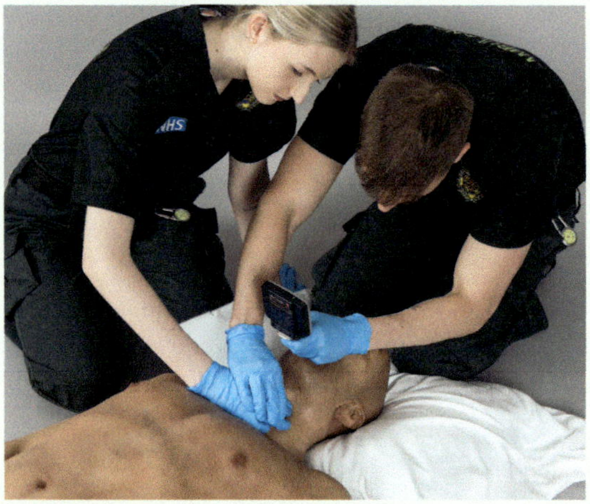	
4.	The intubating clinician instructs the non-intubating clinician to 'keep the pressure and direction' applied to the larynx.	
5.	The non-intubating clinician maintains the position and steady pressure until instructed to remove their hand by the intubating clinician. If a video laryngoscope is being used, monitor the view to ensure that the correct pressure continues to be maintained.	Premature release may result in loss of view and abandonment of the intubation attempt.
6.	Document the procedure.	You must keep full, clear and accurate records for everyone you care for, treat, or provide other services to (6).

References

1. Levitan RM, Mickler T, Hollander JE. Bimanual laryngoscopy: a videographic study of external laryngeal manipulation by novice intubators. *Annals of Emergency Medicine*. 2002 Jul;40(1):30–37.
2. Hwang J, Park S, Huh J, et al. Optimal external laryngeal manipulation: modified bimanual laryngoscopy. *American Journal of Emergency Medicine*. 2013 Jan;31(1):32–36.
3. Brown CA, Sakles JC, Mick NW, editors. *The Walls Manual of Emergency Airway Management*. 5th edition. Philadelphia, PA: Wolters Kluwer; 2018.
4. Kovacs G, Law JA. *Airway Management in Emergencies*. 2nd edition. Shelton: McGraw-Hill Medical; 2011.
5. NHS England, NHS Improvement. Standard infection control precautions: national hand hygiene and personal protective equipment policy [Internet]. 2019 [cited 2021 Nov 11]. Available from: https://www.england.nhs.uk/publication/standard-infection-control-precautionsnational-hand-hygiene-and-personal-protectiveequipment-policy/.
6. Health and Care Professions Council. Standards of conduct, performance and ethics [Internet]. 2018 [cited 2019 Dec 29]. Available from: https://www.hcpc-uk.org/standards/standards-of-conduct-performance-and-ethics/.

Airway Foreign-Body Removal with Laryngoscopy

Indications

- To facilitate removal of foreign bodies located in the pharynx in the unconscious patient.

Contraindications

- Any patient who has an effective cough.
- Any patient who is not unconscious.

Advantages

- May be more effective at removing foreign bodies than more basic manoeuvres (although evidence is weak) (1,2).

Disadvantages

- Prolonged laryngoscopy can contribute to hypoxia.
- Aggressive or careless laryngoscopy can damage tissues of the pharynx.
- Manipulating a foreign body (FB) can cause a partial obstruction to become a complete obstruction.

Procedure – Airway Foreign-Body Removal with Laryngoscopy

Take the following steps to remove an FB from the airway with laryngoscopy (3):

Action		Rationale
1.	Don appropriate personal protective equipment (PPE), and undertake appropriate hand hygiene.	This reduces the risk of cross-infection (4).
2.	Prepare your equipment. You will need: • Suction • Laryngoscope and blade • Oxygen • Bag-valve-mask (BVM) • Magill forceps. 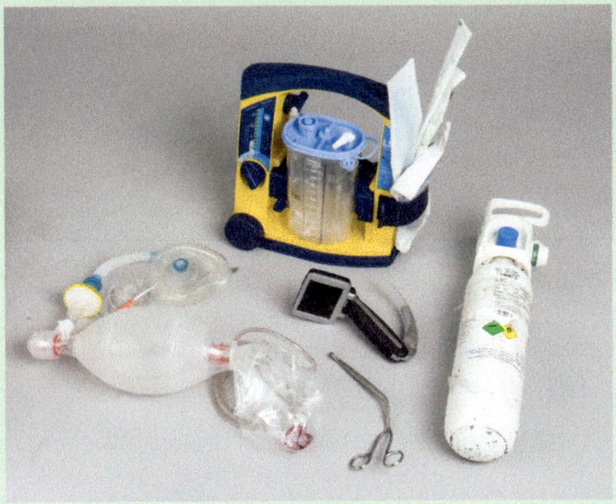	

Action		Rationale
3.	Place the patient on their back (supine) and consider moving them so that you have more space to work.	
4.	Pull down on the chin to inspect the anterior portion of the oropharynx. If an FB is visible, remove with Magill forceps. 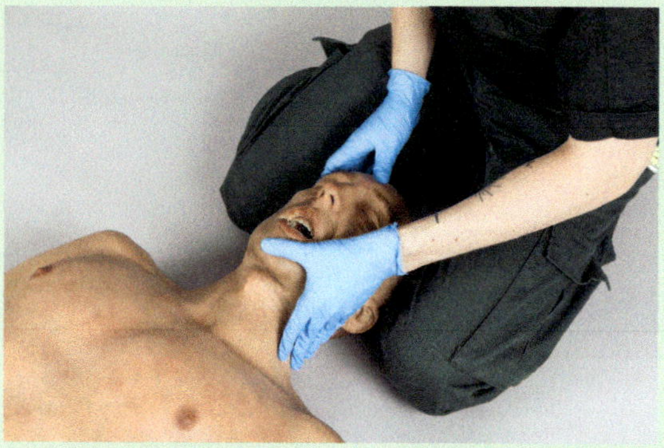	If an FB is present, step 5 may inadvertently cause the FB to move posteriorly. Remember to consider suction at all stages of this procedure.
5.	Place the patient's head and neck in the 'sniffing the morning air' position (head extended and neck flexed). 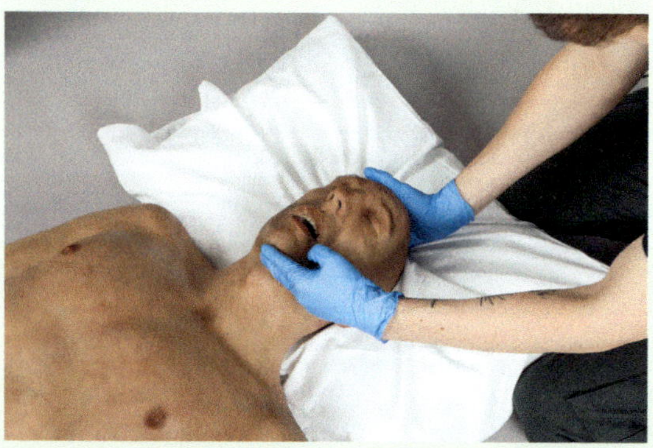	This will help optimise the view of the laryngeal inlet. A pillow is useful if you have one available.
6.	Open the patient's mouth and inspect the oral cavity, using a 'scissor technique', if required. This is achieved by placing the thumb of your right hand on the lower incisors and the middle finger on the upper incisors and scissoring the jaw open.	Some patients, when placed in an appropriate head position, will have a jaw that opens to reveal a gaping chasm, preferably without teeth. If this is not the case, then the 'scissor technique' can assist in visualisation of the oral cavity.

<table>
<tr><th></th><th>Action</th><th>Rationale</th></tr>
<tr><td></td><td>Remove dentures if present, to give yourself more room to work.
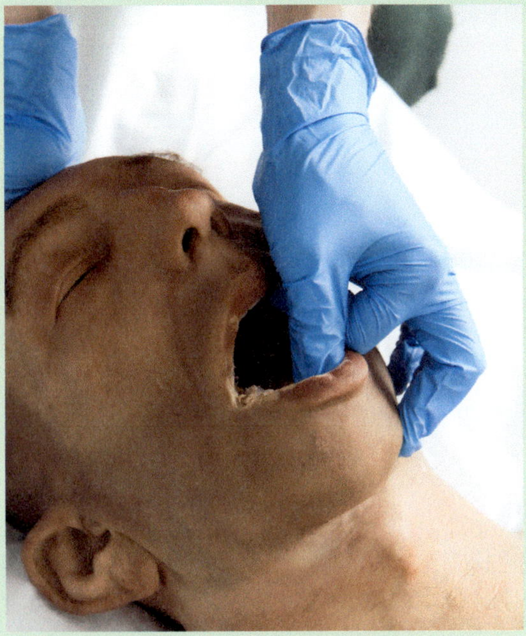</td><td></td></tr>
<tr><td>7.</td><td>Grip the laryngoscope low down on the handle, such that the proximal end of the blade pushes into the thenar or hypothenar eminence of your left hand.
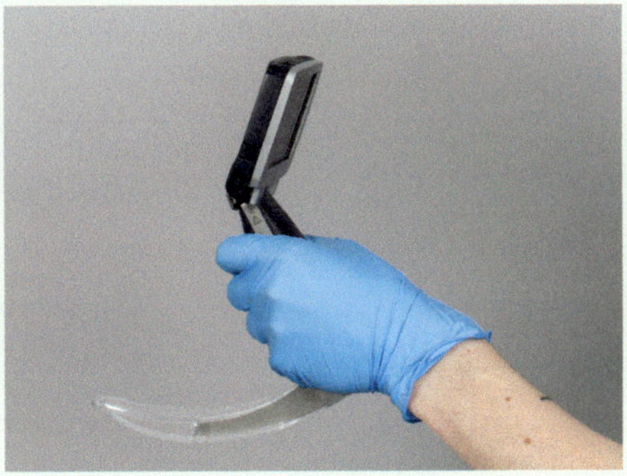</td><td></td></tr>
<tr><td></td><td>Insert the blade along the right mandibular (lower) molars and gently sweep the tongue to the left (5).</td><td>Only insert the laryngoscope as far as required to remove the foreign body. This will reduce the chance of oropharyngeal or laryngeal injury.</td></tr>
</table>

Action		Rationale
	With the mouth open, check to see whether suction is required, but take care only to suction the oropharynx that you can see. 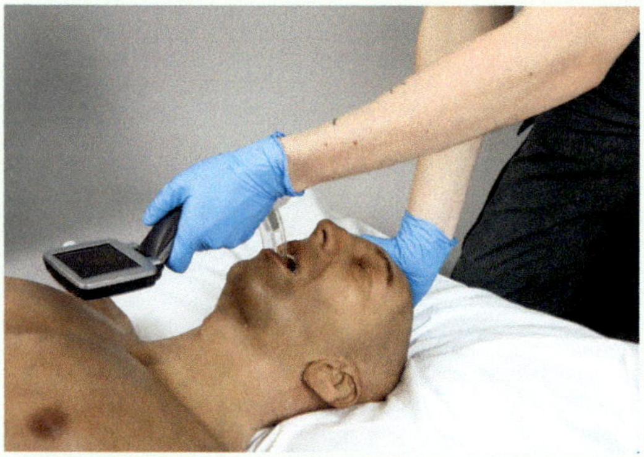	Keeping the suction tip in view will help minimise any damage to soft tissues or laryngeal structures.
8.	With the laryngoscope blade in the midline, slowly advance the blade until the epiglottis comes into view. Then advance the laryngoscope to the vallecula. 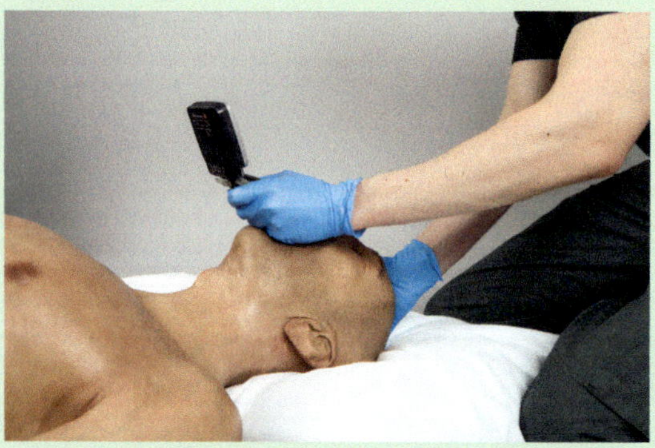	The epiglottis is reliably located at the base of the tongue, making it easier to orientate yourself (6).
9.	Lift the blade at an angle of 45° (or parallel to the handle) until you can see the posterior or arytenoid cartilages and the inter-arytenoid notch (7).	This should provide a good view of the entire laryngeal inlet and surrounding structures.
10.	Grasp the forceps in your right hand, inserting your thumb and either ring or middle finger into the ring handles. You can use your index finger to guide the forceps by resting it on the shaft of the forceps. Insert the closed forceps into the patient's mouth.	This will ensure your hands do not obstruct your view while retrieving the FB.

Action		Rationale
	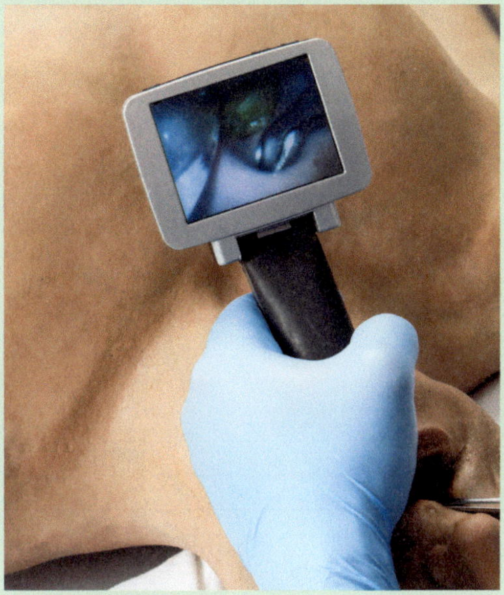	
11.	Under direct vision, open the forceps to grasp the FB, taking care not to grab any pharyngeal structures or the epiglottis in the process, and remove. 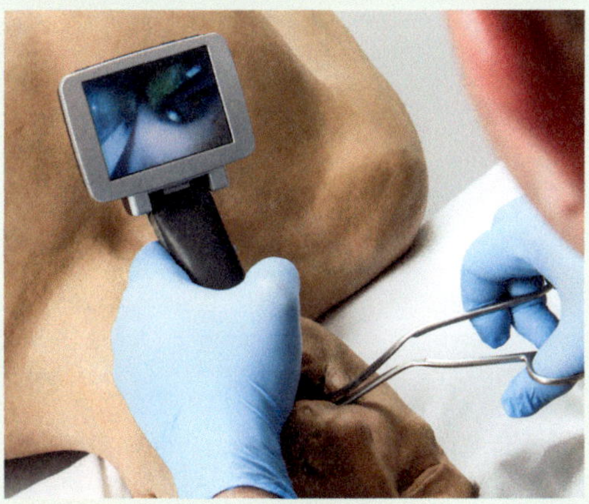 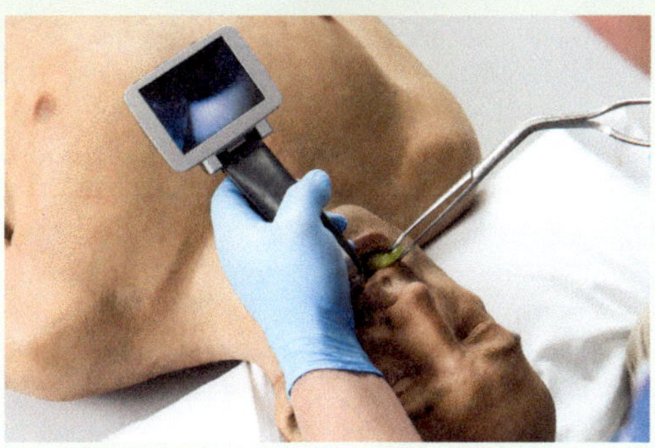	While the priority is to obtain a patent airway, you should try not to damage delicate airway structures.

Action		Rationale
12.	Attempt to oxygenate your patient, with assisted ventilations if required. 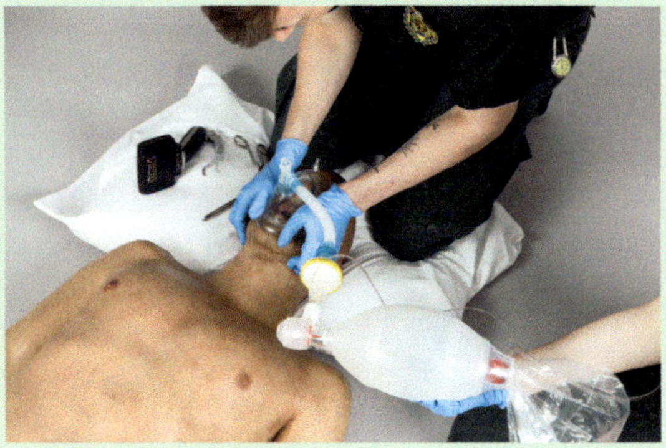	Choking is a hypoxic event.
13.	If the FB has not been fully removed, repeat this procedure once more.	You are likely to have to repeat this procedure to retrieve a foreign body. However, if you cannot remove the foreign body after two attempts, concentrate on chest compressions instead (8). As always, follow local guidance.
14.	Document the procedure.	You must keep full, clear and accurate records for everyone you care for, treat, or provide other services to (9).

References

1. Sakai T, Kitamura T, Iwami T, et al. Effectiveness of prehospital Magill forceps use for out-of-hospital cardiac arrest due to foreign body airway obstruction in Osaka City. *Scandinavian Journal of Trauma, Resuscitation and Emergency Medicine* [Internet]. 2014 Sep 4 [cited 2015 Oct 14];22. Available from: http://www.ncbi.nlm.nih.gov/pmc/articles/PMC4156961/.
2. Soroudi A, Shipp HE, Stepanski BM, et al. Adult foreign body airway obstruction in the prehospital setting. *Prehospital Emergency Care*. 2007 Jan;11(1):25–29.
3. Queensland Ambulance Service. Clinical practice manual [Internet]. 2021 [cited 2022 Jan 2]. Available from: https://ambulance.qld.gov.au/clinical.html.
4. NHS England, NHS Improvement. Standard infection control precautions: national hand hygiene and personal protective equipment policy [Internet]. 2019 [cited 2021 Nov 11]. Available from: https://www.england.nhs.uk/publication/standard-infection-control-precautions-national-hand-hygiene-and-personal-protective-equipment-policy/.
5. Brown CA. *The Walls Manual of Emergency Airway Management*. 5th edition. Sakles JC, Mick NW, editors. Philadelphia, PA: Lippincott Williams and Wilkins; 2017.
6. Levitan RM, Sather SD, Ochroch EA. Demystifying direct laryngoscopy and intubation. *Hospital Physician*. 2000;36(5):47–56.
7. Schmitt HJ, Mang H. Head and neck elevation beyond the sniffing position improves laryngeal view in cases of difficult direct laryngoscopy. *Journal of Clinical Anesthesia*. 2002 Aug;14(5):335–338.
8. Olasveengen TM, Mancini ME, Perkins GD, et al. Adult basic life support: 2020 international consensus on cardiopulmonary resuscitation and emergency cardiovascular care science with treatment recommendations. *Circulation*. 2020 Oct 20;142(16 Suppl 1):S41–91.
9. Health and Care Professions Council. Standards of conduct, performance and ethics [Internet]. 2018 [cited 2019 Dec 29]. Available from: https://www.hcpc-uk.org/standards/standards-of-conduct-performance-and-ethics/.

Suctioning with a Rigid Suction Catheter

Indications

- Patients who cannot maintain and clear their own airway and in whom vomit, blood or secretions are at risk of entering the lower respiratory tract.

Contraindications

- Patients who can maintain and clear their own airway.

Advantages

- Reduces risk of aspiration of vomit, blood and secretions.
- Supports maintenance of a clear airway.

Disadvantages

- Suctioning removes air as well as secretions.
- Might not be possible to use with patients who have limited mouth opening.
- May not be sufficient to overcome continuous emesis or haemorrhage.

Procedure – Suctioning with a Rigid Suction Catheter

Take the following steps to suction an airway with a rigid suction catheter (1,2):

Action		Rationale
1.	Don appropriate PPE, including respiratory protective equipment (RPE) if suctioning beyond the oropharynx (3), and undertake appropriate hand hygiene.	This reduces the risk of cross-infection (4).
2.	Prepare your equipment. You will need: • Suction unit • Rigid wide-bore and soft-tip catheters and suction tubing • Oxygen. 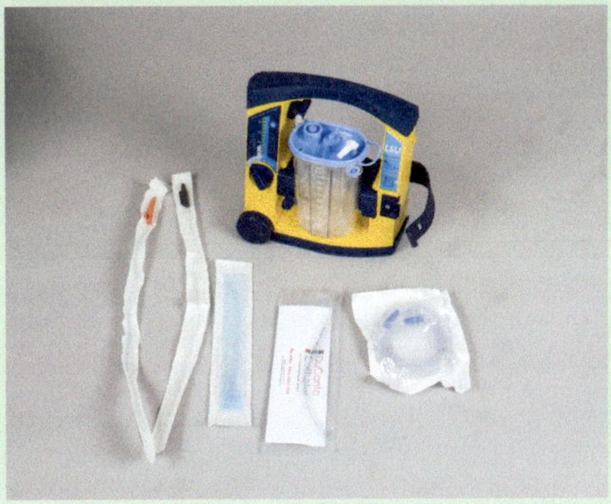	

	Action	Rationale
3.	Consider adjusting the patient position to allow for postural drainage and pre-oxygenate the patient, if you have time.	In cases of severe bleeding or active vomiting, positioning the patient to allow for postural drainage is important. This can be achieved by turning the patient on their side and positioning the trolley into a head-down position (5). Suctioning (especially prolonged) may cause hypoxia so supplemental oxygen is useful.
4.	Attach suction tubing and catheter and switch on the suction unit. Adjust the suction pressure based on the volume and viscosity of airway contaminant to be cleared. 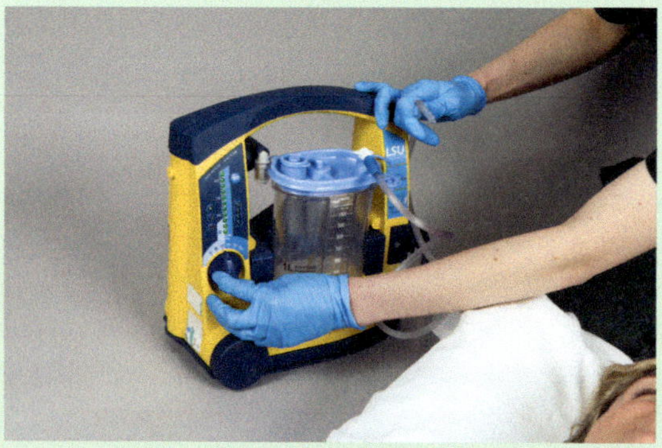	If you only need to clear small amounts of saliva, then a suction pressure of 100–150 mmHg is sufficient (1). However, in cases where there is a large amount of blood or vomit, turn the suction up to maximum initially and adjust downwards, as required.
5.	Open the patient's mouth and insert the catheter into their mouth without suctioning. Make sure you can always visualise the end of the suction catheter. 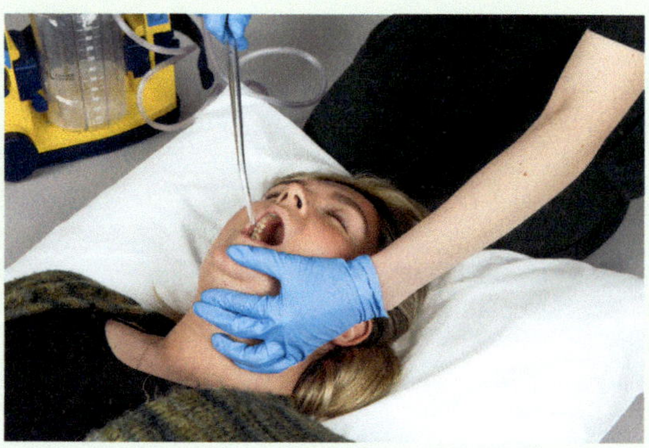	This is not possible with suction catheters that have no vent hole. Take care not to damage soft tissue, particularly when using high-pressure suction. Visualising the tip will ensure you do not inadvertently insert the suction catheter too far.

Action		Rationale
6.	Apply suction by occluding the vent hole on the catheter and gently withdraw the catheter. Suction for no more than 10 seconds (6). 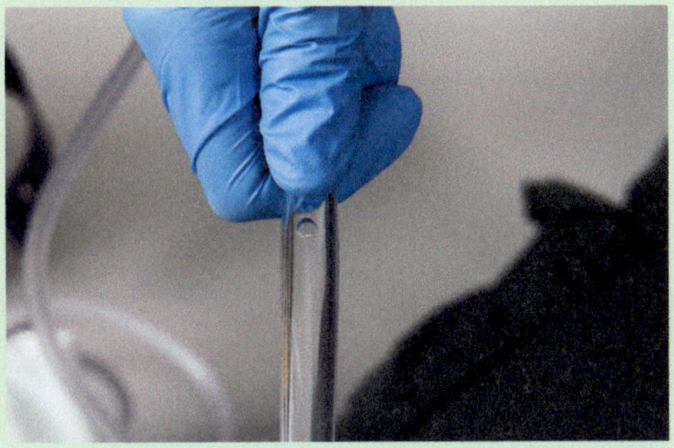	Although prolonged suctioning will cause hypoxia (which is why suctioning for no more than 10 seconds is suggested), an airway obstructed by blood or vomit will not allow any air exchange and is likely to result in aspiration. In this case, patient positioning and aggressive suctioning will be required until the airway is at least partially clear, even if this takes more than 10 seconds (7).
7.	Re-oxygenate the patient and reassess the airway. Further suction attempts may be required.	This helps to prevent and address hypoxia (2).
8.	Document the procedure.	You must keep full, clear and accurate records for everyone you care for, treat, or provide other services to (8).

References

1. Randle J, Coffey F, Bradbury M. *Oxford Handbook of Clinical Skills in Adult Nursing*. Oxford: Oxford University Press; 2009.
2. Roberts J et al. *Roberts and Hedges' Clinical Procedures in Emergency Medicine and Acute Care*, 7th edition. Philadelphia, PA: Elsevier; 2018.
3. UK Health Security Agency, NHS England, Public Health Agency (Northern Ireland), Public Health Wales. Infection prevention and control for seasonal respiratory infections in health and care settings (including SARS-CoV-2) for winter 2021 to 2022 [Internet]. 2021 [cited 2022 Jan 16]. Available from: https://www.gov.uk/government/publications/wuhan-novel-coronavirus-infection-prevention-and-control/covid-19-guidance-for-maintaining-services-within-health-and-care-settings-infection-prevention-and-control-recommendations.
4. NHS England, NHS Improvement. Standard infection control precautions: national hand hygiene and personal protective equipment policy [Internet]. 2019 [cited 2021 Nov 11]. Available from: https://www.england.nhs.uk/publication/standard-infection-control-precautions-national-hand-hygiene-and-personal-protective-equipment-policy/.
5. Nutbeam T, Boylan M. *ABC of Prehospital Emergency Medicine*. Chichester: John Wiley & Sons; 2013.
6. National Tracheostomy Safety Project (Great Britain). *Comprehensive Tracheostomy Care: The National Tracheostomy Safety Project Manual*. McGrath BA, editor. Chichester: John Wiley & Sons; 2014.
7. National Association of Emergency Medical Technicians (US), editor. *PHTLS: Prehospital Trauma Life Support*. 9th edition. Burlington, MA: Jones & Bartlett Learning; 2020.
8. Health and Care Professions Council. Standards of conduct, performance and ethics [Internet]. 2018 [cited 2019 Dec 29]. Available from: https://www.hcpc-uk.org/standards/standards-of-conduct-performance-and-ethics/.

Suctioning with a Flexible Suction Catheter

Indications

- Patients who cannot maintain and clear their own airway and in whom secretions are at risk of entering the lower respiratory tract or have already done so.

Contraindications

- Patients who can maintain and clear their own airway.

Advantages

- Reduces risk of aspiration of secretions.
- Can provide suction through airway adjuncts, supraglottic airways, and tracheostomy and tracheal tubes.
- Less likely to cause soft-tissue injury than using a rigid suction catheter.

Disadvantages

- Suctioning removes air as well as secretions.
- Not suitable for thick liquids and solids.

Procedure – Suctioning with a Flexible Suction Catheter

Take the following steps to suction an airway with a flexible suction catheter (1,2):

Action		Rationale
1.	Don appropriate PPE, including respiratory protective equipment (RPE) if suctioning beyond the oropharynx (3), and undertake appropriate hand hygiene.	This reduces the risk of cross-infection (4).
2.	Prepare your equipment. You will need: • Suction unit • Rigid wide-bore and soft-tip catheters and suction tubing • Oxygen.	
3.	Explain the procedure to the patient and obtain consent if appropriate to do so.	You must make sure that you have valid consent from service users or other appropriate authority before you provide care, treatment or other services (5,6).
4.	Consider adjusting the patient position to allow for postural drainage if you have time.	In cases of severe bleeding or active vomiting, positioning the patient to allow for postural drainage is important. This can be achieved by turning the patient on their side and positioning the trolley into a head-down position (7). Suctioning (especially prolonged) may cause hypoxia so supplemental oxygen is useful.

Action		Rationale
5.	Attach suction tubing and catheter and switch on the suction unit. Adjust the suction pressure based on the type of fluid. 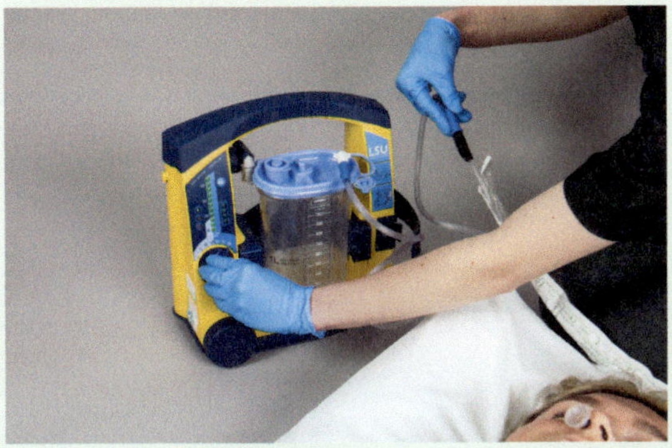	If you only need to clear small amounts of saliva, then a suction pressure of 100–150 mmHg is sufficient (1). However, in cases where there is a large amount of blood or vomit, turn the suction up to maximum initially and adjust downwards, as required.
6.	With your thumb clear of the suction port, insert the catheter no further than the end of the airway adjunct or tracheostomy tube. This can be achieved by measuring the catheter against another (uninserted) adjunct or tube. 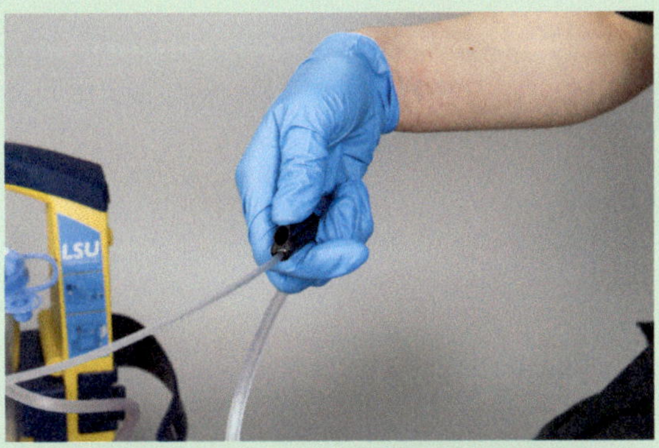 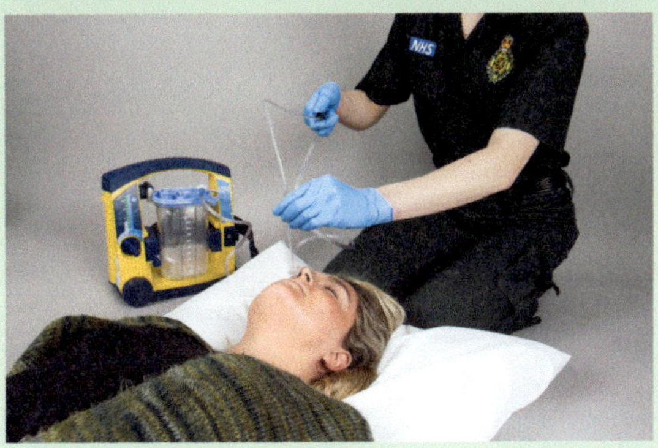	This will ensure you do not inadvertently insert the suction catheter too far. Note: Tracheostomy suctioning should be performed with a non-fenestrated inner tube in situ (8).

Action		Rationale
7.	Occlude the suction port, apply suction and gently withdraw the catheter. Suction for no more than 10 seconds (8). 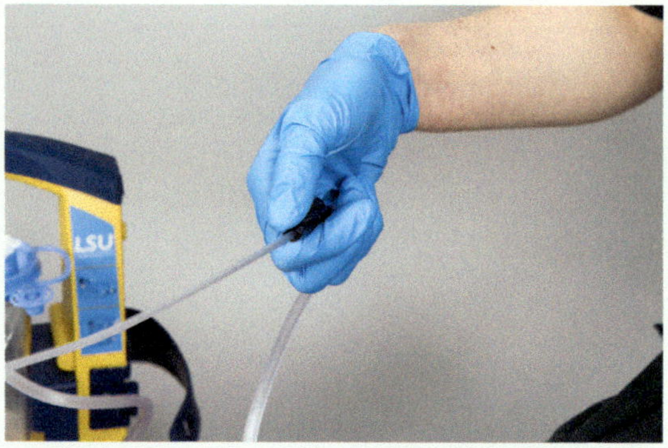 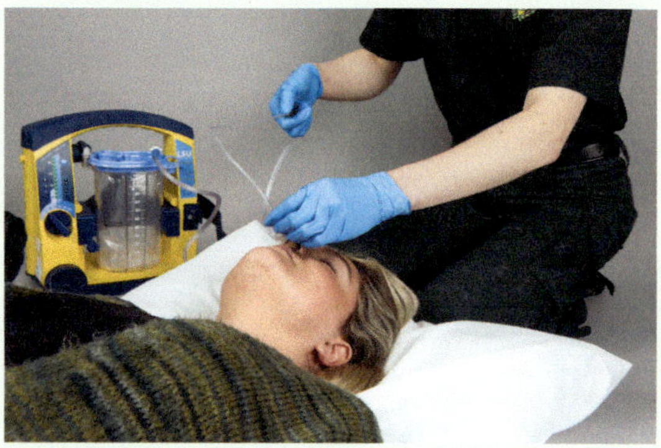	Although prolonged suctioning will cause hypoxia (which is why suctioning for no more than 10 seconds is suggested), an airway obstructed by blood or vomit will not allow any air exchange to take place and is likely to result in aspiration. In this case, patient positioning and aggressive suctioning will be required until the airway is at least partially clear, even if this takes more than 10 seconds (9).
8.	Re-oxygenate the patient and reassess the airway. Further suction attempts may be required.	This helps to prevent and/or address hypoxia (2).
9.	Document the procedure.	You must keep full, clear and accurate records for everyone you care for, treat, or provide other services to (6).

References

1. Randle J, Coffey F, Bradbury M. *Oxford Handbook of Clinical Skills in Adult Nursing*. Oxford: Oxford University Press; 2009.
2. Roberts J. *Roberts and Hedges' Clinical Procedures in Emergency Medicine and Acute Care*. 7th edition. Philadelphia, PA: Elsevier; 2018.
3. UK Health Security Agency, NHS England, Public Health Agency (Northern Ireland), Public Health Wales. Infection prevention and control for seasonal respiratory infections in health and care settings (including SARS-CoV-2) for winter 2021 to 2022 [Internet]. 2021 [cited 2022 Jan 16]. Available from: https://www.gov.uk/government/publications/wuhan-novel-coronavirus-infection-prevention-and-control/covid-19-guidance-for-maintaining-services-within-health-and-care-settings-infection-prevention-and-control-recommendations.
4. NHS England, NHS Improvement. Standard infection control precautions: national hand hygiene and personal protective equipment policy [Internet]. 2019 [cited 2021 Nov 11]. Available from: https://www.england.nhs.uk/publication/

standard-infection-control-precautions-national-hand-hygiene-and-personal-protective-equipment-policy/.

5. British Medical Association. General information [Internet]. 2018 [cited 2019 Dec 29]. Available from: https://www.bma.org.uk/advice/employment/ethics/consent/consent-tool-kit/2-general-information.
6. Health and Care Professions Council. Standards of conduct, performance and ethics [Internet]. 2018 [cited 2019 Dec 29]. Available from: https://www.hcpc-uk.org/standards/standards-of-conduct-performance-and-ethics/.
7. Nutbeam T, Boylan M. *ABC of Prehospital Emergency Medicine*. Chichester: John Wiley & Sons; 2013.
8. National Tracheostomy Safety Project (Great Britain). *Comprehensive Tracheostomy Care: The National Tracheostomy Safety Project Manual*. McGrath BA, editor. Chichester: John Wiley & Sons; 2014.
9. National Association of Emergency Medical Technicians (US), editor. *PHTLS: Prehospital Trauma Life Support*. 9th edition. Burlington, MA: Jones & Bartlett Learning; 2020.

Oropharyngeal Airway

Indications

- An unresponsive patient with an absent gag reflex.
- Patient requires bag-valve-mask ventilation.

Contraindications

- Patient has a gag reflex.

Advantages

- Easy to place.
- Technique is simple and minimally invasive.

Disadvantages

- Tongue can be pushed back during insertion, making obstruction worse.
- Does not protect against vomiting or aspiration.

Procedure – Oropharyngeal Airway Insertion

Take the following steps to insert an oropharyngeal airway (OPA) (1):

Action		Rationale
1.	Don appropriate personal protective equipment (PPE), and undertake appropriate hand hygiene.	This reduces the risk of cross-infection (2).
2.	Select the correctly sized OPA by measuring the vertical distance between the patient's incisors and the angle of the jaw. 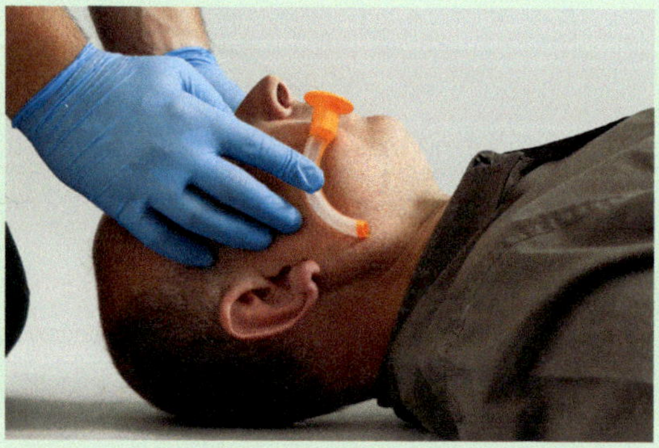	OPAs that are too small may not prevent obstruction by the tongue, whereas OPAs that are too large can be obstructed by the vallecula or epiglottis. However, a slightly larger OPA is better than one that is too small.

Action		Rationale
3.	Open the patient's mouth and check it is clear of foreign bodies, vomit, blood or secretions. Suction if required. 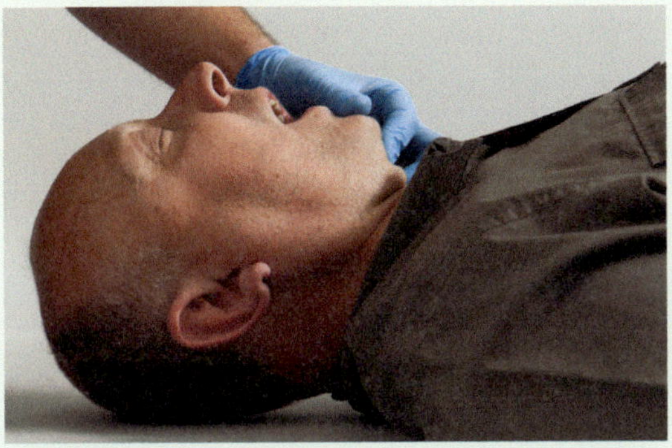	The OPA may push foreign bodies into the larynx if they are not removed prior to insertion.
4.	Insert the airway 'upside down' along the roof of the mouth until it reaches the soft palate. 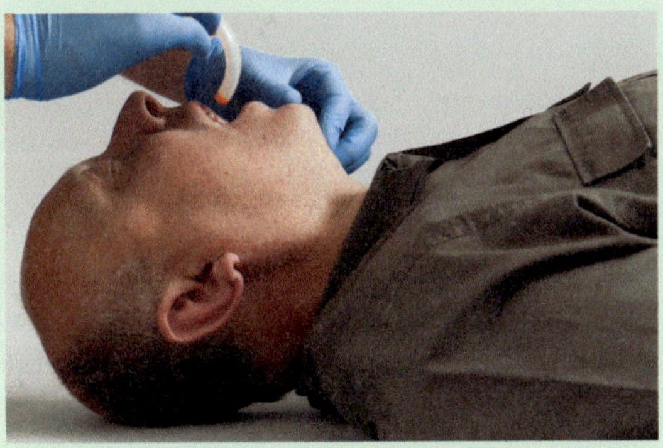	This reduces the chances of tongue displacement during insertion.
5.	Rotate the OPA through 180°. 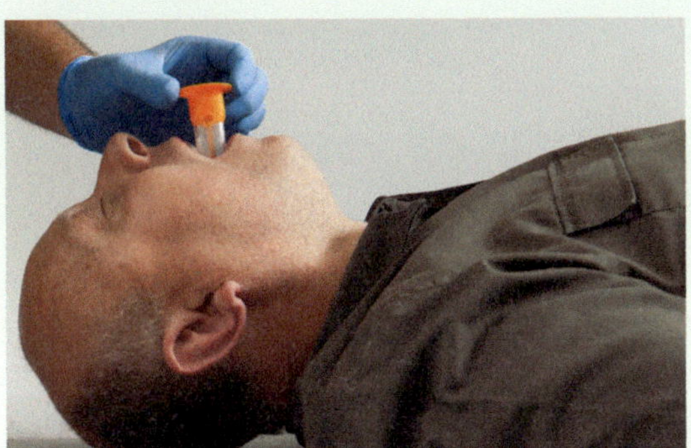	This places the OPA in its correct anatomical position.

Action		Rationale
6.	Advance the OPA until it rests in the pharynx. Consider using a jaw thrust to assist with final seating of the OPA. Remove immediately if the patient gags. 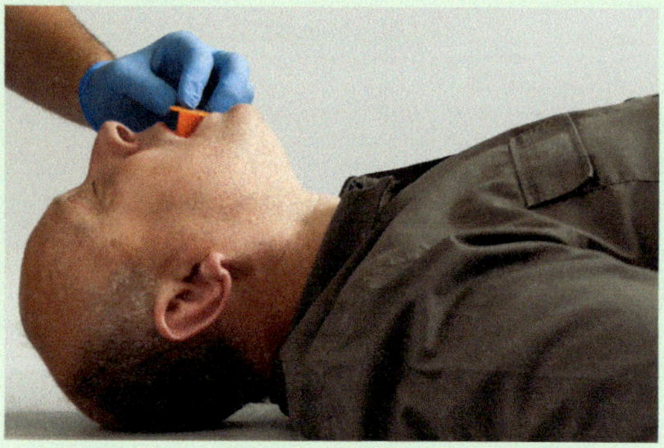	OPA insertion can cause vomiting or laryngospasm in patients with an intact gag reflex. A jaw thrust can aid final placement and help seat OPA in correct position. The correct position should be evident by an improvement in airway patency.
7.	Continue to provide manual manoeuvres such as head tilt–chin lift or jaw thrust as appropriate.	These may help with the improvement or maintenance of airway patency.
8.	Document the procedure.	You must keep full, clear and accurate records for everyone you care for, treat, or provide other services to (3).

References

1. Resuscitation Council (UK). *Advanced Life Support*. London: Resuscitation Council (UK); 2021.
2. NHS England, NHS Improvement. Standard infection control precautions: national hand hygiene and personal protective equipment policy [Internet]. 2019 [cited 2021 Nov 11]. Available from: https://www.england.nhs.uk/publication/standard-infection-control-precautions-national-hand-hygiene-and-personal-protective-equipment-policy/.
3. Health and Care Professions Council. Standards of conduct, performance and ethics [Internet]. 2018 [cited 2019 Dec 29]. Available from: https://www.hcpc-uk.org/standards/standards-of-conduct-performance-and-ethics/.

Nasopharyngeal Airway

Indications

- An unresponsive patient, or a patient with a reduced level of consciousness (LOC) who has an intact gag reflex.

Contraindications

- Patients who do not tolerate the procedure.

Cautions

- Patients who have a suspected basal skull fracture or other serious head injury (oropharyngeal airways are preferred, unless these are not possible to insert because of trismus, for example).
- Patients with nasal polyps.

Advantages

- Can be suctioned through.
- Can be tolerated by patients who are not unconscious.
- Does not require the mouth to open.

Disadvantages

- Can cause bleeding.
- Does not protect against aspiration.

Procedure – Nasopharyngeal Airway Insertion

Take the following steps to insert a nasopharyngeal airway (NPA) (1,2):

Action		Rationale
1.	Don appropriate personal protective equipment (PPE), and undertake appropriate hand hygiene.	This reduces the risk of cross-infection (3).
2.	Prepare the following: • An appropriately sized NPA, which is generally considered to be a 7 for an average adult male and 6 for an average adult female • Water-soluble gel • Suction. If the NPA you are using comes with a safety pin, insert it through the non-bevelled end. 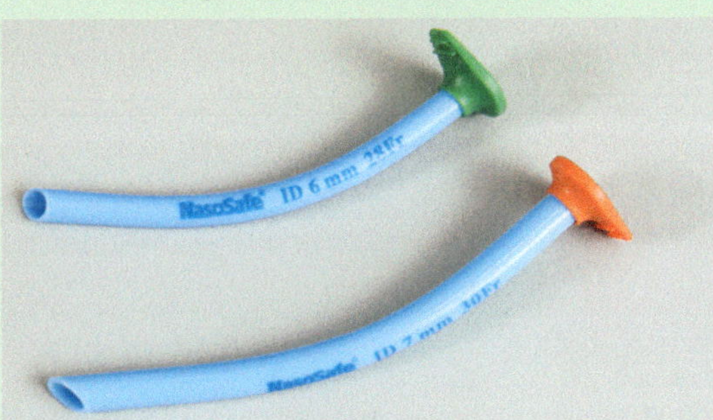	Previous sizing measures, such as using the diameter of the nares or the patient's little finger, or the distance from the patient's nose tip to ear lobe, are unreliable and should not be used (1,4). The safety pin will prevent inserting the NPA too far.

	Action	Rationale
3.	Lubricate the NPA, ensuring that the gel does not go over the open ends of the airway. 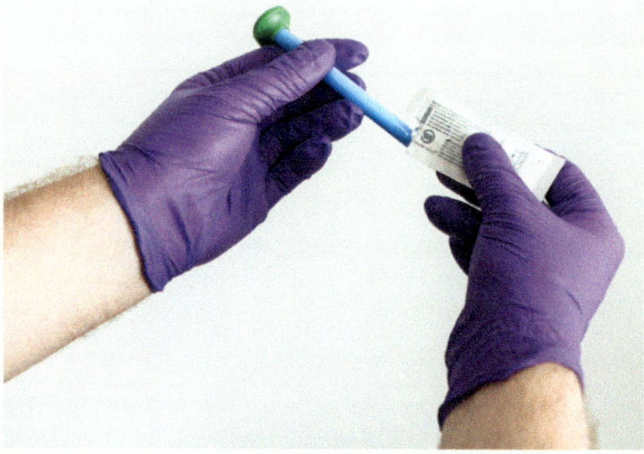	Lubricant will help reduce resistance and ease insertion, but it should not end up in the lumen of the NPA as it may get aspirated.
4.	Insert the NPA posteriorly and with the bevel facing the nasal septum. This means that the right nostril is usually used, although if the left is clearly larger, then this can be used. 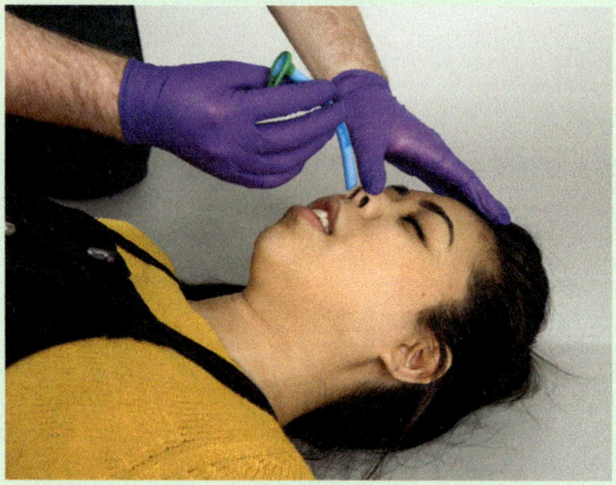	Aiming upwards could direct the NPA towards the vascular middle turbinate and thin bone of the cribriform plate (2). The bevel should help the NPA pass under the inferior turbinate more easily (5).

	Action	Rationale
5.	If resistance is felt when inserting the NPA, twist the device a little; if it still cannot be advanced, consider changing nostrils or using a smaller-size NPA. Check for blanching of the patient's nostrils. If this occurs, the NPA should be removed and a smaller-diameter NPA inserted instead. 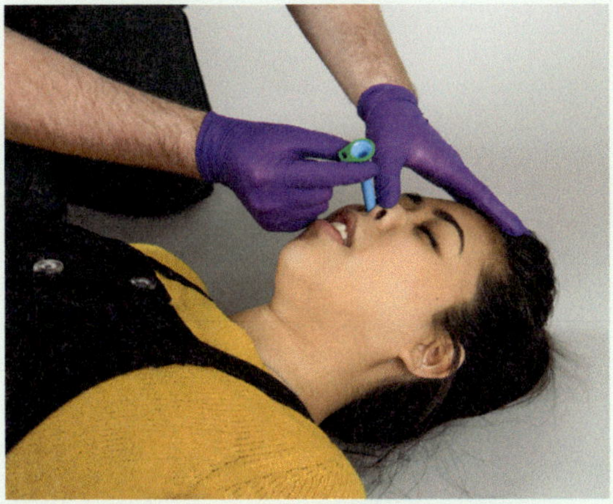	The correct technique will minimise the risk of bleeding, but if this occurs, have suction ready.
6.	Confirm position by listening for breath sounds and ensuring the chest rises and falls. 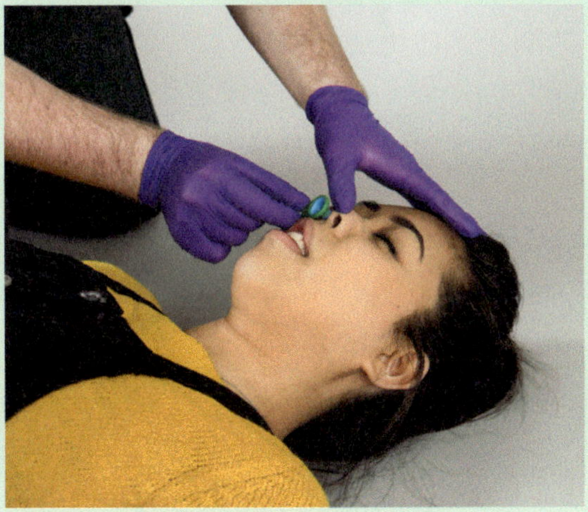	
7.	Document the procedure.	You must keep full, clear and accurate records for everyone you care for, treat, or provide other services to (6).

References

1. Roberts K, Porter K. How do you size a nasopharyngeal airway. *Resuscitation*. 2003;56(1):19–23.
2. Kovacs G, Law JA. *Airway Management in Emergencies*. 2nd edition. Shelton: McGraw-Hill Medical; 2011.
3. NHS England, NHS Improvement. Standard infection control precautions: national hand hygiene and personal protective equipment policy [Internet]. 2019 [cited 2021 Nov 11]. Available from: https://www.england.nhs.uk/publication/standard-infection-control-precautions-national-hand-hygiene-and-personal-protective-equipment-policy/.
4. Resuscitation Council (UK). *Advanced Life Support*. London: Resuscitation Council (UK); 2021.
5. Atanelov Z, Aina T, Amin B, et al. Nasopharyngeal airway. In: StatPearls [Internet]. Treasure Island, FL: StatPearls Publishing; 2022 [cited 2022 Jan 14]. Available from: http://www.ncbi.nlm.nih.gov/books/NBK513220/.
6. Health and Care Professions Council. Standards of conduct, performance and ethics [Internet]. 2018 [cited 2019 Dec 29]. Available from: https://www.hcpc-uk.org/standards/standards-of-conduct-performance-and-ethics/.

i-gel® Supraglottic Airway Device

Indications

- Airway of choice in cardiac arrest.
- When bag-valve-mask (BVM) ventilation with an oropharyngeal airway (OPA) is not effective or prolonged ventilation is required.
- A rescue device when tracheal intubation fails.

Contraindications

- Any patient who has a gag reflex.
- Any patient who is not deeply unconscious.

Advantages

- Easy to insert and position correctly.
- No need to maintain continuous manual airway seal.
- Easier than tracheal intubation and does not require laryngoscopy.
- Can be used in conjunction for waveform capnography for improved monitoring of efficacy of ventilation.

Disadvantages

- Does not protect against vomiting.
- May leak when high ventilatory pressures are required, such as in obese, asthmatic or chronic obstructive pulmonary disease (COPD) patients.

Procedure – i-gel® Supraglottic Airway Device Insertion

Take the following steps to insert an i-gel® (1,2):

Action		Rationale
1.	Don appropriate personal protective equipment (PPE), and undertake appropriate hand hygiene.	This reduces the risk of cross-infection (3).
2.	Ensure the airway is clear and prepare your equipment (**Figure 2.1**).	If you are inserting an i-gel®, the patient is highly likely to have ineffective or absent ventilation and will develop hypoxia quickly. It is therefore important that appropriate ongoing care is provided, for example ventilation or chest compressions.
3.	Choose the correct size i-gel®: 3 for small adults, 4 for medium adults and 5 for large adults. Weight ranges are provided on the i-gel®.	The correct size will increase the likelihood that you obtain a good seal.

Action		Rationale
4.	Open the packaging and remove the i-gel® from its cradle. Place a small amount of water-based lubricant in the small pit on the cradle. 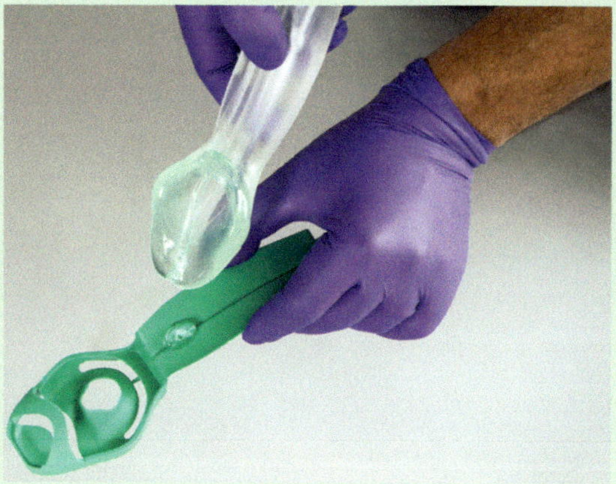	
5.	Lubricate the back, sides and front tip of the i-gel®.	Lubricant will help reduce resistance to insertion.
6.	If you suspect a foreign body may be present, perform laryngoscopy.	Inserting an i-gel® can lead to impaction of a foreign body and subsequent inability to ventilate (4).
7.	With the patient in the 'sniffing the morning air' position, hold the i-gel® by the integrated bite block, gently pull down on the patient's chin and introduce the green tip into the patient's mouth, directed at the hard palate. 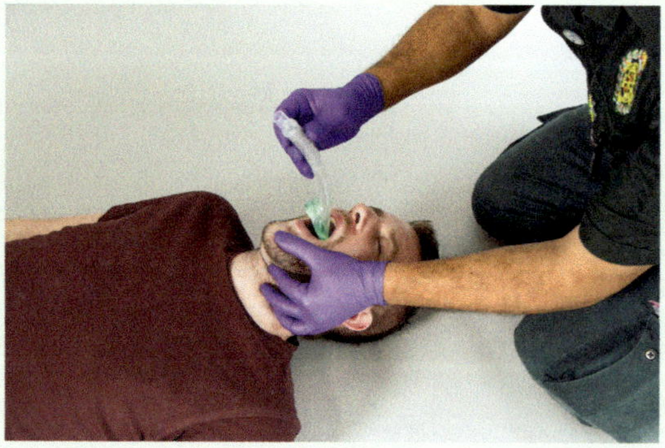	This will help prevent the tongue from causing an obstruction during insertion.

	Action	Rationale
8.	Glide the device downwards and backwards along the hard palate with a continuous but gentle push until a definitive resistance is felt. As a rough guide, the bite block should end up at the level of the incisors. You will also see anterior displacement of the larynx when the i-gel® is seated. Any early resistance to insertion may be resolved by slightly twisting the i-gel® or instructing an assistant to provide a jaw thrust. 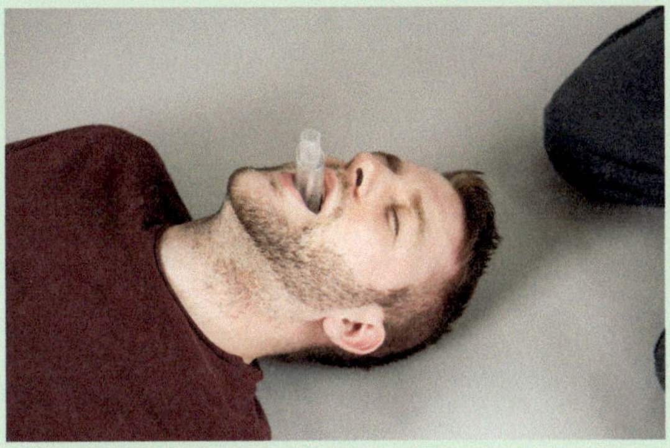	Because the end of the i-gel® is quite wide, it may be held up by the faucial pillars. Applying a jaw thrust or gently twisting the i-gel® should enable it to pass and continue until it sits over the laryngeal inlet.
9.	Connect the i-gel® to an 'airway tree', consisting of a catheter mount, filter and waveform capnography, which in turn should be connected to the bag-valve-mask. Check for end-tidal carbon dioxide and bilateral chest air entry and movement on ventilating the patient. 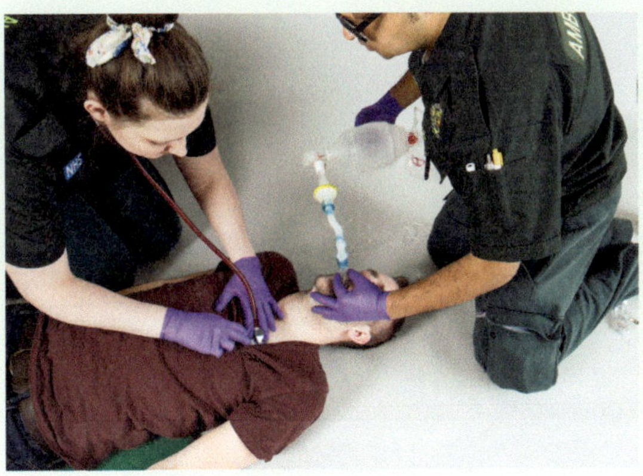	Effective ventilation consists of oxygenation and expiration of waste gases (mostly carbon dioxide). Waveform capnography will confirm correct placement. It is good practice to auscultate since a capnography trace will be generated even if the patient has a pneumothorax, which is preventing ventilation of one lung.

Action		Rationale
10.	Secure the device appropriately. 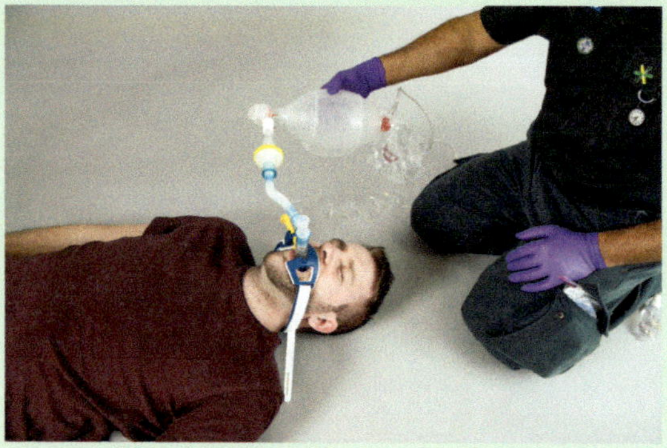	This prevents inadvertent dislodgement, particularly when moving the patient.
11.	Re-check placement after moving or when there is any change in patient condition, for example after loss of capnography trace.	
12.	Document the procedure.	You must keep full, clear and accurate records for everyone you care for, treat, or provide other services to (5).

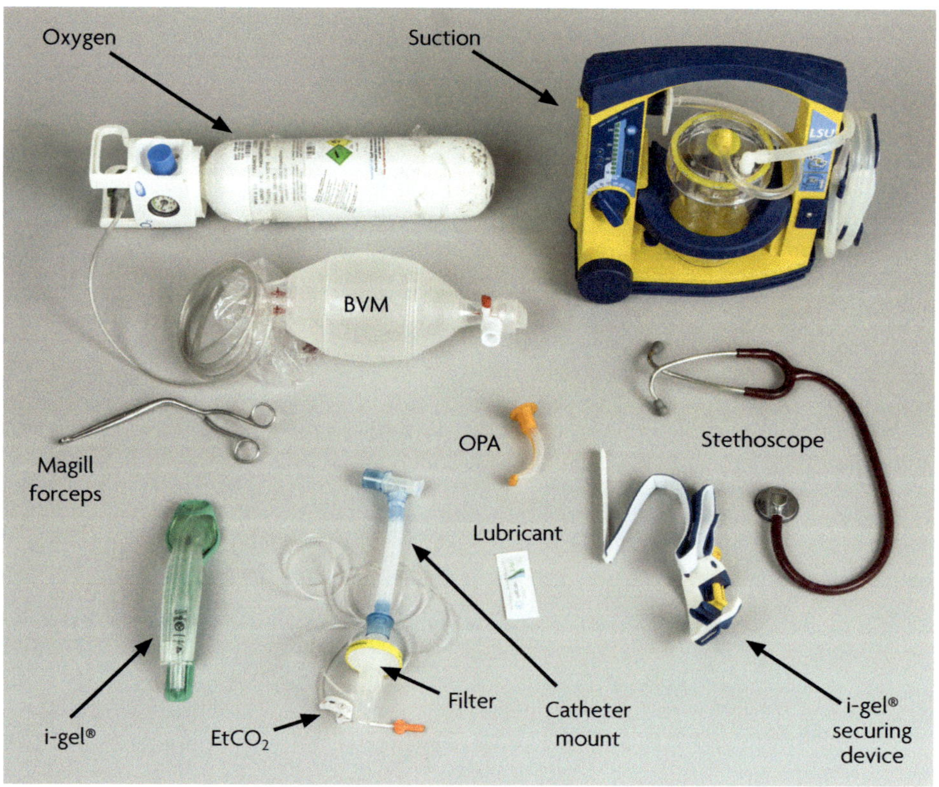

Figure 2.1 Equipment for i-gel® insertion.

References

1. intersurgical. i-gel® supraglottic airway from Intersurgical: an introduction [Internet]. 2017 [cited 2022 Apr 30]. Available from: https://www.youtube.com/watch?v=Z0962B8axAY.
2. Resuscitation Council (UK). *Advanced Life Support*. London: Resuscitation Council (UK); 2021.
3. NHS England, NHS Improvement. Standard infection control precautions: national hand hygiene and personal protective equipment policy [Internet]. 2019 [cited 2021 Nov 11]. Available from: https://www.england.nhs.uk/publication/standard-infection-control-precautions-national-hand-hygiene-and-personal-protective-equipment-policy/.
4. Edwards T. Complications associated with supraglottic airway use in an urban ambulance service: a case series. *Emergency Medicine Journal*. 2016 Sep;33(9):e8.2-e8.
5. Health and Care Professions Council. Standards of conduct, performance and ethics [Internet]. 2018 [cited 2019 Dec 29]. Available from: https://www.hcpc-uk.org/standards/standards-of-conduct-performance-and-ethics/.

Tracheal Intubation

Indications

- In cardiac arrest where despite effective problem-solving a supraglottic airway is proving ineffective.

Contraindications

- Clinician not experienced and competent at prehospital intubation.
- In the first few minutes of a cardiac arrest (chest compressions have priority and a supraglottic device should be attempted initially).
- When supraglottic airway device (SGA) is providing effective ventilation.

Advantages

- Improved protection from airway secretions/blood/vomit.
- Allows for ventilation at higher airway pressures.
- Can be used in conjunction for waveform capnography for improved monitoring of efficacy of ventilation.

Disadvantages

- Requires significant experience and frequent practice to develop and maintain competence.
- Bypasses physiological functions of the upper airway (filtering, warming and humidifying).
- Difficult to perform in the prehospital environment and catastrophic for the patient if an incorrect placement is missed.

Procedure – Tracheal Intubation

Take the following steps to intubate the trachea:

Action		Rationale
1.	Don appropriate personal protective equipment (PPE), and undertake appropriate hand hygiene.	This reduces the risk of cross-infection (1).
2.	Make an early assessment about the scene and the patient's position within it. If possible, consider moving the patient to gain 360° access. 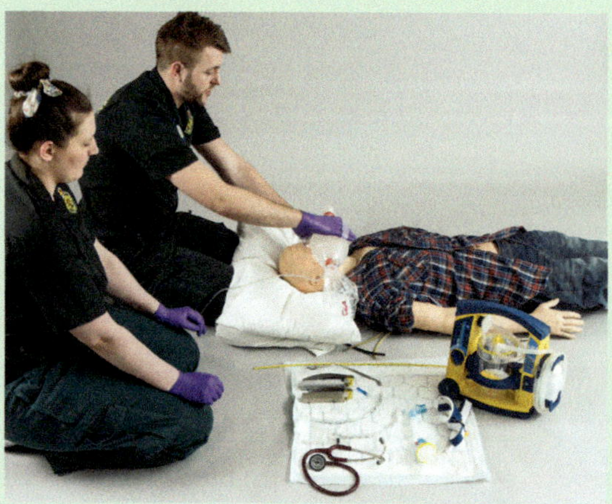	Ideally, your patient will be on a bed or ambulance trolley where you can adjust the height so that the patient's head is your focal length away (usually 12–18 cm or the distance you would hold a book to read). However, most of your patients are likely to be on the floor, but you can potentially move them so that you have more space to work. There are several positions that are advocated when intubating, including supine, kneeling, straddling and left and right lateral positions. None of them have clinically important differences in time to intubate, so it will be up to you to determine the position that ensures you are able to visualise the glottis and still affords enough mechanical advantage to be able to lift the jaw (2–4).

Action		Rationale
3.	Ensure the airway is clear and provide ventilation and oxygenation with a bag-valve-mask (BVM) and supraglottic airway (if effective) while an assistant prepares your equipment (**Figure 2.2**), including the selection of an appropriate laryngoscope blade and tracheal tube size. 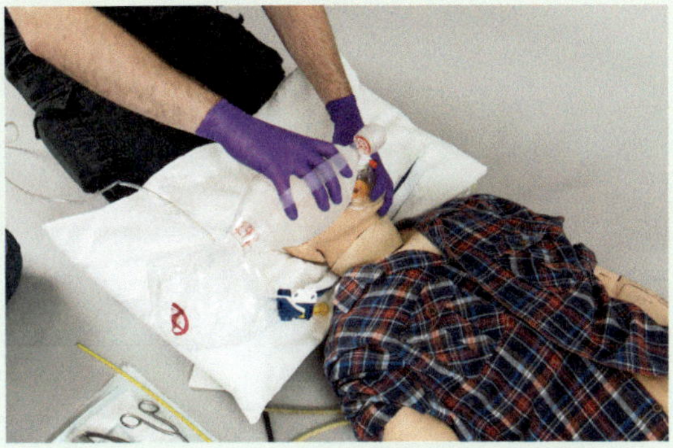	It is generally recommended to use a curved (Macintosh) size 4 blade as it is the longest, so will almost certainly reach the vallecula of your patient, and the curved blade generally allows better control of the tongue (5). Also, it is recommended that you use a size 7 mm tube for females and an 8 mm tube for males. However, use your clinical judgement to determine the correct size for the patient that you are intubating (6).
4.	Consider the mnemonic LEMON to assess the patient to identify any indications that they might be a difficult intubation (5): • Look externally • Evaluate 3-3-2 • Mallampati scale • Obstruction • Neck mobility.	Pre-empting potential difficulties will help optimise the attempt and potentially lower the threshold at which an attempt is considered futile and a rescue technique be utilised instead. In the context of cardiac arrest, some of the steps, including the 3-3-2 and Mallampati, will not be possible to complete, but having an awareness of the principles nonetheless will help in identifying a potentially challenging intubation.
5.	Make and communicate your intubation procedure plan, including actions to take in the event the attempt is unsuccessful. This should follow a standard difficult-airway algorithm already established by your service. Establish who your skilled assistant (someone who is familiar with the process and equipment required) will be and confirm the steps of the procedure and what equipment you will require.	Intubation is a team activity. Sharing your mental model will help the attempt go to plan and for assistant(s) to know what you are likely to need next in the event of difficulty occurring (7). A difficult-airway plan is a structured method for approaching a difficult airway that helps to identify and mange challenging situations. A standard plan ensures everyone has a shared mental model on the steps to take. Any service where intubation is performed should have an agreed difficult-airway plan.

Action		Rationale
6.	Position the patient's head into the 'sniffing the morning air' position (head extended and neck flexed). Use pillows, cushions, towels or anything else similar in the vicinity of your patient to maintain this position, by placing the items under the patient's head and shoulders. For large and obese patients, a large quantity of padding may be required.	This should give the best view, but consider whether the patient has a cervical injury or pre-existing injury or disease of the vertebrae in the neck. In this case, the risk vs benefit of movement of the head and neck should be considered. A good position will have been achieved when the external auditory meatus ('earhole') is at the same level as the sternal notch ('neck hole') (8).
7.	Open the mouth and inspect the oropharynx. Have an assistant with suction ready. Remove ill-fitting dentures.	This provides an opportunity to identify any foreign bodies and remove them in case insertion of the tracheal tube displaces them. Vomit and blood will obscure a view of the oropharyngeal and laryngeal inlets.
8.	Utilise a checklist to ensure that all essential equipment is present and the team are appropriately prepared.	Intubation in an emergency is a potentially difficult skill, made more complex by the clinical urgency of the situation, the forming of an ad hoc team on scene and working in an environment which has not been specifically prepared for that purpose. Use of a safety checklist can help to reduce errors and ensure all equipment is present (9).
9.	Gently insert the laryngoscope blade along the right mandibular (lower) molars and gently sweep the tongue to the left. 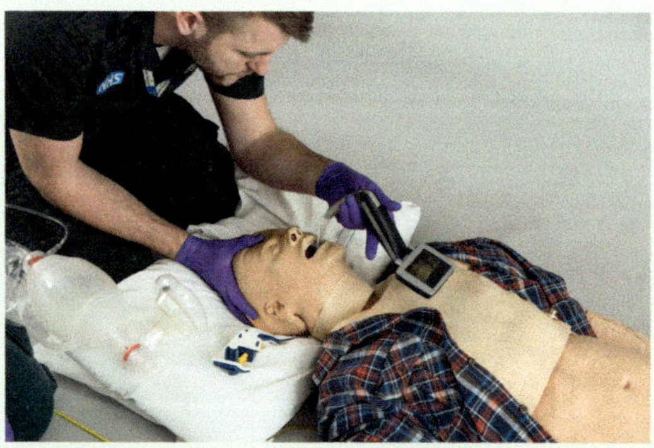	Displacing the tongue will improve the chance of an unobstructed view of the laryngeal inlet. When using a video laryngoscope, it can sometimes be difficult to get the blade inserted initially due to the video unit coming into contact with the patient. If this happens, start with the blade rotated 90° to the side and turn back towards the normal position once the tip of the blade has been inserted.
10.	With the blade now in the midline, slowly advance the blade down the tongue until the epiglottis comes into view.	The epiglottis is reliably located at the base of the tongue, making it easier to orientate yourself (10). If you cannot locate the epiglottis, consider using suction if the airway is soiled. Alternatively, you may have inserted the blade too far and it is easy to become 'lost' in a sea of soft tissue that makes up the posterior pharynx and oesophagus. In this case, withdraw the laryngoscope, ventilate, communicate your plan and consider trying again.

Action		Rationale
11.	With the epiglottis located, convert the potential space of the vallecula into an actual space by applying pressure with the tip of your laryngoscope blade.	This should make it straightforward to insert the tip of the blade into the vallecula. If this is proving challenging, then external laryngeal manipulation (see Bimanual Laryngoscopy with External Laryngeal Manipulation procedure) can assist in improving the view.
12.	Now lift the blade at an angle of 45° (or parallel to the handle). Do not lever backwards on the handle (think pulling a pint) as this may not only damage the upper teeth, but also worsen the view. Keep lifting until you can see the posterior or arytenoid cartilages and the inter-arytenoid notch (11).	If you can only see the epiglottis or, worse, only the soft palate, you are unlikely to be able to successfully intubate. Consider abandoning the technique and think about how you could improve the view, for example by changing operator position or using a difficult-airway blade. You must be able to view these structures, otherwise you are likely to intubate the oesophagus.
13.	While maintaining your view of the glottic opening, request your assistant pass you the bougie. It should have a 40° bend at the distal end, which looks a bit like a hockey stick (Coudé tip). Do not pre-load the tube on to the bougie.	The Coudé tip will help keep the distal end of the bougie in contact with the underside of the epiglottis until it finds the laryngeal inlet. This will result in it becoming top-heavy and you will lose control.
14.	Insert the bougie into the right-hand side of the patient's mouth. 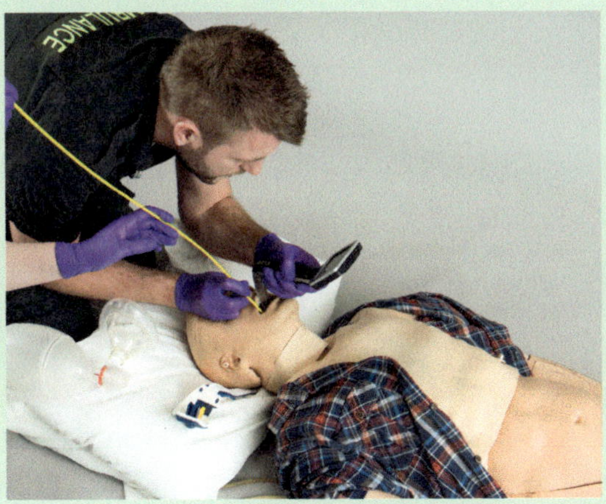 Guide the bougie so it passes through the vocal cords. You must visualise the tip of the bougie passing between the vocal cords. Normally this is easiest to confirm on the screen of the video laryngoscope.	This prevents the bougie from obstructing your view. Your assistant can hook an index finger in the corner of the patient's mouth to pull the corner of the mouth laterally and improve your view, if required. Beyond 22–24 cm your assistant may not be able to hold the end of the bougie once the tube has been passed over it.

	Action	Rationale
	As the bougie passes through the cords, the Coudé tip will rub against the tracheal rings, which can be felt as a series of clicks (12). Once approximately 22–24 cm of the bougie is in the patient's mouth, do not advance any further. 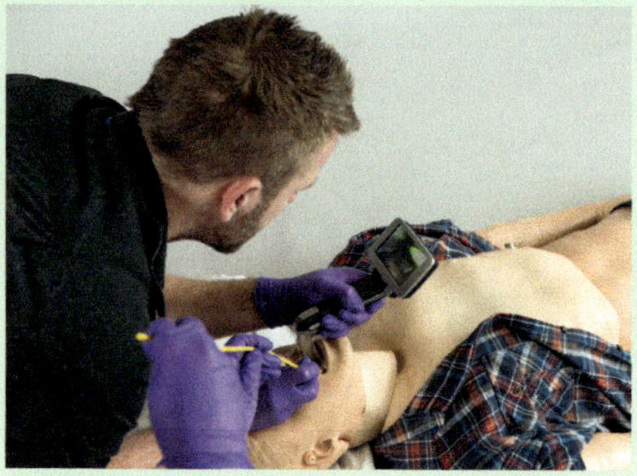	
15.	Ask your assistant to thread the tube over the bougie and slide it down. When the tube reaches your hand (holding the bougie), ask your assistant to take firm grasp of the bougie at the distal end. Once your assistant confirms they have control of the bougie by stating 'I have the bougie', release your grip of the bougie and take hold of the tube.	Clear communication will help ensure that the bougie is held in position at all times during this stage of the procedure.
	Gently advance the tube into the mouth and through the vocal cords, giving it a 90° anti-clockwise twist as you approach the glottic opening.	This anti-clockwise twist is advisable, because it is not uncommon for the tube to 'hang up' on the posterior structures of the glottis. If this does happen, withdraw the tube 2 cm and rotate it 90° anti-clockwise and then try advancing the tube again (13,14).
	Visualise the tube going through the cords and stop when the depth-marker black line reaches the level of the vocal cords. 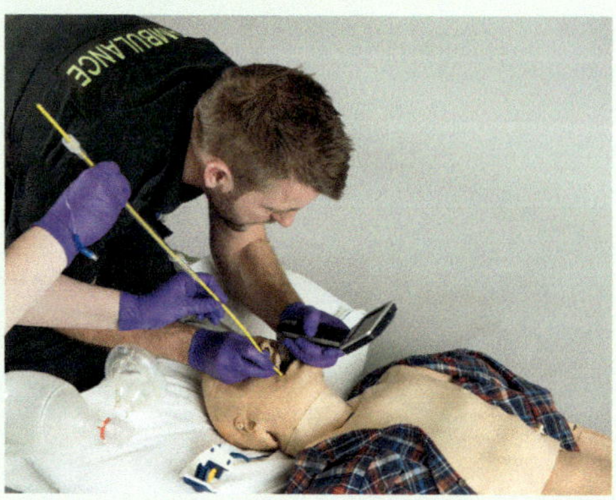	The black line is positioned so that the opening of the tube will sit below the vocal cords, but it should be above the carina and therefore avoid endobronchial intubation.

Action		Rationale
16.	Once the tube is in situ, ask your assistant to remove the bougie. Do not remove the laryngoscope from the patient's vallecula. 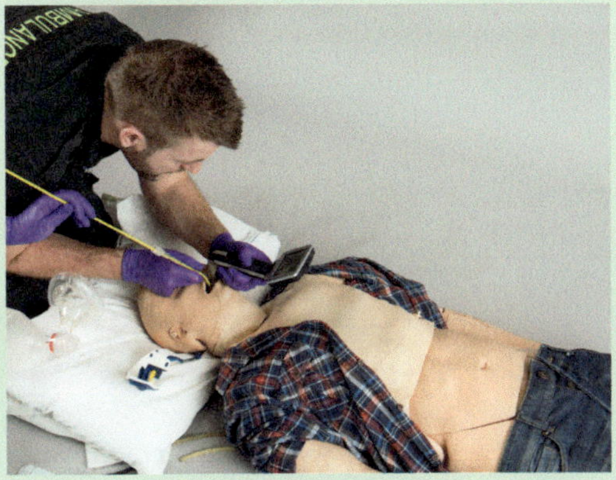	Until you have confirmation of correct tube placement, it is helpful to maintain a view of the laryngeal inlet.
17.	Ask your assistant to inflate the tube cuff by injecting 6–8 ml of air into the inflation valve with a 10 ml syringe. 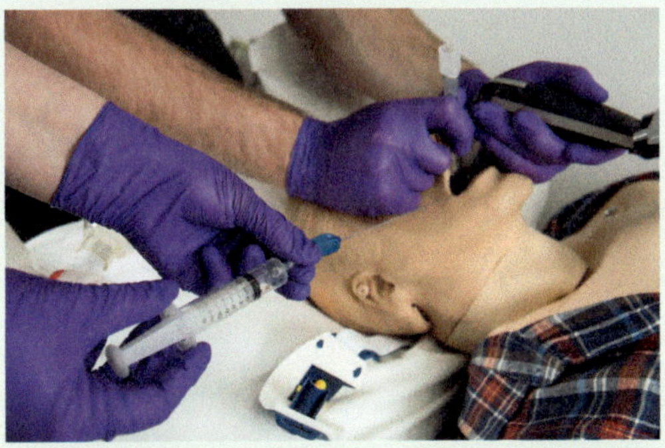	This should be enough air to inflate the baloon but avoid putting excess pressure on the tracheal wall, which, if prolonged, can lead to ischaemia.
18.	Attach the capnography, filter and catheter mount (sometimes referred to as the 'airway tree') on to the tracheal tube and gently ventilate the patient. 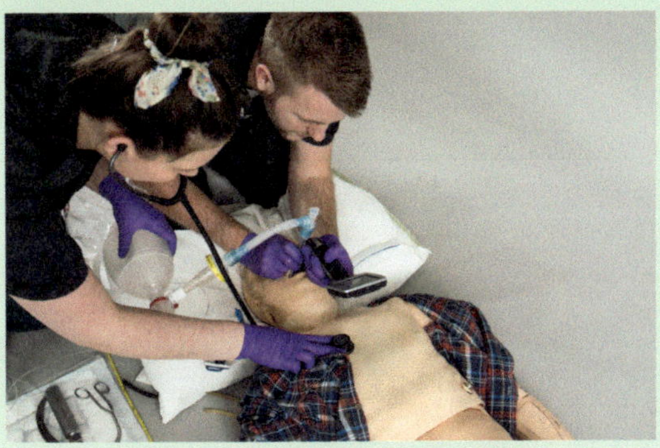	Ventilation is required to see a capnography waveform.

Action		Rationale
19.	Confirm placement by observing for a consistent capnography trace and bi-lateral rise and fall of the chest and auscultate both lungs in the lateral positions.	Waveform capnography is the best confirmation of correct tube placement and is mandatory to confirm endotracheal (ET) tube placement, but it is important to auscultate as capnography will not detect an endobronchial intubation.
20.	Once correct tube placement has been confirmed, gently remove the laryngoscope from the patient's mouth, keeping a firm hold on the tube.	This prevents inadvertent tube dislodgement.
21.	Secure the tube with a Thomas ET-tube holder, tape or tie, depending on what you have available. 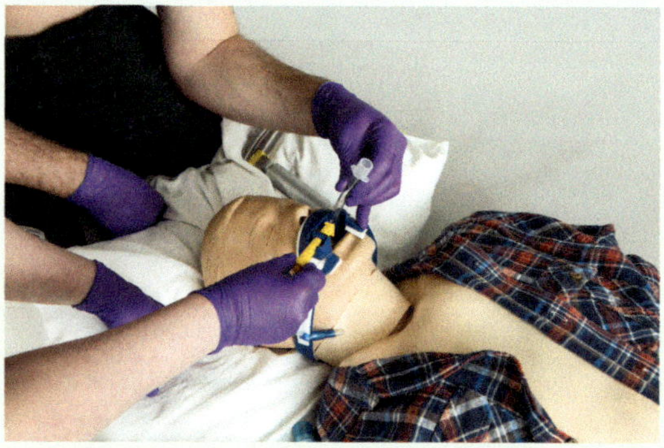	Tight tube ties may reduce venous drainage, increasing intracranial pressure (ICP) and contribute to secondary brain injury in a patient post-return of spontaneous circulation (ROSC), so if it is necessary to use ties (the least preferable option), these should not be overly tight.
22.	Document the procedure.	You must keep full, clear and accurate records for everyone you care for, treat, or provide other services to (15).

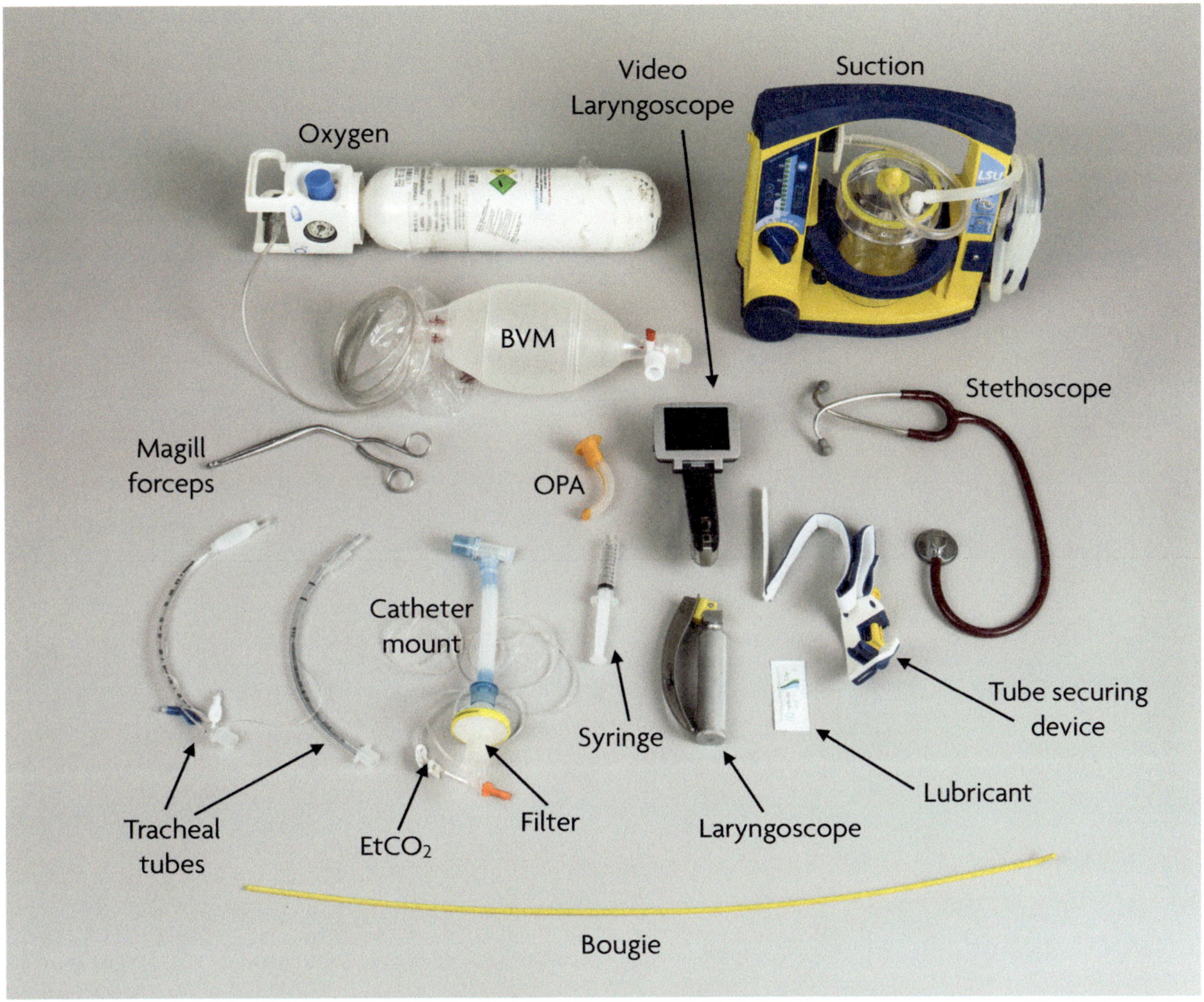

Figure 2.2 Equipment required for an intubation attempt.

References

1. NHS England, NHS Improvement. Standard infection control precautions: national hand hygiene and personal protective equipment policy [Internet]. 2019 [cited 2021 Nov 11]. Available from: https://www.england.nhs.uk/publication/standard-infection-control-precautions-national-hand-hygiene-and-personal-protective-equipment-policy/.
2. Tesler J, Rucker J, Sommer D, et al. Rescuer position for tracheal intubation on the ground. *Resuscitation*. 2003 Jan;56(1):83–89.
3. Adnet F, Cydulka RK, Lapandry C. Emergency tracheal intubation of patients lying supine on the ground: influence of operator body position. *Canadian Journal of Anaesthesia*. 1998 Mar 1;45(3):266–269.
4. Koetter KP, Hilker T, Genzwuerker HV, et al. A randomized comparison of rescuer positions for intubation on the ground. *Prehospital Emergency Care*. 1997 Jan 1;1(2):96–99.
5. Brown CA. *The Walls Manual of Emergency Airway Management*. 5th edition. Sakles JC, Mick NW, editors. Philadelphia, PA: Lippincott Williams and Wilkins; 2017.
6. Benger J, Nolan J, Clancy M, editors. *Emergency Airway Management*. Cambridge: Cambridge University Press; 2009.
7. Rutherford G, editor. *Human Factors in Paramedic Practice* [Internet]. 1st edition. Bridgwater: Class Professional Publishing; 2020 [cited 2022 Feb 20]. Available from: http://search.ebscohost

.com/login.aspx?direct=true&scope=site&db=nlebk&db=nlabk&AN=2633378.

8. Alimian M, Zaman B, Seyed Siamdoust SA, et al. Comparison of RAMP and new modified RAMP positioning in laryngoscopic view during intubation in patients with morbid obesity: a randomized clinical trial. *Anesthesia and Pain Medicine*. 2021 Jun 29;11(3):e114508.
9. The National Institute of Academic Anaesthesia. NAP4 report [Internet]. 2011 [cited 2022 May 8]. Available from: https://www.niaa.org.uk/NAP4-Report?newsid=513#pt.
10. Levitan RM, Sather SD, Ochroch EA. Demystifying direct laryngoscopy and intubation. *Hospital Physician*. 2000;36(5):47–56.
11. Schmitt HJ, Mang H. Head and neck elevation beyond the sniffing position improves laryngeal view in cases of difficult direct laryngoscopy. *Journal of Clinical Anesthesia*. 2002 Aug;14(5):335–338.
12. Kovacs G, Law JA. *Airway Management in Emergencies*. 2nd edition. Shelton: McGraw-Hill Medical; 2011.
13. McGill J. The Bougie [Internet]. HQMedEd.com. 2008 [cited 2022 Feb 20]. Available from: https://hqmeded.com/the-bougie-2/.
14. McGill J. Difficulty passing the bougie [Internet]. HQMedEd.com. 2012 [cited 2022 Feb 20]. Available from: https://hqmeded.com/difficulty-passing-the-bougie-2/.
15. Health and Care Professions Council. Standards of conduct, performance and ethics [Internet]. 2018 [cited 2019 Dec 29]. Available from: https://www.hcpc-uk.org/standards/standards-of-conduct-performance-and-ethics/.

Needle Cricothyroidotomy

Indications
- All basic and advanced airway interventions unsuccessful in providing ventilation and oxygenation.
- Clinician unable to perform surgical airway.

Contraindications
- Inability to locate landmarks required to perform procedure.

Advantages
- May provide time for definitive airway management to be undertaken.

Disadvantages
- Can distract from other time-sensitive patient management.
- Not shown to be an effective technique outside of hospital to prevent death.
- Does not allow expiration of carbon dioxide.
- Only provides temporary oxygenation of patient.
- Evidence that oxygenation is poor when using low-pressure oxygenation, for example providing 15 l/min rather than jet ventilation (which is not commonly available in the out-of-hospital setting).
- Likely to be performed with makeshift equipment (non-commercial device).

Procedure – Needle Cricothyroidotomy

Take the following steps to perform a needle cricothyroidotomy (1):

Action		Rationale
1.	Don appropriate personal protective equipment (PPE), and undertake appropriate hand hygiene.	This reduces the risk of cross-infection (2).
2.	If not already undertaken, communicate your intention to perform the procedure with the team.	Needle cricothyroidotomy is a team activity. Sharing your mental model will help the attempt go to plan (3).
3.	Prepare your equipment. This might be a commercial device if you have one, but a needle cricothyroidotomy can be undertaken with the following: • Large-bore cannula (14 gauge) • 3-way tap with extension tubing • Oxygen tubing • 10 or 20 ml syringe • Sharps container • Saline flush (optional).	A commercial device is probably preferable. However, we have outlined a DIY solution here. If you do not have a 3-way tap, cut a small hole into one side of the oxygen tubing, which you can occlude with your thumb or fingers.

Action		Rationale
	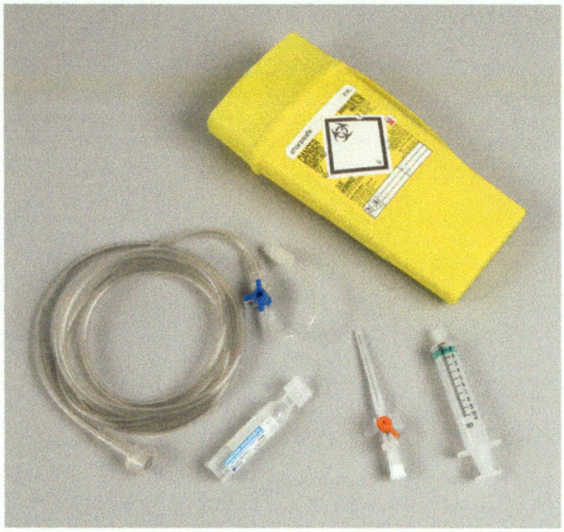	
4.	Attach oxygen tubing to the 3-way tap and open all the ports. Remove any port covers if present.	This aids with intermittent administration of oxygen in the later steps of this procedure. Check that the oxygen tubing fits on the 3-way taps that you use in your clinical setting.
5.	Set the oxygen flow rate to 15 l/min.	Setting it now may help prevent forgetting to do it after the procedure has been performed.
6.	Extend the patient's head to hyperextend the neck. Padding under the shoulders can be used to assist with this.	This enables better identification of landmarks and unobstructed access for the catheter/syringe assembly.
7.	If possible, position yourself so the patient is on your non-dominant side and then identify the cricothyroid membrane by palpating down from the thyroid.	This aids accurate placement. Identification may be more challenging with excess adipose tissue around the neck.
8.	Immobilise the larynx using the thumb, middle and ring fingers of your non-dominant hand, allowing the index finger to palpate the cricothyroid membrane. 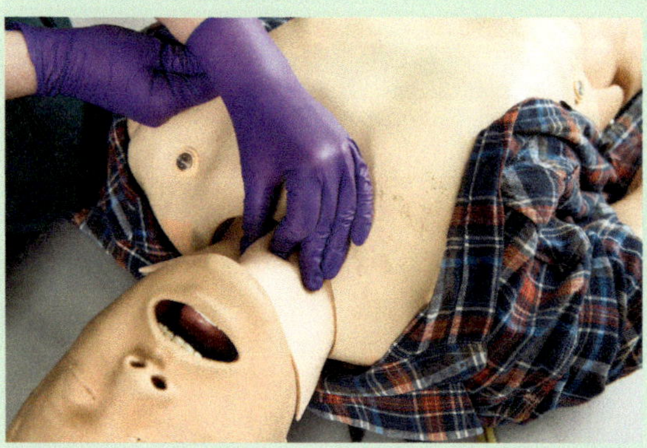	The larynx and trachea are highly mobile; keeping them stationary will help to ensure accurate needle placement.

Action		Rationale
9.	Ask an assistant to pass you the cannula affixed to the 10 or 20 ml syringe (partially filled with saline if it does not delay the procedure).	Air bubbles in the saline-filled syringe may provide an early indication that you are within the lumen of the trachea and help avoid inadvertent posterior tracheal wall puncture.
10.	Hold the cannula with syringe in your dominant hand and direct it caudally along the long axis of the trachea at an angle of 30° to the skin. 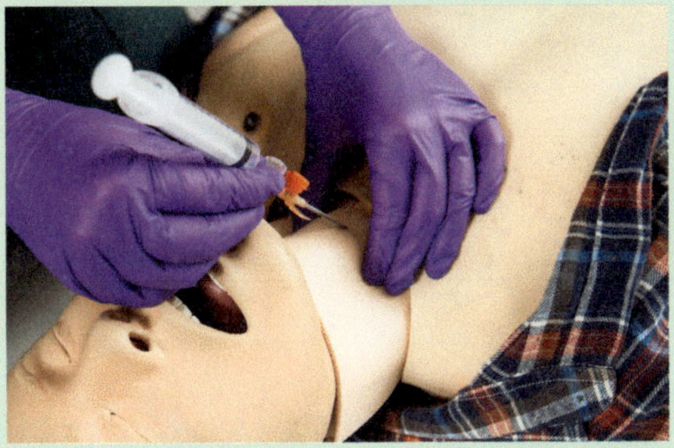	This will help direct the needle into the trachea and not into other structures around it.
11.	Insert the cannula, aspirating the syringe as you advance. Stop once you can easily aspirate air into the syringe (bubbles will appear if the syringe is partially filled with saline).	This may help avoid inadvertent posterior tracheal wall puncture.
12.	Hold the needle and syringe stationary and advance the catheter into the trachea. 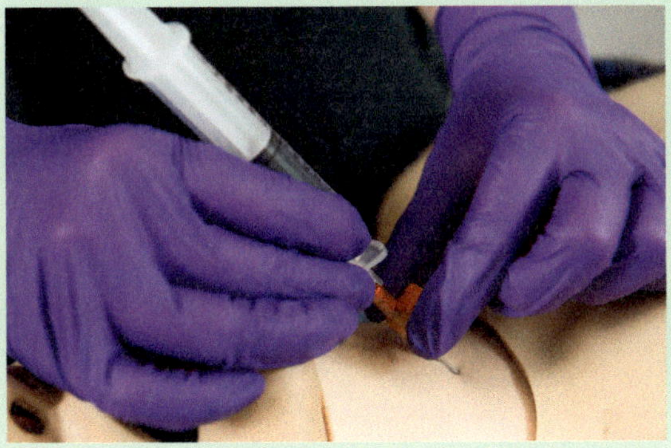	

Action		Rationale
13.	Remove the catheter needle and syringe, and attach the port at the end of the 3-way tap tubing on to the cannula. 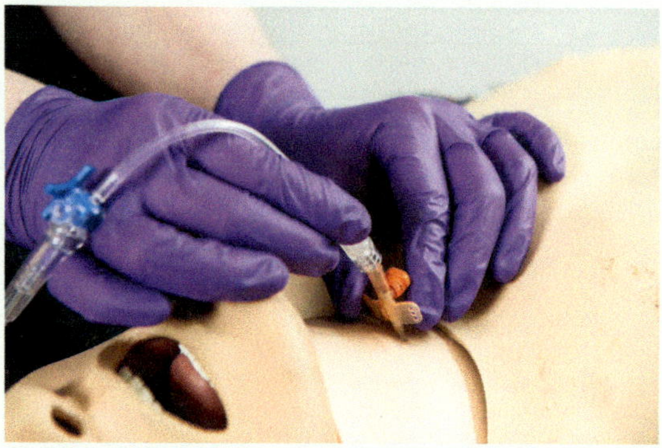	
14.	Attempt to ventilate at ratio of 1 second inspiration to 3 seconds expiration. Look for surgical emphysema developing around the cannula. 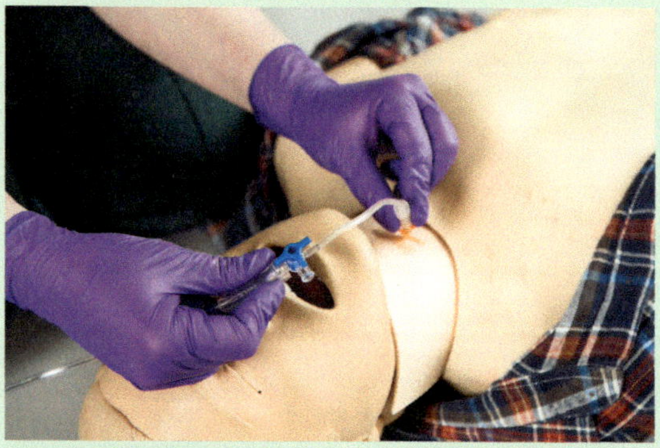	Surgical emphysema will indicate that the cannula has been incorrectly placed. Remove and consider another attempt.
15.	If possible, manually hold the cannula in position. If this is not possible, tape the cannula in situ, but frequently reassess.	
16.	Document the procedure.	You must keep full, clear and accurate records for everyone you care for, treat, or provide other services to (4).

References

1. Brown CA. *The Walls Manual of Emergency Airway Management*. 5th edition. Sakles JC, Mick NW, editors. Philadelphia, PA: Lippincott Williams and Wilkins; 2017.
2. NHS England, NHS Improvement. Standard infection control precautions: national hand hygiene and personal protective equipment policy [Internet]. 2019 [cited 2021 Nov 11]. Available from: https://www.england.nhs.uk/publication/standard-infection-control-precautions-national-hand-hygiene-and-personal-protective-equipment-policy/.
3. Rutherford G, editor. *Human Factors in Paramedic Practice*. 1st edition. Bridgwater: Class Professional Publishing; 2020.
4. Health and Care Professions Council. Standards of conduct, performance and ethics [Internet]. 2018 [cited 2019 Dec 29]. Available from: https://www.hcpc-uk.org/standards/standards-of-conduct-performance-and-ethics/.

Scalpel Cricothyroidotomy (Emergency Front of Neck Access)

Indications

- Emergency ventilation when all other airway options have been exhausted and proven ineffective (cannot intubate, cannot oxygenate).

Contraindications

- Less invasive ventilation techniques are effective.
- Inability to identify landmarks.
- In paediatrics, where the landmarks cannot be identified or the anatomy is too small to be successful (typically aged below ten years of age).

Advantages

- Can provide an effective method of ventilation when other techniques fail.

Disadvantages

- Requires regular training to develop and maintain competence (1).
- Associated with a high rate of failure (2).
- Identification of surface anatomy is often inaccurate (3).

Procedure – Scalpel Cricothyroidotomy

Take the following steps to perform a scalpel cricothyroidotomy (4):

Note: This procedure is also referred to as a surgical cricothyroidotomy or surgical airway.

Action		Rationale
1.	Don appropriate personal protective equipment (PPE), and undertake appropriate hand hygiene.	This reduces the risk of cross-infection (5).
2.	Gather the necessary equipment, which includes: • Size 10 scalpel • Size 10 fr bougie • 6 mm cuffed tracheal tube • 10 ml syringe • Tape for securing the tube • Bag-valve-mask and ventilation circuit including catheter mount, heat and moisture exchanger (HME) filter and capnography • Stethoscope for confirming placement • Gauze.	
3.	Place a small amount of padding (for example a pillow) under the patient's shoulders, causing a slight extension of the head.	This increases the area of the front of the neck and provides some tension to the skin.

Action		Rationale
4.	Position yourself on the side of the patient opposite to your dominant hand (for example, if you are right-handed stand on the patient's left side). Ensure your assistant is positioned so they can pass you equipment.	This positioning will make it easier for you to perform the procedure.
5.	Grasp the patient's trachea between your thumb and index finger, slowly move your fingers up, with your thumb on one side of the trachea and the middle finger on the other side. Use your index finger to palpate the midline, feeling for the cricothyroid membrane. Once identified, use your thumb and middle finger to anchor the cricoid cartilage and the index finger to mark the position of the cricothyroid membrane. 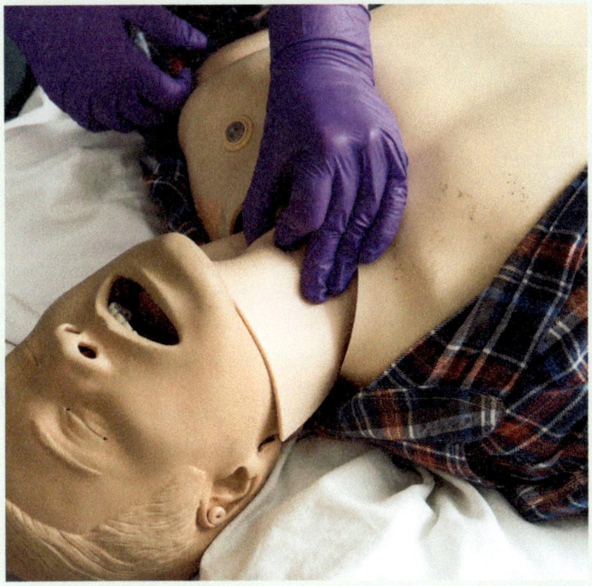	Moving up from the sternal notch to find the cricothyroid membrane is more effective than moving down from the top (6). This is called the 'laryngeal handshake' and is used to anchor the cricoid and laryngeal cartilages.

Action		Rationale
6.	Using a size 10 scalpel, make a stab incision horizontally through the centre of the cricoid membrane (4). 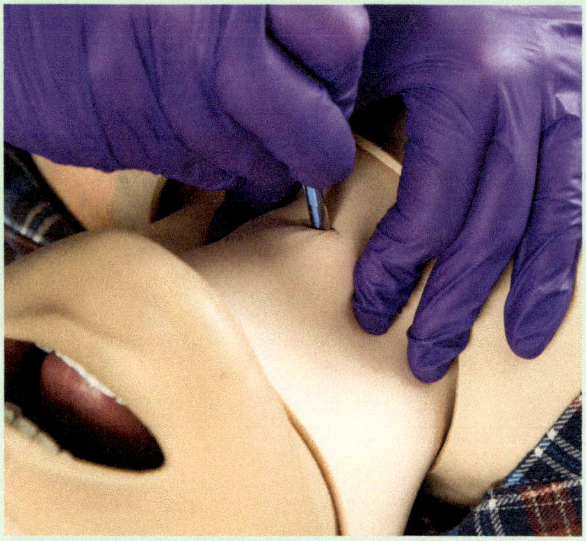	You may feel a pop as the blade goes through the membranes.
7.	Turn the blade 90° so the blade on the knife faces towards the patient's feet (4). 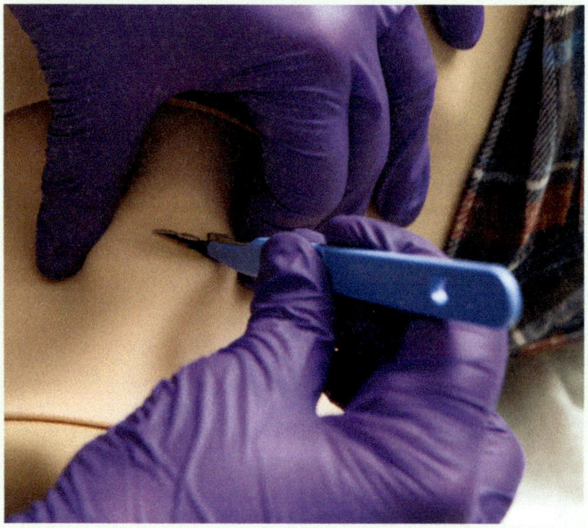	Turning the blade opens a gap to allow the bougie to be inserted. Turning the blade towards the feet reduces the chance of the bougie being damaged when inserted.

Action		Rationale
8.	Ask your assistant to pass you the bougie. Insert the Coudé tip of the bougie along the side of the scalpel into the trachea. Once the bougie is in the trachea, remove the scalpel. 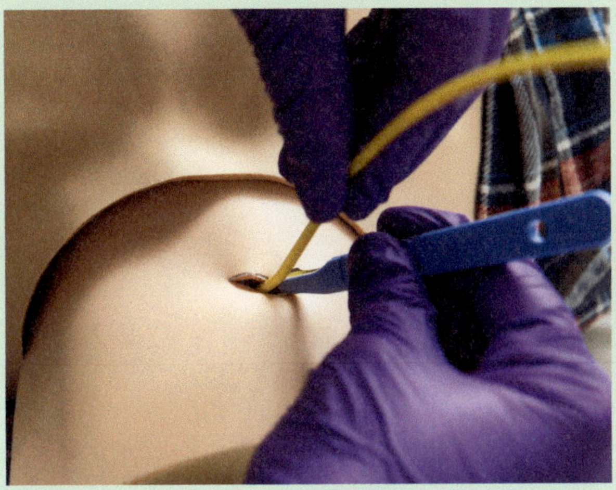	To make the insertion of the 6 mm tracheal tube a 10 fr bougie should be used. Do not remove the scalpel until the bougie is in situ. This will ease the passage of the bougie into the trachea and also ensure the hole created by the scalpel is not lost.
9.	Ask your assistant to place the tracheal tube on the bougie and slide the tube over the bougie down to your hand. Confirm your assistant has a firm hold on the distal end of the bougie. Railroad the tube over the bougie into the trachea until the tube is inserted to the level of the depth marker line. 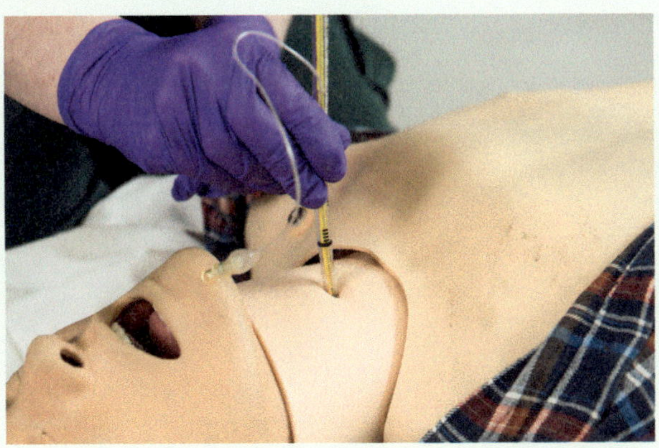	You should keep a firm hold of the bougie with your hand close to the patients' mouth, to ensure it stays firmly in the trachea while the tracheal tube is placed on the bougie. As the tube is inserted directly into the trachea, it can easily be advanced too far and become endobronchial, so care must be taken not to insert beyond the marking line.
10.	With a firm hold on the tracheal tube, ask your assistant to gently remove the bougie.	

Action		Rationale
11.	Attach a bag-valve-mask and ventilation circuit with capnography. 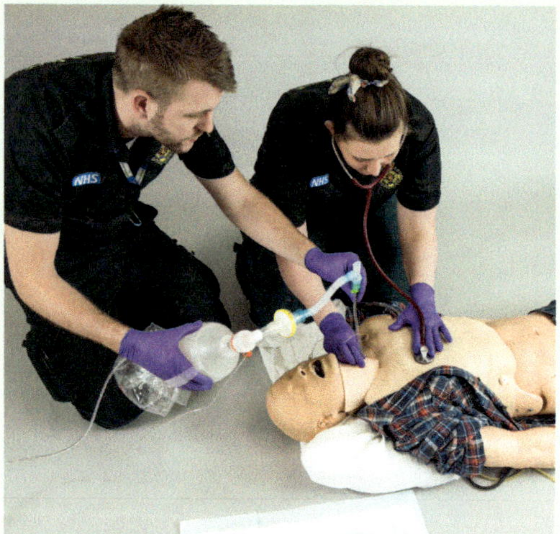 Inflate the cuff and gently ventilate. Confirm placement by a combination of observing for chest rise, capnography and bilateral auscultation (4).	Capnography is an essential component for confirming effective ventilation is occurring.
12.	Note the length and secure the tube with tape.	Even once secure, the tube can easily be displaced, especially during movement. Every time the patient is moved, the person coordinating the move should also hold the tube.
13.	Document the procedure.	You must keep full, clear and accurate records for everyone you care for, treat, or provide other services to (7).

References

1. Timmermann A, Chrimes N, Hagberg CA. Need to consider human factors when determining first-line technique for emergency front-of-neck access. *British Journal of Anaesthesia* [Internet]. 2016 Jul 1;117(1):5–7. Available from: https://doi.org/10.1093/bja/aew107.
2. The Royal College of Anaesthetists and the Difficult Airway Society. Major complications of airway management in the United Kingdom [Internet]. 2011 [cited 2022 Jun 19]. Available from: https://www.nationalauditprojects.org.uk/downloads/NAP4%20Full%20Report.pdf.
3. Law JA. Deficiencies in locating the cricothyroid membrane by palpation: we can't and the surgeons can't, so what now for the emergency surgical airway? *Canadian Journal of Anesthesia/Journal canadien d'anesthésie* [Internet]. 2016;63(7):791–796. Available from: https://doi.org/10.1007/s12630-016-0648-4.
4. Difficult Airway Society. Scalpel cricothyroidotomy [Internet]. 2015 [cited 2022 Jun 19]. Available from: https://das.uk.com/guidelines/das_intubation_guidelines.
5. NHS England. Standard infection control precautions: national hand hygiene and personal protective equipment policy [Internet]. 2019 [cited 2022 Feb 13]. Available from: www.england.nhs.uk/publication/standard-infection-control-precautions-national-hand-hygiene-and-personal-protective-equipment-policy/.
6. Chang JE, Kim H, Won D, et al. Comparison of the conventional downward and modified upward laryngeal handshake techniques to identify the cricothyroid membrane: a randomized, comparative study. *Anesthesia & Analgesia* [Internet]. 2021;133(5):1288–1295.
7. Health and Care Professions Council. Standards of conduct, performance and ethics [Internet]. 2018 [cited 2019 Dec 29]. Available from: www.hcpc-uk.org/standards/standards-of-conduct-performance-and-ethics/.

Chapter

3 Breathing

After the airway, ensuring your patient is ventilating properly is vital. This short chapter describes the most important skills to master.

In this book we have emphasised the use of a two-person bag-valve-mask (BVM) technique, since maintaining a patent airway is usually easier than with the single-handed technique, and always using an oropharyngeal and nasopharyngeal airway(s) with a BVM. Of course, we understand that in some cases the number of available personnel at the scene may make this difficult. However, in these cases it is probably better to upgrade the airway to a supraglottic airway device, for example, so that only careful squeezing of the bag is required.

We have described two techniques for needle thoracentesis. While commercial devices are probably preferable (although evidence is lacking) (1), the reality is that you may have to use a large-bore cannula. However, it is important that you understand the potential pitfalls of this approach (2).

References

1. Leech C, Porter K, Steyn R, et al. The pre-hospital management of life-threatening chest injuries: a consensus statement from the Faculty of Pre-Hospital Care, Royal College of Surgeons of Edinburgh. *Trauma*. 2017 Jan 1;19(1):54–62.
2. Laan DV, Vu TDN, Thiels CA, et al. Chest wall thickness and decompression failure: a systematic review and meta-analysis comparing anatomic locations in needle thoracostomy. *Injury*. 2016 Apr 1;47(4):797–804.

Single-Handed Bag-Valve-Mask Ventilation

Indications
- Patient requiring ventilation.

Contraindications
- None in the emergency situation.

Advantages
- Can be performed by one clinician.
- No need for complex equipment.
- Supplemental oxygen is easy to administer.

Disadvantages
- Difficult technique to master and maintain.
- Challenging to perform in some patient groups, for example obese or bearded patients, or those with a maxillofacial injury.

Procedure – Single-Handed Bag-Valve-Mask Ventilation

Take the following steps to perform single-handed bag-valve-mask (BVM) ventilation:

Action		Rationale
1.	Don appropriate personal protective equipment (PPE), and undertake appropriate hand hygiene.	This reduces the risk of cross-infection (1).
2.	Open the airway and position the patient's head into the 'sniffing the morning air' position (head extended and neck flexed) unless they have a suspected cervical spine injury. In this case a jaw thrust can be used to minimise movement. 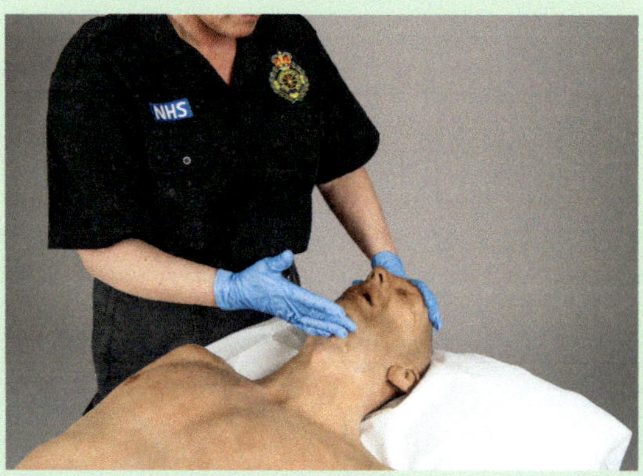	This elevates the tongue and epiglottis away from the posterior pharyngeal wall, resulting in a patent airway (2).

Action		Rationale
3.	Perform a quick visual check of the oropharynx to detect a foreign body, unless there is an indication in the history that a foreign body might be present, in which case laryngoscopy should be performed. 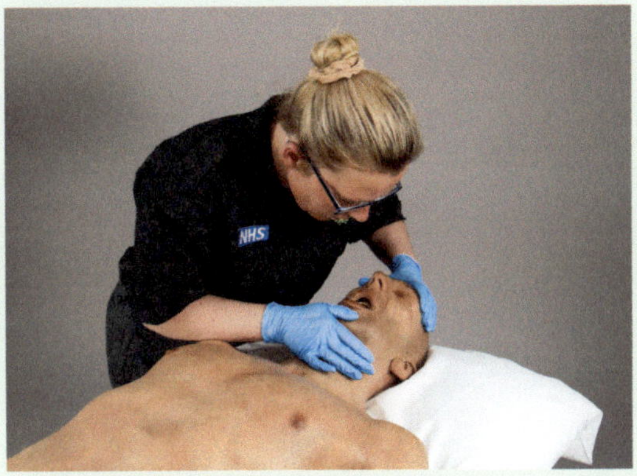 	Foreign bodies in the oropharynx may be aspirated when ventilation commences.
4.	The ventilating clinician should locate themselves at the head of the patient, facing the feet. 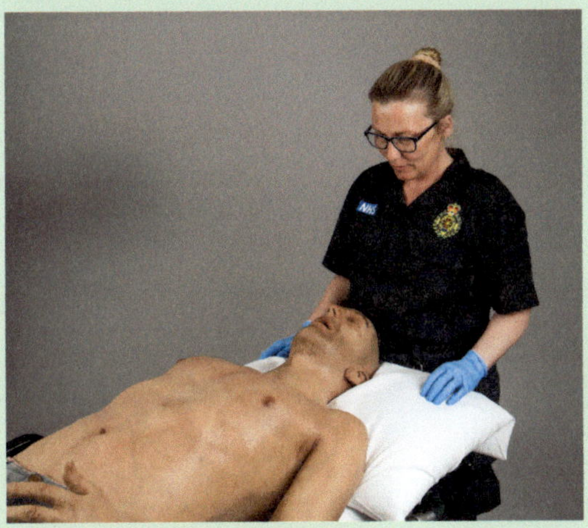	This position should enable the clinician to provide an adequate mask seal while allowing ventilation of the patient.
5.	Use the mnemonic ROMAN to assess the patient for signs that they may be difficult to ventilate with a BVM (3,4): • Radiation/restriction • Obesity/obstruction/obstructive sleep apnoea • Mask seal/Mallampati/male sex • Age more than 55 years • No teeth.	Pre-empting potential difficulties can help ensure that effective ventilation is provided. In the emergency situation it will not be possible to assess all of these factors, but having a good understanding of the potential challenges will help you to adapt and overcome any problems you encounter.

Action		Rationale
6.	Insert an appropriately sized oropharyngeal airway (OPA), or nasopharyngeal airway(s) (NPA) if an OPA cannot be used for any reason. 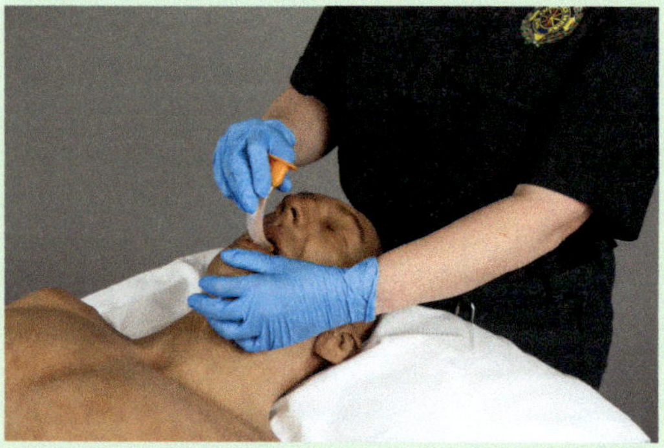	The BVM works best with airway adjuncts. This helps maintain a patent airway by preventing the tongue from causing an obstruction.
7.	Select the most appropriately sized mask. The lower edge of the mask should rest in the groove between the patient's chin and lower lip, and the upper edge should rest across the bridge of the nose. 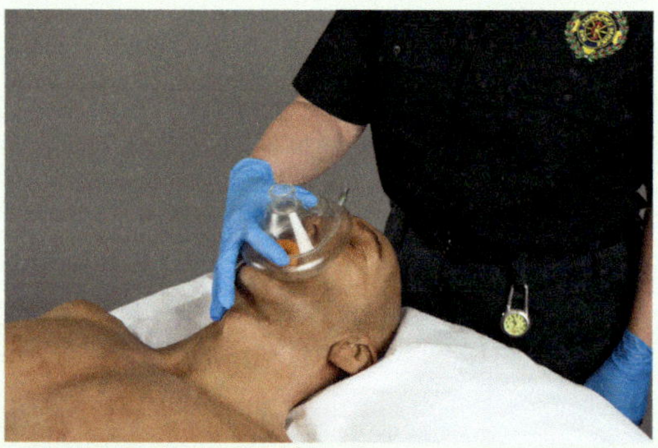	This helps to ensure a good seal and thus minimise air leaks.
8.	Connect mask to bag, capnography (where available) and oxygen supply.	Some texts advise fitting the mask first. However, ensuring the mask fits onto the bag firmly, to avoid it falling off during use, takes precedence.
9.	Position the mask on the patient's face and ensure an adequate seal. Apply the mask to the groove formed by the chin and lower lip first, and then the bridge of the nose (2).	This should ensure that the mask completely covers the mouth and nose, and the cuff of the mask is supported by the bony structures of the skull and mandible (3).
10.	Form a 'C' shape with the thumb and index finger and rest this on top of the mask; place the middle and ring fingers on the ridge of the jaw and the little finger behind the angle of the jaw.	This enables the clinician to keep the mask in position with the thumb and index finger while **lifting the jaw to meet the mask**. Pressing down on the mask may worsen functional obstruction (2).

Action		Rationale
11.	Gently squeeze the bag just enough to see the chest rise. Each ventilation should consist of an inspiratory component lasting 1 second. If capnography is available, aim for a ventilatory rate that results in normal end-tidal carbon dioxide (normocapnia). Otherwise, ventilate at a rate of 10–12 ventilations per minute. 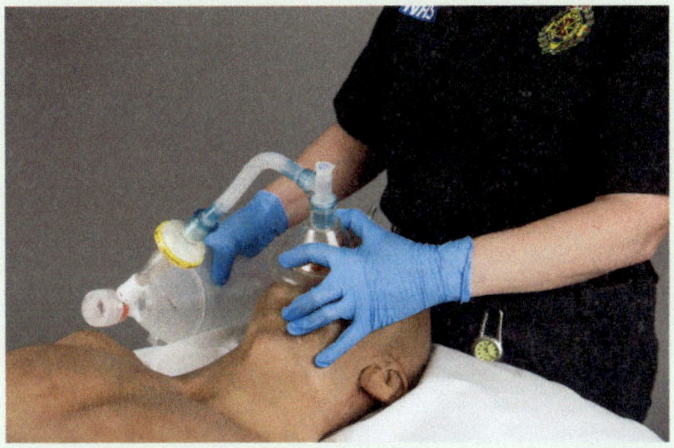	Excessive ventilatory pressures will result in air entering the stomach, increasing the risk of passive regurgitation. It can also result in barotrauma to the lungs (2,3).
12.	If ventilation is difficult, try gently flexing and extending the airway until you can successfully ventilate. If this fails, consider upgrading the airway to a supraglottic airway device.	Every patient has slightly different anatomy. Small positional changes can help improve airway patency.
13.	Frequently reassess the adequacy of the ventilation and escalate airway management if required.	Single-handed BVM ventilation is fatiguing. If prolonged ventilation is required, consider alternatives such as two-handed BVM or escalating the airway adjunct.
14.	Document the procedure.	You must keep full, clear and accurate records for everyone you care for, treat, or provide other services to (5).

References

1. NHS England, NHS Improvement. Standard infection control precautions: national hand hygiene and personal protective equipment policy [Internet]. 2019 [cited 2021 Nov 11]. Available from: https://www.england.nhs.uk/publication/standard-infection-control-precautions-national-hand-hygiene-and-personal-protective-equipment-policy/.
2. Kovacs G, Law JA. *Airway Management in Emergencies*. 2nd edition. Shelton: McGraw-Hill Medical; 2011.
3. Brown CA. *The Walls Manual of Emergency Airway Management*. 5th edition. Sakles JC, Mick NW, editors. Philadelphia: Lippincott Williams and Wilkins; 2017.
4. Kheterpal S, Healy D, Aziz MF, Shanks AM, Freundlich RE, Linton F, et al. Incidence, predictors, and outcome of difficult mask ventilation combined with difficult laryngoscopy: a report from the Multicenter Perioperative Outcomes Group. *Anesthesiology*. 2013 Dec 1;119(6):1360–1369.
5. Health and Care Professions Council. Standards of conduct, performance and ethics [Internet]. 2018 [cited 2019 Dec 29]. Available from: https://www.hcpc-uk.org/standards/standards-of-conduct-performance-and-ethics/.

Two-Handed Bag-Valve-Mask Ventilation

Indications

- Patient requiring ventilation.

Contraindications

- None in the emergency situation.

Advantages

- Maintaining a patent airway is usually easier than with the single-handed technique.
- No need for complex equipment.
- Supplemental oxygen is easy to administer.

Disadvantages

- Difficult technique to master and maintain.
- Challenging to perform in some patient groups, for example obese or bearded patients, or those with a maxillofacial injury.
- Requires two clinicians.

Procedure – Two-Handed Bag-Valve-Mask Ventilation

Take the following steps to perform two-handed bag-valve-mask (BVM) ventilation:

Action		Rationale
1.	Don appropriate personal protective equipment (PPE), and undertake appropriate hand hygiene.	This reduces the risk of cross-infection (1).
2.	Open the airway and position the patient's head in the 'sniffing the morning air' position (head extended and neck flexed) unless they have a suspected cervical spine injury. In this case a jaw thrust can be used to minimise movement. 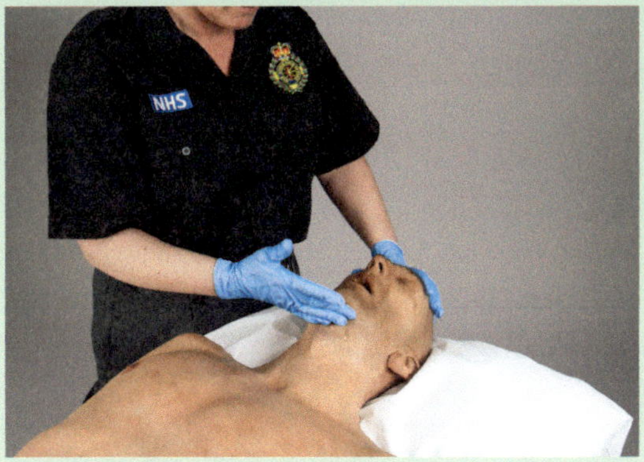	This elevates the tongue and epiglottis away from the posterior pharyngeal wall, resulting in a patent airway (2).

	Action	Rationale
3.	Perform a quick visual check of the oropharynx to detect a foreign body, unless there is an indication in the history that a foreign body might be present, in which case laryngoscopy should be performed. 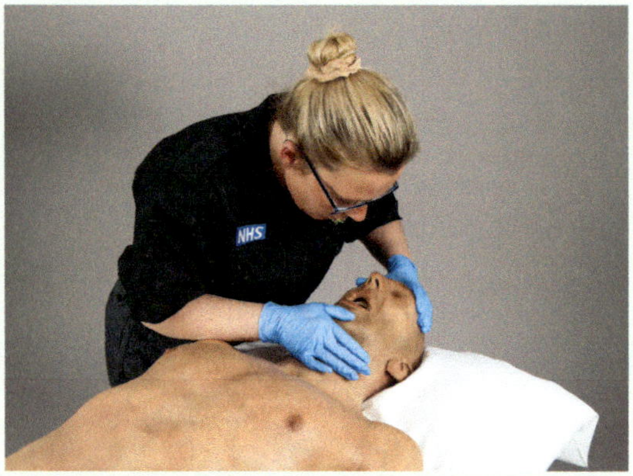 	Foreign bodies in the oropharynx may be aspirated when ventilation commences.
4.	The clinician responsible for holding the mask in position should be located at the head of the patient, facing the feet. 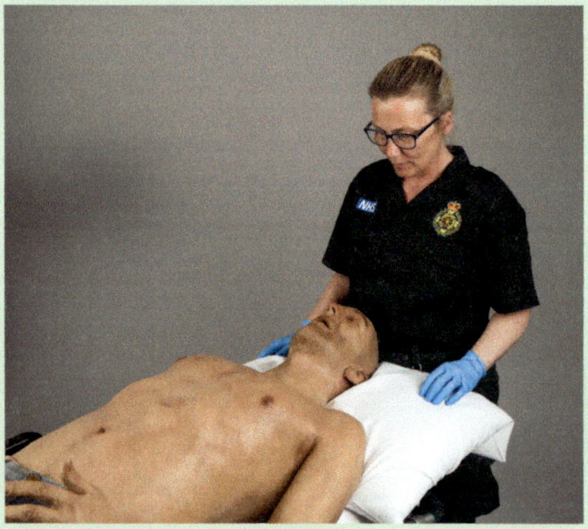	This position should enable the clinician to maintain a good mask seal while simultaneously providing jaw thrust.
5.	Use the mnemonic ROMAN to assess the patient for signs that they may be difficult to ventilate with a BVM (3,4): • Radiation/restriction • Obesity/obstruction/obstructive sleep apnoea • Mask seal/Mallampati/male sex • Age more than 55 years • No teeth.	Pre-empting potential difficulties can help ensure that effective ventilation is provided.

Action		Rationale
6.	Insert an appropriately sized oropharyngeal airway (OPA) or nasopharyngeal airway(s) (NPA) if an OPA cannot be used for any reason. 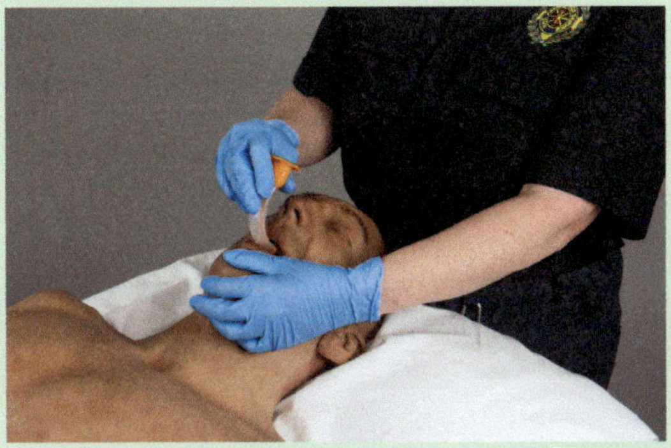	BVM works best with airway adjuncts. This helps maintain a patent airway by preventing the tongue causing obstruction.
7.	Select the most appropriately sized mask. The lower edge of the mask should rest in the groove between the patient's chin and lower lip, and the upper edge should rest across the bridge of the nose. 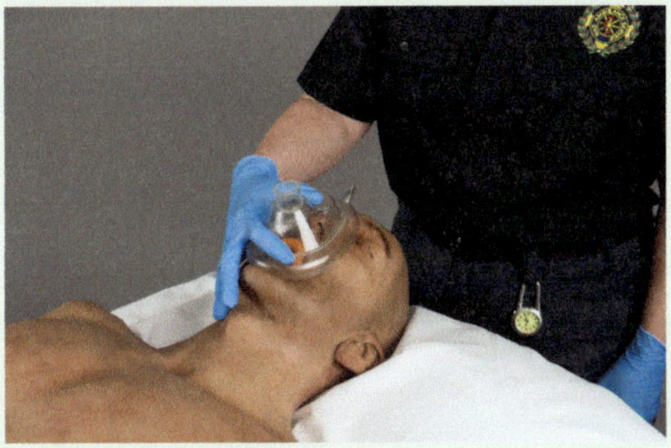	This helps to ensure a good seal and thus minimise air leaks.
8.	Connect mask to bag, capnography (where available) and oxygen supply.	Some texts advise fitting the mask first. However, ensuring the mask fits onto the bag firmly, to avoid it falling off during use, takes precedence.
9.	Position the mask on the patient's face and ensure an adequate seal. Apply the mask to the groove formed by the chin and lower lip first, and then the bridge of the nose (2).	This should ensure that the mask completely covers the mouth and nose, and the cuff of the mask is supported by the bony structures of the skull and mandible (3).

	Action	Rationale
10.	The mask-holding clinician should place both thenar eminences on top of the mask with their thumbs facing the patient's feet (caudally). The fingers should then grasp the mandible and pull it forward to meet the mask. 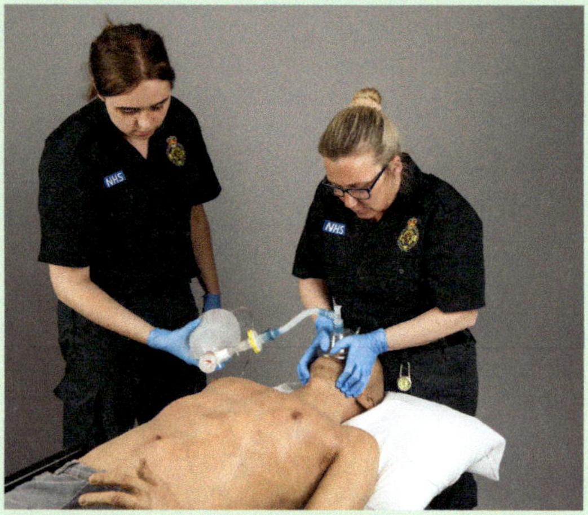	This method provides a better seal and is less likely to lead to a failure to ventilate. In addition, it is less fatiguing (3).
11.	The clinician who is not holding the mask should gently squeeze the bag just enough to see the chest rise. Each ventilation should consist of an inspiratory component lasting 1 second. If capnography is available, aim for a ventilatory rate that results in normal end-tidal carbon dioxide (normocapnia). Otherwise, ventilate at a rate of 10–12 ventilations per minute. 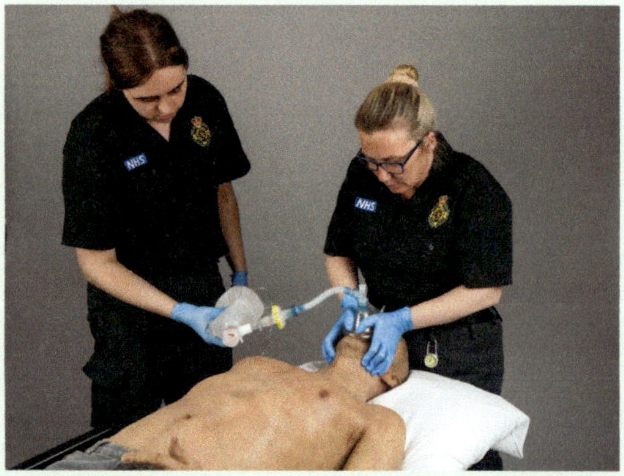	Excessive ventilatory pressures will result in air entering the stomach, increasing the risk of passive regurgitation. It can also result in barotrauma to the lungs (2,3).
12.	If ventilation is difficult, try gently flexing and extending the airway until you can successfully ventilate. If this fails, consider upgrading the airway to a supraglottic airway device.	Every patient has slightly different anatomy. Small positional changes can help improve airway patency.

Action		Rationale
13.	Frequently reassess the adequacy of the ventilation and escalate airway management if required.	
14.	Document the procedure.	You must keep full, clear and accurate records for everyone you care for, treat, or provide other services to (5).

References

1. NHS England, NHS Improvement. Standard infection control precautions: national hand hygiene and personal protective equipment policy [Internet]. 2019 [cited 2021 Nov 11]. Available from: https://www.england.nhs.uk/publication/standard-infection-control-precautions-national-hand-hygiene-and-personal-protective-equipment-policy/.
2. Kovacs G, Law JA. *Airway Management in Emergencies*. 2nd edition. Shelton: McGraw-Hill Medical; 2011.
3. Brown CA. *The Walls Manual of Emergency Airway Management*. 5th edition. Sakles JC, Mick NW, editors. Philadelphia: Lippincott Williams and Wilkins; 2017.
4. Kheterpal S, Healy D, Aziz MF, Shanks AM, Freundlich RE, Linton F, et al. Incidence, predictors, and outcome of difficult mask ventilation combined with difficult laryngoscopy: a report from the Multicenter Perioperative Outcomes Group. *Anesthesiology*. 2013 Dec 1;119(6):1360–1369.
5. Health and Care Professions Council. Standards of conduct, performance and ethics [Internet]. 2018 [cited 2019 Dec 29]. Available from: https://www.hcpc-uk.org/standards/standards-of-conduct-performance-and-ethics/.

Bag-Valve-Mask Ventilation with Positive End-Expiratory Pressure

Indications

- Ventilated patients where positive end-expiratory pressure (PEEP) may be of benefit to improve oxygenation.

Contraindications

- Suspected pneumothorax.
- Asthma.

Advantages

- An appropriate amount of PEEP can:
  - improve oxygenation
  - reduce atelectasis.

Disadvantages

- If set incorrectly can worsen haemodynamic stability, worsen oxygenation and cause trauma to the lungs (1).
- PEEP can only be used by clinicians trained and experienced in safely setting the correct pressure based on individual patient needs.

Procedure – Bag-Valve-Mask Ventilation with Positive End-Expiratory Pressure

Take the following steps to ventilate using a bag-valve-mask (BVM) with positive end-expiratory pressure (PEEP):

Note: Different valves and different manufacturers may have specific instructions or requirements. Ensure that you consult manufacturer instructions for the specific device you are using.

Action		Rationale
1.	PEEP can be added to a BVM breathing circuit at any time it is felt to be clinically appropriate. Follow the appropriate one- or two-handed procedure for other steps relating to BVM ventilation. In addition, you will require a disposable PEEP valve.	
2.	Inspect the valve for damage or debris and set the correct initial PEEP prior to connecting to the BVM.	This prevents inadvertently connecting the valve to the breathing circuit with a setting higher than intended.

Action		Rationale
3.	Remove the outlet cap from the BVM. 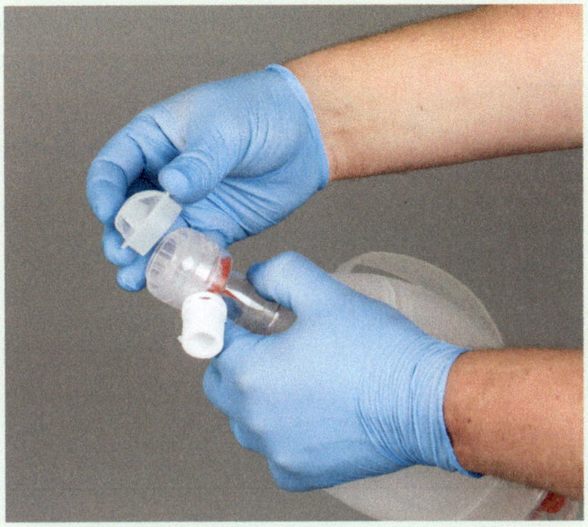	
4.	Attach the PEEP valve by pushing it firmly into the exhaust valve (2). 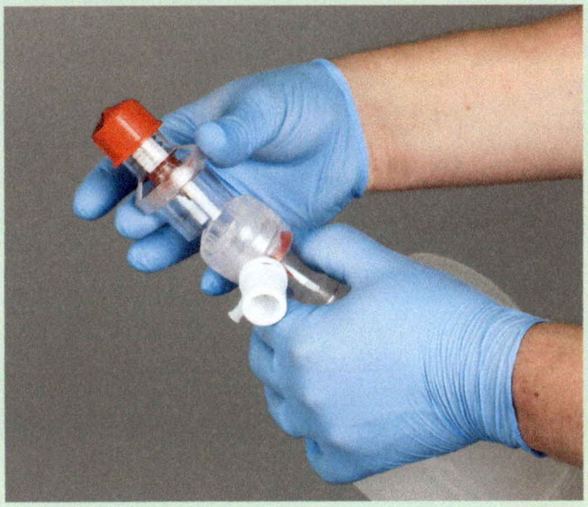	If using the correct device, the valve is designed to fit into this position. Pushing it in firmly, creates a good seal and reduces the risk of the valve becoming dislodged or an air leak occurring.

Action		Rationale
5.	If necessary, adjust the amount of pressure by turning the end of the device. Observe the marker for determining the set level of PEEP (3). 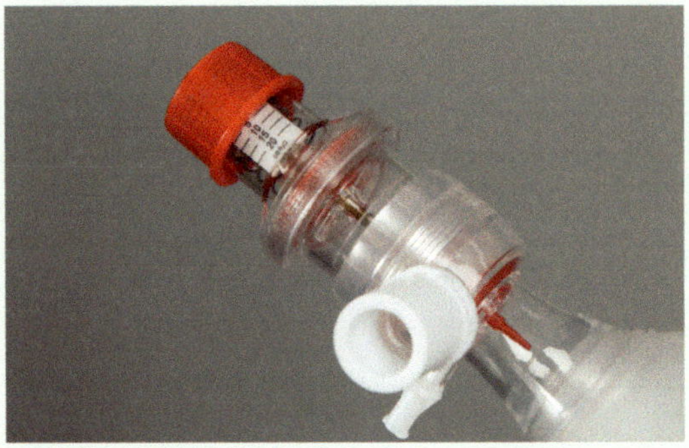	PEEP may need to be adjusted to an optimum setting for individual patients.
6.	Frequently recheck the set level of PEEP.	During patient care and handling, the valve can be inadvertently turned. Recheck regularly to ensure the pressure set is correct.
7.	Document the procedure.	You must keep full, clear and accurate records for everyone you care for, treat, or provide other services to (4).

References

1. Nickson C. Positive End-Expiratory Pressure (PEEP) Life In the fast lane [Internet]. 2021 [cited 2022 Jul 16]. Available from: https://litfl.com/positive-end-expiratory-pressure/#3-disadvantages-of-peep.
2. Ambu. Instructions for use: Ambu SPUR II [Internet]. 2022 [cited 2022 Jul 16]. Available from: https://www.ambu.co.uk/Admin/Public/DWSDownload.aspx?File=%2fFiles%2fFiles%2fDownloads%2fAmbu+UK%2fAnaesthesia%2fResuscitators%2fSPUR+II+-+Disposable+Resuscitator%2fDirections+for+Use%2fSPUR_II_DFU.pdf.
3. Ambu. Instructions for use Ambu PEEP 10 valve [Internet]. 2020 [cited 2022 Jul 16]. Available from: https://www.ambu.it/Admin/Public/Download.aspx?file=Files%2fFiles%2fDownloads%2fAmbu+IT%2fCure-di-emergenza%2fPalloni+rianimatori%2fPEEP+Valves+-+Disposable+and+Reusable%2fIstruzioni+per+l%27uso%2f492203140_-Ambu-Peep-Valve_-Multi_10797_Multi.pdf.
4. Health and Care Professions Council. Standards of conduct, performance and ethics [Internet]. 2016 [cited 2022 Jul 16]. Available from: https://www.hcpc-uk.org/standards/standards-of-conduct-performance-and-ethics/.

Needle Thoracentesis (Cannula Method)

Indications
- Patient with suspected tension pneumothorax showing signs of decompensation (1).
- Cardiac arrest where tension pneumothorax is a credible reversible cause.

Contraindications
- Patient without suspected tension pneumothorax, for example simple pneumothorax.

Advantages
- Does not require specialised kit.
- Can provide prompt decompression of a tension pneumothorax, 'buying time' for definitive care.

Disadvantages
- Standard cannulas may not be long enough to puncture the pleura (2).
- Likely to be performed with makeshift equipment (non-commercial device).
- Less effective than a finger thoracostomy, which, when available, should be the first-line treatment for a ventilated patient with suspected tension pneumothorax (3).

Procedure – Needle Thoracentesis (Cannula Method)

Take the following steps to perform a needle thoracentesis with a cannula (1):

Action		Rationale
1.	Don appropriate personal protective equipment (PPE), and undertake appropriate hand hygiene.	This reduces the risk of cross-infection (4).
2.	Prepare your equipment: • Large-bore cannula • 10 ml syringe • Saline flush • Skin-cleansing wipe • Roll of tape • Chest seal • Sharps container. 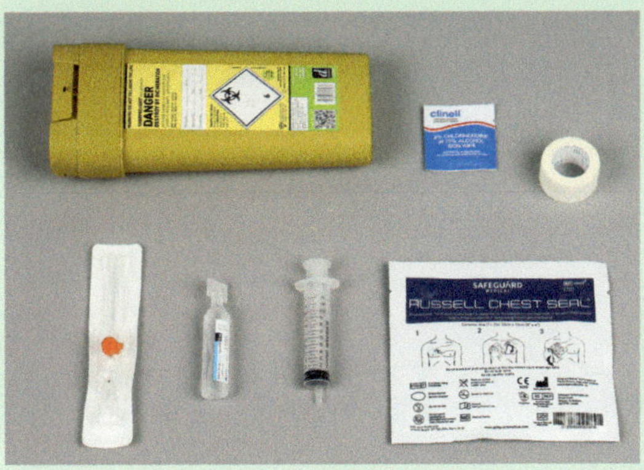	

Action		Rationale
3.	Locate where the mid-clavicular line (MCL) intersects with the second intercostal space. 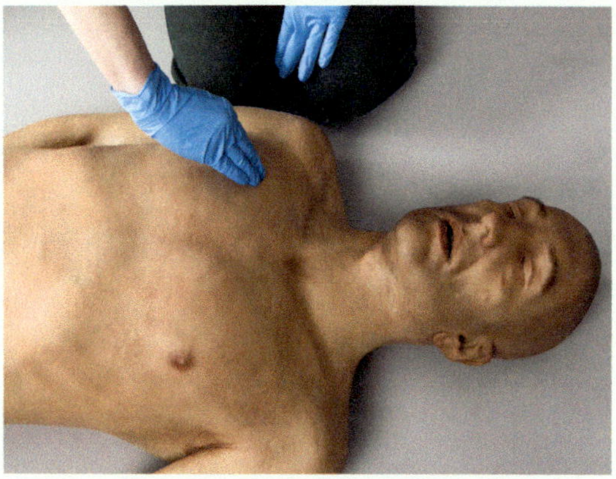	Incorrect placement is the most significant factor in complications arising as a result of the procedure (1).
4.	Clean the site and allow to dry. 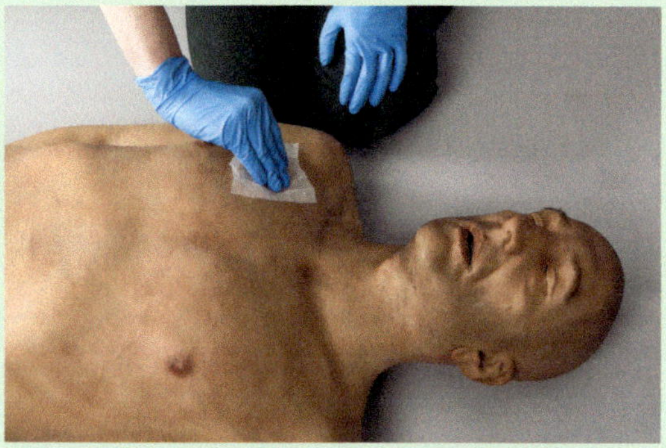	This may help reduce infection risk, but evidence to support this is limited.
5.	Draw up 3–4 ml of saline into the syringe and attach the cannula. 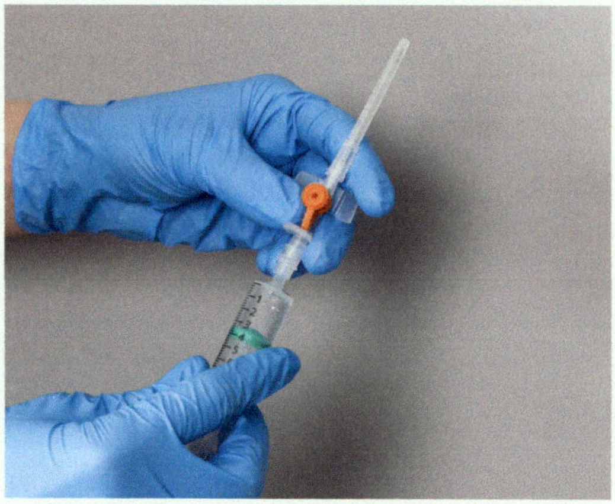	This is optional, but may provide a clearer indication of successful penetration of the pleura.

Action		Rationale
6.	Place your non-dominant hand on the patient's chest.	This will help stabilise the chest and give you better control as the needle is inserted.
7.	Insert the cannula perpendicular (90°) to the patient's back, just above the third rib. 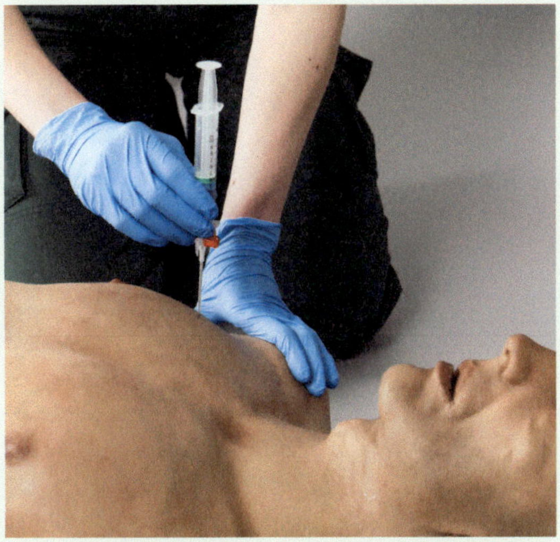	The neurovascular bundle is positioned on the inferior aspect of each rib. Inserting close to the superior aspect of the third rib should avoid the neurovascular bundle of the second rib.
8.	Advance the cannula while gently pulling back on the plunger, until either a sudden loss of resistance or 'give' is felt, or you see bubbles in the syringe. 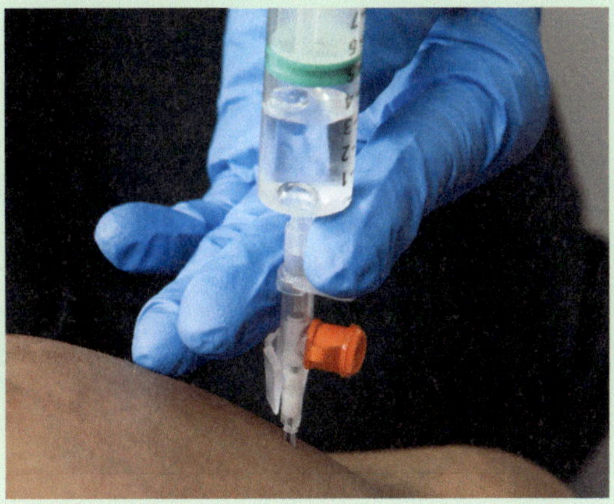	These signs indicate that you have successfully punctured the pleura. The needle could damage structures if advanced further.

Action		Rationale
9.	Anchor the syringe and cannula needle with your dominant hand and advance the cannula to the patient's chest. 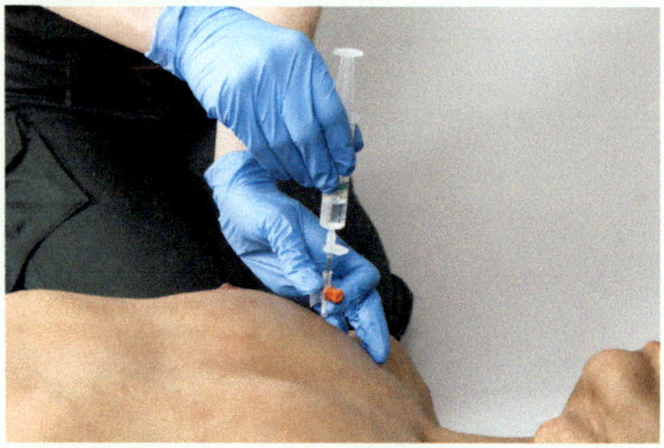	This should prevent inadvertent advancement of the needle.
10.	Remove the syringe and needle and dispose into a sharps container. 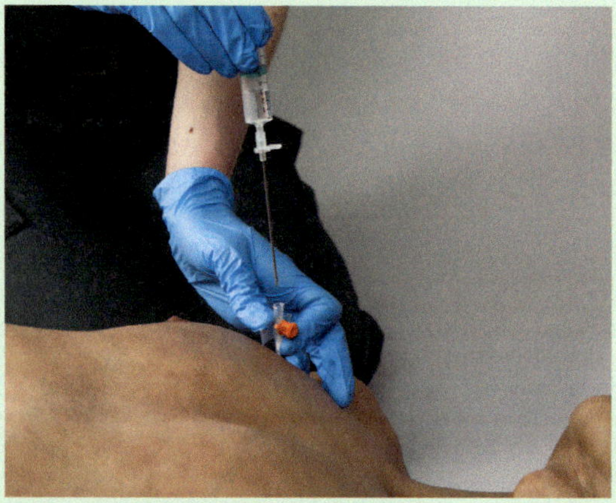	This reduces the risk of needle-stick injury and/or infection.
11.	Reassess the patient.	Improvement in symptoms or physiological measurements, should occur fairly soon after aspiration of air from the pleura. However, the relatively small diameter of the cannula will limit the escape of air, and is at risk of blockage through kinking and obstruction with blood, for example.

Action		Rationale
12.	If the attempt is unsuccessful, repeat the procedure but use a lateral approach (fifth intercostal space just anterior to the mid-axillary line). 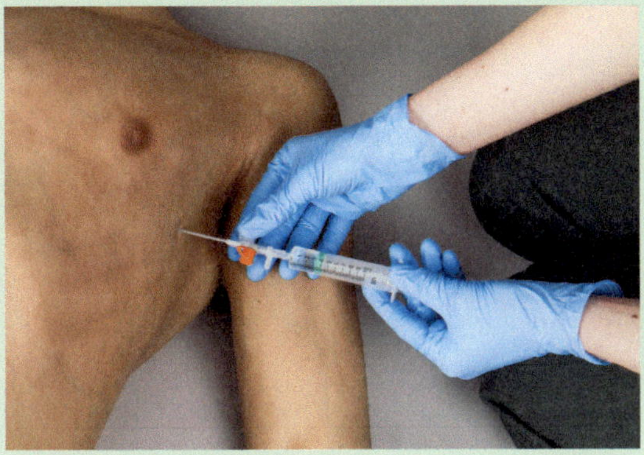	The chest wall is thinner here, although there are varying reports of success with this approach. Also bear in mind that the patient's arm will need to be elevated above their head using this approach, which will make transporting the patient difficult and the cannula may be more likely to kink in this position.
13.	Secure the cannula. Here, a roll of tape, covered with a chest seal that has had a hole cut in the centre of it, has been used. 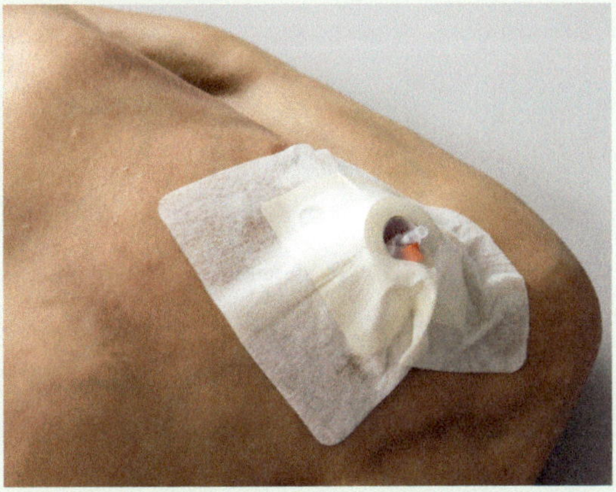	This should help reduce the likelihood of the cannula kinking or being inadvertently removed.
14.	Document the procedure.	You must keep full, clear and accurate records for everyone you care for, treat, or provide other services to (5).

References

1. Leech C, Porter K, Steyn R, et al. The pre-hospital management of life-threatening chest injuries: a consensus statement from the Faculty of Pre-Hospital Care, Royal College of Surgeons of Edinburgh. *Trauma*. 2017 Jan 1;19(1):54–62.
2. Laan DV, Vu TDN, Thiels CA, et al. Chest wall thickness and decompression failure: a systematic review and meta-analysis comparing anatomic locations in needle thoracostomy. *Injury*. 2016 Apr 1;47(4):797–804.
3. Resuscitation Council (UK). *Advanced Life Support*. London: Resuscitation Council (UK); 2021.
4. NHS England, NHS Improvement. Standard infection control precautions: national hand hygiene and personal protective equipment policy [Internet]. 2019 [cited 2021 Nov 11]. Available from: www.england.nhs.uk/publication/standard-infection-control-precautions-national-hand-hygiene-and-personal-protective-equipment-policy/.
5. Health and Care Professions Council. Standards of conduct, performance and ethics [Internet]. 2018 [cited 2019 Dec 29]. Available from: https://www.hcpc-uk.org/standards/standards-of-conduct-performance-and-ethics/.

Needle Thoracentesis (PneumoDart Method)

Indications

- Patient with suspected tension pneumothorax showing signs of decompensation (1).
- Cardiac arrest where tension pneumothorax is a credible reversible cause.

Contraindications

- Patient without suspected tension pneumothorax, for example simple pneumothorax.

Advantages

- Can provide prompt decompression of a tension pneumothorax, 'buying time' for definitive care.
- More likely to reach the pleural cavity than a needle technique that uses a cannula.

Disadvantages

- Less effective than a finger thoracostomy, which, when available, should be the first-line treatment for a ventilated patient with suspected tension pneumothorax.

Procedure – Needle Thoracentesis (PneumoDart Method)

Take the following steps to perform a needle thoracentesis utilising a PneumoDart (2):

Action		Rationale
1.	Don appropriate personal protective equipment (PPE), and undertake appropriate hand hygiene.	This reduces the risk of cross-infection (3).
2.	Prepare your equipment: • PneumoDart • Skin-cleansing wipe • Materials to secure the needle (check local procedures) • Sharps container.	
3.	Locate where the mid-clavicular line (MCL) intersects with the second intercostal space. 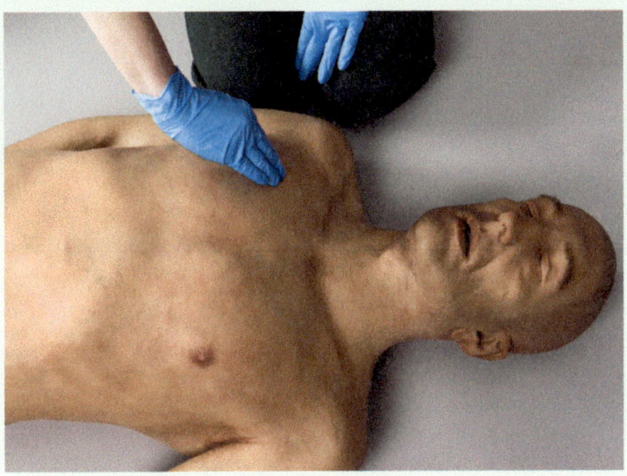	Incorrect placement is the most significant factor in complications arising as a result of the procedure (1).

Action		Rationale
4.	Clean the site and allow to dry. 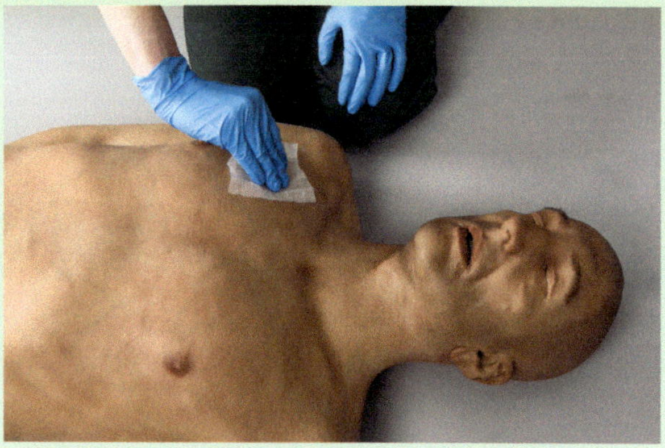	This may help reduce infection risk, but evidence to support this is limited.
5.	Inspect the safety seal on the tube for the PneumoDart and ensure it is still intact.	If the seal is damaged, the device should not be used as it may no longer be sterile.
6.	Remove the PneumoDart from its case.	
7.	Place your non-dominant hand on the patient's chest.	This will help stabilise the chest and give you better control as the needle is inserted.
8.	Insert the needle over the top of the third rib in the MCL at 90° to the chest wall; insertion should not be medial to the nipple. Observe the needle position indicator, which should move backwards in the viewing window as the device makes contact with, and penetrates, the chest wall. 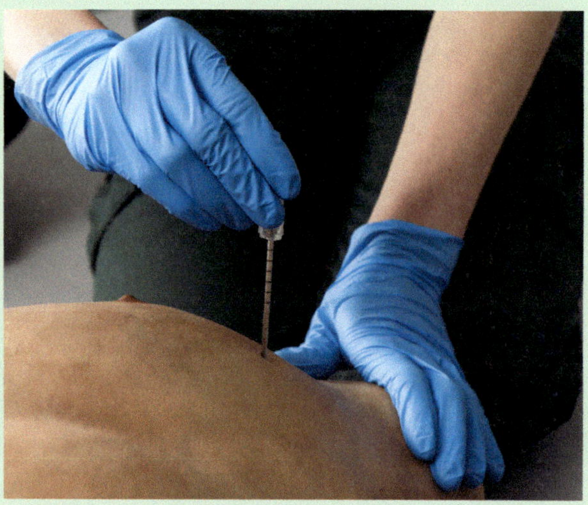	Insertion medial to the nipple increases the risk of damaging underlying structures.

Action		Rationale
9.	Advance the needle directly towards the patient's back, ensuring the tip is not directed towards the heart. Observe the needle position indicator. Once the tip penetrates the pleural cavity, the indicator will move back into the down position and air should be released. 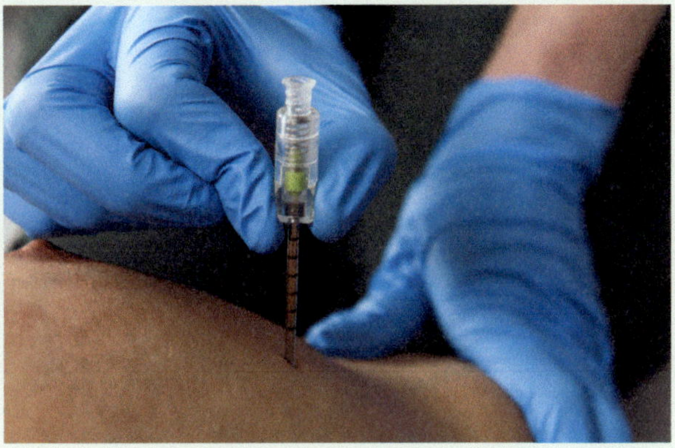	The indicator in the image on the left, shows the needle has reached the pleural space and should not be advanced further as it may damage underlying structures.
10.	Secure the needle in place in accordance with local procedures.	There is no specific guidance from the manufacturer about how to secure this device.
11.	Reassess the patient.	Improvement in symptoms or physiological measurements should occur soon after aspiration of air from the pleura. However, the needle is at risk of blockage, so constant reassessment is required.
12.	Document the procedure.	You must keep full, clear and accurate records for everyone you care for, treat, or provide other services to (4).

References

1. Leech C, Porter K, Steyn R, et al. The pre-hospital management of life-threatening chest injuries: a consensus statement from the Faculty of Pre-Hospital Care, Royal College of Surgeons of Edinburgh. *Trauma*. 2017 Jan 1;19(1):54–62.
2. Tylek Medical. PneumoDart: instructions for trained medical personnel [Internet]. 2022 [cited 2022 Jul 24]. Available from: https://cdn.shopify.com/s/files/1/0508/6196/5469/files/Rev.05042022_PNEUMODART_Instructions_English_Both_Sides_2022.pdf?v=1651661211.
3. NHS England, NHS Improvement. Standard infection control precautions: national hand hygiene and personal protective equipment policy [Internet]. 2019 [cited 2021 Nov 11]. Available from: https://www.england.nhs.uk/publication/standard-infection-control-precautions-national-hand-hygiene-and-personal-protective-equipment-policy/.
4. Health and Care Professions Council. Standards of conduct, performance and ethics [Internet]. 2018 [cited 2019 Dec 29]. Available from: https://www.hcpc-uk.org/standards/standards-of-conduct-performance-and-ethics/.

Finger Thoracostomy in Adults

Indications

- Ventilated patients with suspected tension pneumothorax showing signs of decompensation (1).
- Spontaneously breathing patients with suspected tension pneumothorax showing signs of decompensation, who have not responded to needle thoracentesis (1).
- Cardiac arrest where tension pneumothorax is a credible reversible cause.

Contraindications

- Suspected tension pneumothorax in spontaneously breathing patients where needle thoracentesis has not been attempted.

Advantages

- Provides prompt and effective decompression (typically in under 20 seconds).
- Low complication rate when performed by appropriately trained clinicians (2).

Disadvantages

- Highly invasive and painful in the conscious patient.
- Risk of injury to rescue personnel due to use of sharps or potentially from fractured ribs.
- Potential to cause other iatrogenic injuries to underlying structures (3).
- Can become re-occluded, especially during transport phase.
- Significant risk of serious and potentially life-threatening infection.

Procedure – Finger Thoracostomy

Take the following steps to perform a finger thoracostomy (4,5):

Action		Rationale
1.	If the patient is conscious, explain the procedure and obtain consent if appropriate to do so. In practice, it is unlikely that any patient who is critically unwell enough to require finger thoracostomy will be able to give consent.	You must make sure that you have valid consent from service users or other appropriate authority before you provide care, treatment or other services (6,7).
2.	Don appropriate personal protective equipment (PPE), and undertake appropriate hand hygiene.	This reduces the risk of cross-infection (8).
3.	Prepare your equipment. You will require: • Size 22 scalpel • ChloraPrep™ skin prep (or similar) • Spencer Wells forceps • One-way dressing (for example, Russell Chest Seal®) • Sharps container.	
4.	Position the patient supine, with the arm moved out of the way (imagine the the palm of the patient's hand positioned under their occiput).	This provides good access to the site where the procedure will be performed.

Action		Rationale
5.	If the patient is conscious, then appropriate analgesia, procedural sedation, local anaesthetic, or a combination of these methods, should be administered.	The procedure can be extremely painful so analgesia or local anaesthetic must be used. In the case of cardiac arrest this step must be omitted in preference of speed.
6.	Identify the triangle of safety. This is identified by the lateral border of pectoralis major, the anterior border of latissimus dorsi and the fifth intercostal space. To identify the fifth intercostal space, first find the manubriosternal junction (angle of Louis), which is at the same height as the second rib, and count down. Once the fifth intercostal space has been identified, follow this around the chest wall.	Performing the procedure in the triangle of safety will help to avoid damaging underlying structures. Do not follow a directly horizontal line from the fifth intercostal space on the anterior chest, as this will be too low on the lateral side due to the ribs curling up and around.
7.	Clean the area with ChloraPrep™.	This may help to reduce the risk of infection and empyema, but evidence relating to this is poor. Nonetheless, keeping the incision site as clean as possible for this highly invasive procedure is important.
8.	Using the scalpel, make an incision in the fifth intercostal space, over the top of the inferior rib between the mid-axillary and the anterior axillary lines. The incision should be approximately 3–5 cm long and deep enough to cut through the skin and underlying fat. You should not cut the intercostal muscles with the scalpel. Dispose of the scalpel into a sharps container.	The neurovascular bundle is positioned on the inferior aspect of each rib. An incision close to the superior aspect of the sixth rib should avoid the neurovascular bundle of the fifth rib.
9.	Grip the Spencer Wells forceps 4–5 cm down the shaft and insert into the incision, placing the tip against the intercostal muscle on the superior border of the inferior rib. Using a deliberate and forceful motion, 'punch through' the intercostal muscle.	Holding the forceps at 4–5 cm will prevent them from being inserted too far and damaging underlying structures. This may need to be increased or decreased depending on chest wall thickness. A short, deliberate motion will quickly and easily gain access to the pleural space.
10.	Blunt dissect by gently rotating as you open and close the forceps, while ensuring they do not inadvertently go deeper than necessary into the chest cavity.	Increasing the space will make the insertion of a finger simpler.

Action		Rationale
11.	With the forceps still in the hole, slide your index finger over the top. Once inside the chest cavity, the forceps can be removed. Sweep your finger through 360°, palpating for lung during ventilation.	Initial insertion of a finger can be challenging. Rotating your finger should help position it in the rib space. Do not remove the forceps until your finger has been inserted as you may not be able to find the tract again once the forceps have been removed. Note whether the lung is up or down and ventilating.
12.	If the patient is spontaneously breathing, place a one-way occlusive dressing, such as the Russell Chest Seal®, over the hole.	In spontaneously breathing patients the negative intrathoracic pressure may cause air to be drawn in through the thoracostomy hole, worsening a pneumothorax.
13.	When conveying, try to transport the patient so that their arm does not cover the surgical site.	An arm covering the surgical site can cause it to become occluded and makes reassessment very challenging.
14.	Continually reassess for signs of a tension pneumothorax redeveloping.	If you believe a tension pneumothorax may be redeveloping, you may need to repeat the finger sweep as described in step 11.
15.	Document the procedure.	You must keep full, clear and accurate records for everyone you care for, treat, or provide other services to (7).

References

1. Leech C, Porter K, Steyn R, et al. The pre-hospital management of life-threatening chest injuries: a consensus statement from the Faculty of Pre-Hospital Care, Royal College of Surgeons of Edinburgh. *Trauma*. 2017 Jan 1;19(1):54–62.
2. Sharrock K, Shannon B, Garcia Gonzalez C, et al. Prehospital paramedic pleural decompression: a systematic review. *Injury* [Internet]. 2021;52(10):2778–2786. Available from: www.sciencedirect.com/science/article/pii/S0020138321006860.
3. Hannon L, St Clair T, Smith K, et al. Finger thoracostomy in patients with chest trauma performed by paramedics on a helicopter emergency medical service. *Emergency Medicine Australasia* [Internet]. 2020;32(4):650–656. Available from: https://onlinelibrary.wiley.com/doi/abs/10.1111/1742-6723.13549.
4. Greaves I, Porter K, Wright C. *Trauma Care Pre-hospital Manual*. London: CRC Press; 2019.
5. St John Ambulance Western Australia. Finger thoracostomy [Internet]. 2017 [cited 2022 Jul 16]. Available from: https://clinical.stjohnwa.com.au/clinical-skills/trauma/finger-thoracostomy.
6. British Medical Association. Ethics – general information [Internet]. 2018 [cited 2019 Dec 29]. Available from: www.bma.org.uk/advice/employment/ethics/consent/consent-tool-kit/2-general-information.
7. Health and Care Professions Council. Standards of conduct, performance and ethics [Internet]. 2016 [cited 2022 Jul 16]. Available from: www.hcpc-uk.org/standards/standards-of-conduct-performance-and-ethics/.
8. NHS England. Standard infection control precautions: national hand hygiene and personal protective equipment policy [Internet]. 2019 [cited 2022 Feb 13]. Available from: www.england.nhs.uk/publication/standard-infection-control-precautions-national-hand-hygiene-and-personal-protective-equipment-policy/.

Chapter

4 Circulation

Traditionally, once airway and breathing issues have been resolved, circulation is the next priority. This remains true, though more recent thinking suggests that some aspects of circulation management, such as those associated with arresting catastrophic bleeding (bleeding from which a patient can die in a matter of moments to minutes), should be undertaken as an immediate priority and prior to airway and breathing. In these situations, simple techniques such as placing a torniquet can be lifesaving.

There are numerous skills in this chapter, none of which are necessarily simple to perform well. Whilst applying an arterial torniquet may appear simple, in practice they are often applied incorrectly due to a lack of familiarity, or forgetting a basic step in the heat of the moment. Other techniques such as intravenous cannulation require complex fine motor skills which take time and significant experience to master.

Many of these skills may only be performed on rare occasions, of which intraosseous cannulation is a good example. When required, these skills will likely be undertaken in a stressful situation with a severely unwell patient, so periodically remind yourself of the steps involved and mentally rehearsing, or even better practising on a manikin, can help to keep skills fresh and ready for use.

Epistaxis – Nasal Clip

Indications

- Epistaxis thought to be from an anterior source.

Contraindications

- None.

Advantages

- Maintains continuous pressure without release, making it particularly valuable for young or older and frail patients, who may struggle to maintain pinching with sufficient pressure on their nose.
- Does not rely on patient or healthcare staff to maintain constant pressure (1).

Disadvantages

- Will not stop a posterior bleed.

Procedure – Nasal Clip Application

Take the following steps to apply a nasal clip:

Note: In the example below the RhinoPinch® is used, though other similar products are available.

Action		Rationale
1.	Explain the procedure to the patient and obtain consent if appropriate to do so.	You must make sure that you have valid consent from service users or other appropriate authority before you provide care, treatment or other services (2,3).
2.	Don appropriate personal protective equipment (PPE), and undertake appropriate hand hygiene.	This reduces the risk of cross-infection (4).
3.	Adopt first-aid measures while you prepare to apply a nasal clip: • Instruct the patient to sit, leaning forwards, with their mouth open. • Instruct them to pinch the soft cartilaginous area of the nose firmly.	This is standard first aid for epistaxis and will compress the highly vascular area in the front of the nose, called Little's area, responsible for 95% of all epistaxis (5,6).
4.	Prepare the clip by spreading the padded area wide enough to fit over the nostrils. Place the pads either side of the nose with the pads pointing inwards and upwards.	This placement will ensure the pads are sitting in the correct area to apply the appropriate pressure (7).

Action		Rationale
5.	Pinch the nose with the clip and increase pressure until the patient is unable to breathe through their nose. The ratchet system should maintain this pressure once the clip is released.	The pressure is required to help stem the bleeding. The pressure is maintained for 10–12 minutes to support the formation of a stable clot (7).
6.	If the patient starts to bleed from their mouth or into the oropharynx, consider alternative management according to local guidelines.	Bleeding from the mouth or into the oral pharynx could indicate bleeding is from a posterior, or poorly controlled anterior, source.
7.	After 10–12 minutes the clip should be released and an assessment be made of whether further treatment is required.	Follow local guidelines in the overall management of epistaxis.
8.	Document the procedure, including the time it was undertaken and any complications.	You must keep full, clear and accurate records for everyone you care for, treat, or provide other services to (2).

References

1. Vaghela HM. Using a swimmer's nose clip in the treatment of epistaxis in the A&E department. *Accident and Emergency Nursing*. 2005 Oct 1;13(4):261–263.
2. British Medical Association. Ethics – general information [Internet]. 2018 [cited 2019 Dec 29]. Available from: https://www.bma.org.uk/advice/employment/ethics/consent/consent-tool-kit/2-general-information.
3. Health and Care Professions Council. Standards of conduct, performance and ethics [Internet]. 2016 [cited 2022 Jul 16]. Available from: https://www.hcpc-uk.org/standards/standards-of-conduct-performance-and-ethics/.
4. NHS England. Standard infection control precautions: national hand hygiene and personal protective equipment policy [Internet]. 2019 [cited 2022 Feb 13]. Available from: https://www.england.nhs.uk/publication/standard-infection-control-precautions-national-hand-hygiene-and-personal-protective-equipment-policy/.
5. National Institute for Health and Care Excellence. Acute epistaxis: management [Internet]. 2020 [cited 2022 Feb 13]. Available from: https://cks.nice.org.uk/topics/epistaxis-nosebleeds/management/acute-epistaxis/.
6. BMJ Best Practice. Epistaxis – symptoms, diagnosis and treatment [Internet]. 2020 [cited 2022 Feb 13]. Available from: https://bestpractice.bmj.com/topics/en-gb/3000173.
7. MDTI. RhinoPinch nasal clip [Internet]. 2013 [cited 2022 Feb 13]. Available from: https://media.supplychain.nhs.uk/media/documents/FFE127/Marketing/29664_FFE127.pdf.

Olaes® Modular Bandage

Indications

- Significant haemorrhage from large wounds, not controlled by other simple techniques, particularly useful in the management of wounds in junctional areas.

Contraindications

- None.

Advantages

- Can be rapidly applied.
- Pressure cup and elasticated bandage allow for significant pressure to be directed on to the site of injury.
- Can apply effective pressure in junctional areas if used appropriately.
- The elastic breaks in the bandage prevent it from inadvertently unrolling during application.

Disadvantages

- The elasticated bandage can apply significant pressure leading to a tourniquet effect – be mindful of this when applying the dressing.

Procedure – Olaes® Modular Bandage Application

Take the following steps to apply an Olaes® Modular Bandage (1,2):

Note: This is the specific procedure for the Olaes® Modular Bandage, but other similar emergency dressings are likely to follow similar principles of application.

Action		Rationale
1.	Explain the procedure to the patient and obtain consent if appropriate to do so.	You must make sure that you have valid consent from service users or other appropriate authority before you provide care, treatment or other services (3,4).
2.	Don appropriate personal protective equipment (PPE), and undertake appropriate hand hygiene.	This reduces the risk of cross-infection (5).

Action		Rationale
3.	Open the outer plastic wrapper by starting with one of the pre-formed tear notches. Remove the dressing from the packaging and discard the paper the dressing is wrapped in. 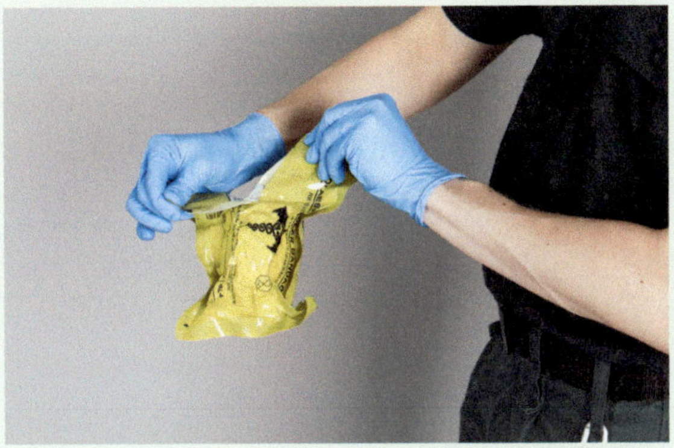	
4.	Ensure the wound is ready to be dressed. Before covering any deep wound, it should be packed with gauze or, if necessary, a haemostatic dressing. If a small amount of gauze is needed, you can open the Olaes® dressing and use the gauze from within it. There is also a plastic sheet inside the dressing.	To help achieve haemostasis, wounds should be packed so there is direct pressure on the site of bleeding. This can be achieved with gauze or haemostatic agents.
5.	Once packed, place the centre of the dressing (the area under the pressure cup) directly over the wound. 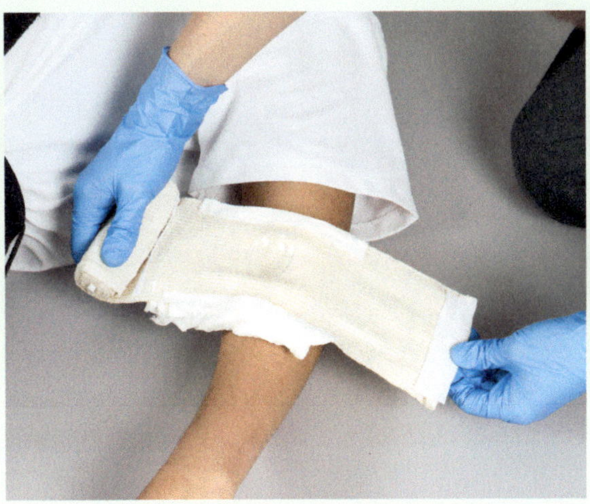	This will ensure that pressure is placed directly onto the wound once the bandage is secured around the dressing.

	Action	Rationale
6.	Wrap the bandage around the dressing, covering both ends of the dressing in the process. The bandage is elasticated, so a small amount of tension on the bandage will help to ensure it applies pressure to the whole site. 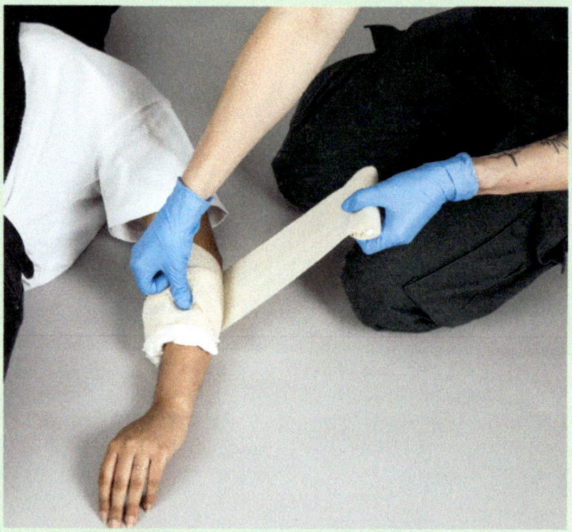	Pressure will help to achieve and maintain haemostasis. Note: Significant pressure may have a tourniquet effect, so consider this when applying the dressing.
7.	To secure, ensure the Velcro on the end of the bandage is stuck down and loop the plastic hooks under one of the previous wraps of material. 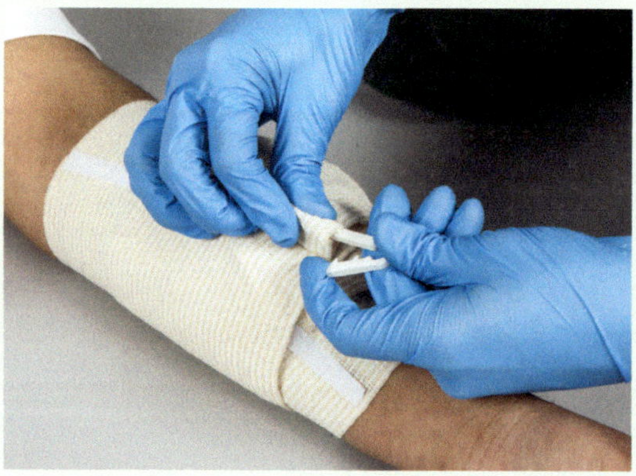	This will secure the end of the bandage in place and reduce the risk of it accidentally becoming undone.

	Action	Rationale
8.	Check the pulse distal to the dressing. 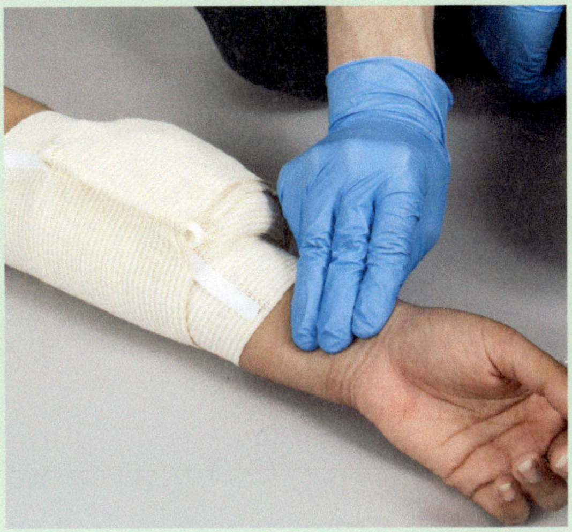	These dressings can become very tight and so a pulse should be checked afterwards to ensure it has not become so tight that it has cut off the arterial supply distal to the injury.
9.	If necessary, further pressure can be applied to the wound by pushing directly on to the top of the dressing.	Further pressure may be required if bleeding continues despite dressing the wound.
10.	Document the procedure, including the time it was undertaken and any complications.	You must keep full, clear and accurate records for everyone you care for, treat, or provide other services to (4).

References

1. Queensland Ambulance Service. Clinical practice procedures: the emergency bandage [Internet]. 2015 [cited 2022 Jan 2]. Available from: https://www.ambulance.qld.gov.au/docs/clinical/cpp/CPP_Bandaging_Emergency%20Bandage.pdf.
2. NAEMT, editor. *PHTLS Prehospital Trauma Life Support*. 9th edition. Burlington, MA: Jones & Bartlett Learning; 2019.
3. British Medical Association. Ethics – general information [Internet]. 2018 [cited 2019 Dec 29]. Available from: https://www.bma.org.uk/advice/employment/ethics/consent/consent-tool-kit/2-general-information.
4. Health and Care Professions Council. Standards of conduct, performance and ethics [Internet]. 2016 [cited 2022 Jul 16]. Available from: https://www.hcpc-uk.org/standards/standards-of-conduct-performance-and-ethics/.
5. NHS England. Standard infection control precautions: national hand hygiene and personal protective equipment policy [Internet]. 2019 [cited 2022 Feb 13]. Available from: https://www.england.nhs.uk/publication/standard-infection-control-precautions-national-hand-hygiene-and-personal-protective-equipment-policy/.

Blast™ Bandage

Indications

- Significant haemorrhage from large wounds not controlled by other, simple techniques.
- Particularly useful in the management of large torso wounds and for dressing the end of an amputated limb.

Contraindications

- None.

Advantages

- Can be rapidly applied.
- Can be used to apply significant pressure to a wound site.
- The elastic breaks in the bandage prevent it from inadvertently unrolling during application.

Disadvantages

- The elasticated bandage can apply significant pressure, leading to a tourniquet effect – be mindful of this when applying the dressing.

Procedure – Blast™ Bandage Application

Take the following steps to apply a Blast™ Bandage (1,2):

Note: This is the specific procedure for the Blast™ Bandage, but other similar emergency dressings are likely to follow similar principles of application.

Action		Rationale
1.	Explain the procedure to the patient and obtain consent if appropriate to do so.	You must make sure that you have valid consent from service users or other appropriate authority before you provide care, treatment or other services (3,4).
2.	Don appropriate personal protective equipment (PPE), and undertake appropriate hand hygiene.	This reduces the risk of cross-infection (5).

	Action	Rationale
3.	Open the outer plastic wrapper by starting with one of the pre-formed tear notches. Remove the dressing from the packaging and discard the paper the dressing is wrapped in. 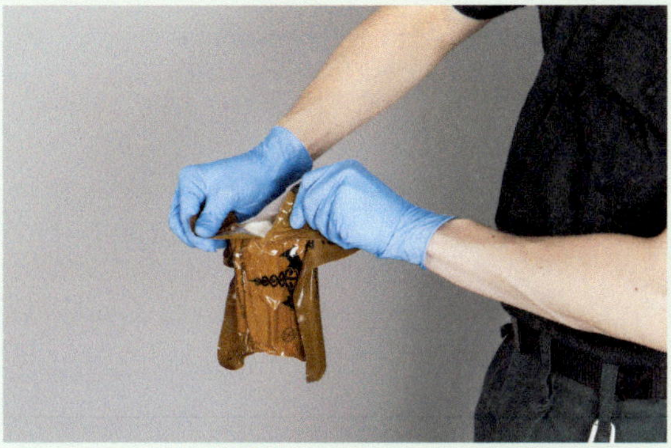	
4.	Ensure the wound is ready to be dressed. For an amputated limb, a tourniquet may need to be applied to gain control of bleeding.	Amputated limbs can experience significant arterial bleeding, which a Blast™ bandage alone will not be able to control.
5.	Gather the end of the amputated limb up into the dressing so all loose tissue is inside it, and wrap the dressing around the end of the limb. 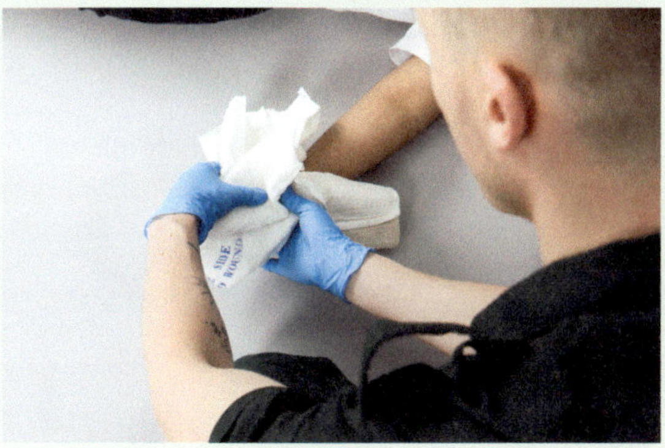	This will ensure that pressure is placed directly onto the wound once the bandage is secured around the dressing.

	Action	Rationale
6.	Place a single wrap of bandage around the dressing over the remaining limb. 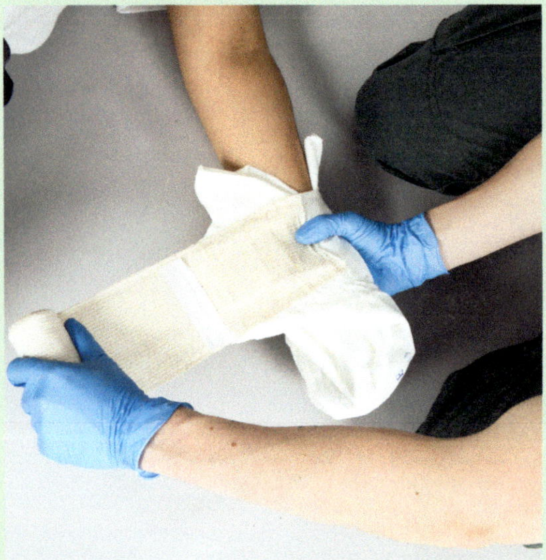	This helps to keep the dressing in place while the remainder of the bandage is applied.
7.	Wrap the bandage around the end of the dressing. At each turn pull the elasticated bandage so that once in place, it applies pressure. Wrap the bandage so that pressure is directed up into the end of the wound, not just around the remaining limb. 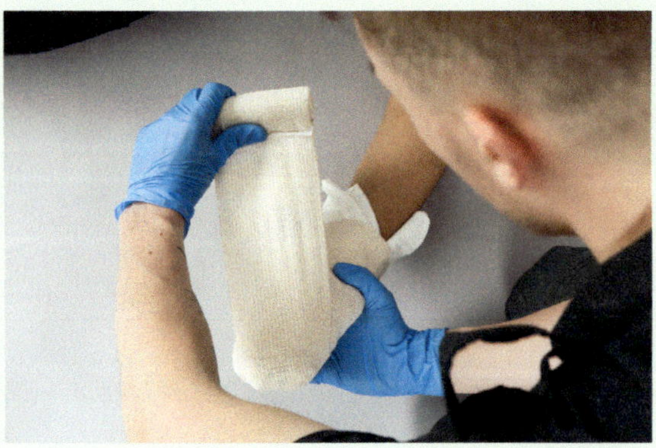	 Pressure will help to achieve and maintain haemostasis. Note: Significant pressure may have a tourniquet effect, so consider this when applying the dressing. In the case of amputation, the main wound is the end of the limb, not the remaining limb, so pressure should be applied to the wound itself where possible.

Action		Rationale
8.	To finish the bandage, ensure the Velcro on the end of the bandage is stuck down and loop the plastic hooks under one of the previous wraps of material. 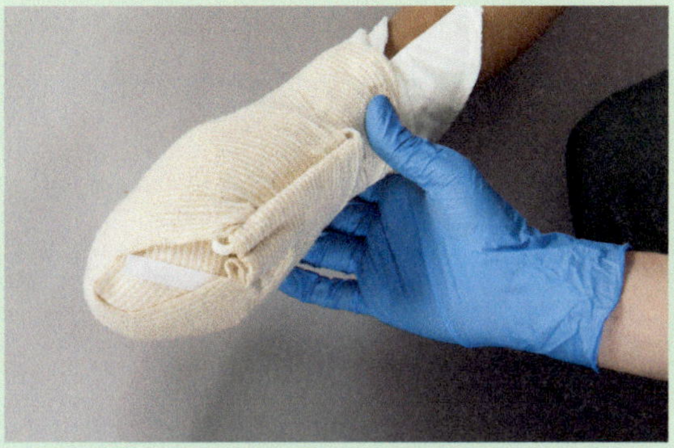	This will secure the end of the bandage in place and reduce the risk of it accidentally becoming undone.
9.	If necessary, further pressure can be applied to the wound by pushing directly on the top of the dressing or by placing a further Blast™ bandage over the top.	Further pressure may be required if bleeding continues despite dressing the wound.
10.	Document the procedure, including the time it was undertaken and any complications.	You must keep full, clear and accurate records for everyone you care for, treat, or provide other services to (4).

References

1. Queensland Ambulance Service. Clinical practice procedures: the emergency bandage [Internet]. 2015 [cited 2022 Jan 2]. Available from: https://www.ambulance.qld.gov.au/docs/clinical/cpp/CPP_Bandaging_Emergency%20Bandage.pdf.
2. NAEMT, editor. *PHTLS Prehospital Trauma Life Support*. 9th edition. Burlington: Jones & Bartlett Learning; 2019.
3. British Medical Association. Ethics – general information [Internet]. 2018 [cited 2019 Dec 29]. Available from: https://www.bma.org.uk/advice/employment/ethics/consent/consent-tool-kit/2-general-information.
4. Health and Care Professions Council. Standards of conduct, performance and ethics. [Internet]. 2016 [cited 2022 Jul 16]. Available from: https://www.hcpc-uk.org/standards/standards-of-conduct-performance-and-ethics/.
5. NHS England. Standard infection control precautions: national hand hygiene and personal protective equipment policy [Internet]. 2019 [cited 2022 Feb 13]. Available from: https://www.england.nhs.uk/publication/standard-infection-control-precautions-national-hand-hygiene-and-personal-protective-equipment-policy/.

Haemostatic Dressings

Indications

- Life-threatening haemorrhage from wounds which can be packed with a dressing. Haemostatic dressings are of particular value in areas that are hard to compress, including the thorax and junctional areas around the groin, arms and neck.

Contraindications

- Do not apply over the eyes.
- Do not apply close to the spine.

Advantages

- The clotting mechanism works independently of clotting factors in the blood so is not impacted by coagulopathy or use of anticoagulants (1).

Disadvantages

- Are commonly misapplied, due to not being packed deeply enough into the wound.

Procedure – HemCon ChitoGauze® XR Pro Application

Follow the procedure below to apply HemCon ChitoGauze® XR Pro (2):

Note: While this procedure is specific for HemCon ChitoGauze® XR Pro, it is likely that other haemostatic agents will be applied using similar principles.

Action		Rationale
1.	Explain the procedure to the patient and obtain consent if appropriate to do so.	You must make sure that you have valid consent from service users or other appropriate authority before you provide care, treatment or other services (3,4).
2.	Don appropriate personal protective equipment (PPE), and undertake appropriate hand hygiene.	This reduces the risk of cross-infection (5).

	Action	Rationale
3.	Open the packet and remove the ChitoGauze®, keeping it folded up. Take care not to drop the gauze or allow it to become contaminated prior to use. 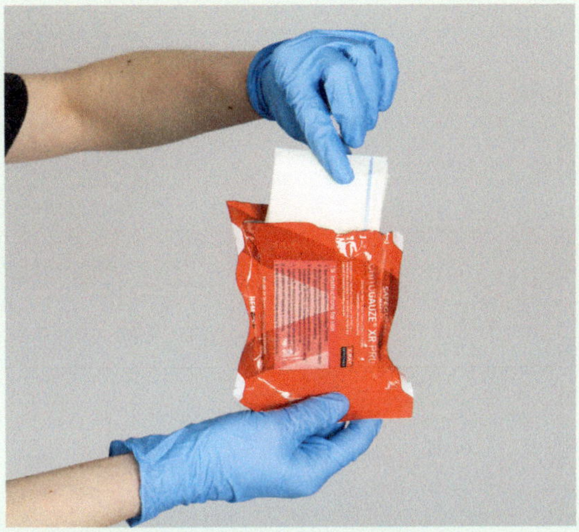	This helps to minimise risk of wound infection.
4.	Pack the gauze deep into the wound. Note: This should not be laid over a wound as it will not work if used like this – it must be packed deep into a wound. More than one pack of gauze may be required. 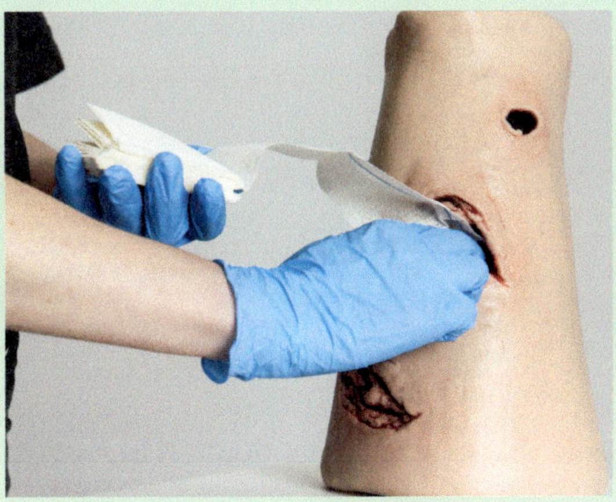	Fill the wound with gauze so it is in contact with all bleeding surfaces. This ensures the active components of the gauze are in contact with the site(s) of bleeding. Filling the wound also has a tamponade effect, which helps to apply direct pressure.
5.	If there is excess dressing after packing the wound, cut off the remaining dressing, ensuring that what remains includes some X-ray-translucent strip (the thin blue line).	The presence of the X-ray strip means the dressing can be seen on imaging, which helps to ensure no dressing is accidentally left in the patient.

	Action	Rationale
6.	Maintain direct pressure until bleeding is controlled. 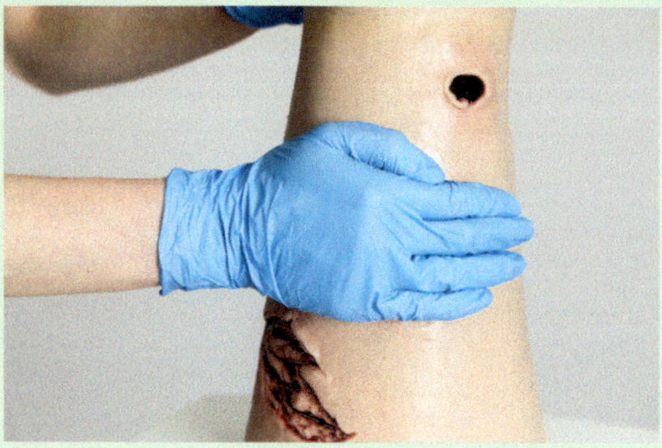	Direct pressure should be applied to help the coagulation reaction to occur.
7.	Dress the wound, ensuring that the dressing continues to apply pressure. 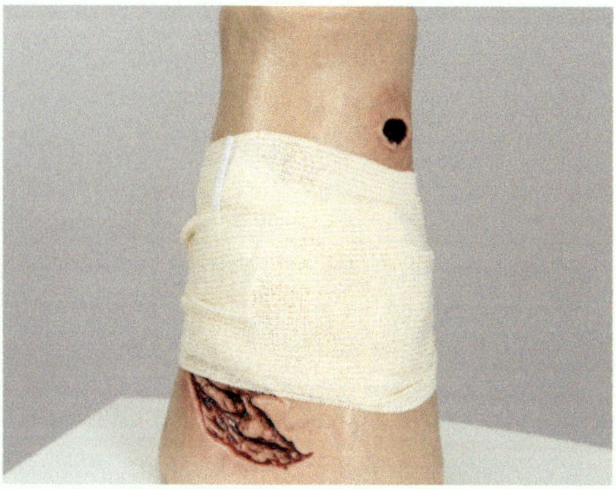	Pressure should be maintained with the dressing to ensure the clot that develops is as stable as possible.
8.	Continually reassess the wound area and dressing.	Movement can lead to the dressing becoming loose and bleeding restarting.
9.	Document the procedure, including the time it was undertaken and any complications.	You must keep full, clear and accurate records for everyone you care for, treat, or provide other services to (4).

References

1. Greaves I, Porter K, Wright C. *Trauma Care Pre-hospital Manual*. London: CRC Press; 2019.
2. Tricol Medical. HemCon ChitoGauze® XR Pro [Internet]. 2021 [cited 2021 Dec 19]. Available from: https://tricolbiomedical.com/wp-content/uploads/2021/06/MMF-RM7255-Rev-5.pdf.
3. British Medical Association. Ethics – general information [Internet]. 2018 [cited 2019 Dec 29]. Available from: https://www.bma.org.uk/advice/employment/ethics/consent/consent-tool-kit/2-general-information.
4. Health and Care Professions Council. Standards of conduct, performance and ethics [Internet]. 2016 [cited 2022 Jul 16]. Available from: https://www.hcpc-uk.org/standards/standards-of-conduct-performance-and-ethics/.
5. NHS England. Standard infection control precautions: national hand hygiene and personal protective equipment policy [Internet]. 2019 [cited 2022 Feb 13]. Available from: https://www.england.nhs.uk/publication/standard-infection-control-precautions-national-hand-hygiene-and-personal-protective-equipment-policy/

Arterial Tourniquets (CAT)

Indications
- Life-threatening limb haemorrhage unable to be controlled by simple techniques alone.

Contraindications
- Absence of bone inside the limb in cases of extreme trauma (tourniquet requires a bone to compress against).

Advantages
- Can be rapidly applied.
- Improves survival from peripheral vascular injury when applied early (1).

Disadvantages
- Causes significant pain; strong analgesia likely to be required (2).
- Can worsen bleeding if applied incorrectly (increases venous bleeding if not applied tightly enough) (3).
- Can cause soft-tissue injury around the site of application.

Procedure – Combat Application Tourniquet

Take the following steps to apply a Combat Application Tourniquet (CAT) (3–5):

Action		Rationale
1.	Explain the procedure to the patient (including that the procedure may be painful) and obtain consent if appropriate to do so. If possible, arrange for analgesia to be administered.	You must make sure that you have valid consent from service users or other appropriate authority before you provide care, treatment or other services (6,7). Application of tourniquets can be extremely painful and analgesia should be given.
2.	Don appropriate personal protective equipment (PPE), and undertake appropriate hand hygiene.	This reduces the risk of cross-infection (8).

Action		Rationale
3.	Place the tourniquet around the limb, around 5–8 cm above the site of bleeding and directly on to the skin. This can be on a single- or double-bone limb but should not be immediately over a joint. 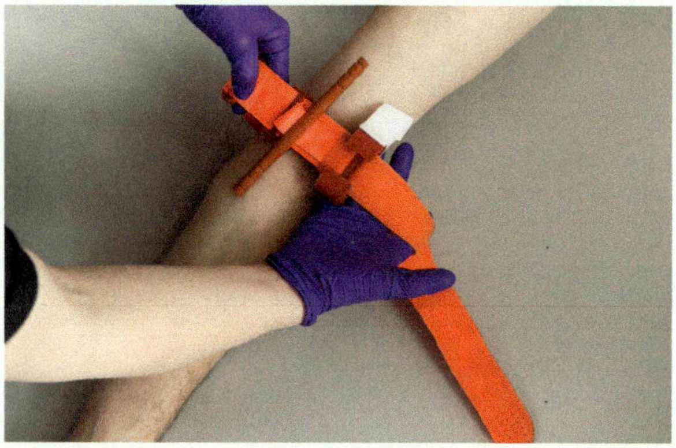	Clothing, etc. should not be trapped under the tourniquet as it may reduce the tourniquet's efficacy and may potentially cause more soft-tissue damage. Tourniquets can be effective over single- or double-bone limbs (3).
4.	Pull the band of material so it pulls through the buckle and becomes tight on the limb. Once tight, stick it back to itself around the limb. It may help to hold the body of the tourniquet in place while you do this. The band should be tight enough that three fingers cannot be slid between the band and the limb. 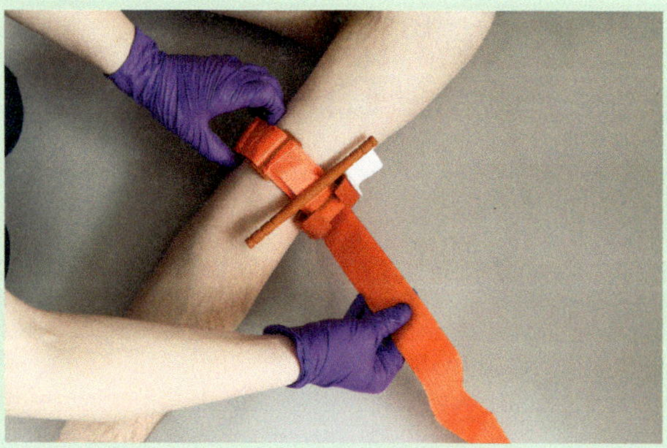	It is important the band is stuck back to itself to prevent it from slipping when tension is applied. If the tourniquet is loose before tension is applied, it may not tighten enough to stop the bleeding.

Action		Rationale
5.	Turn the rod until the bleeding stops. 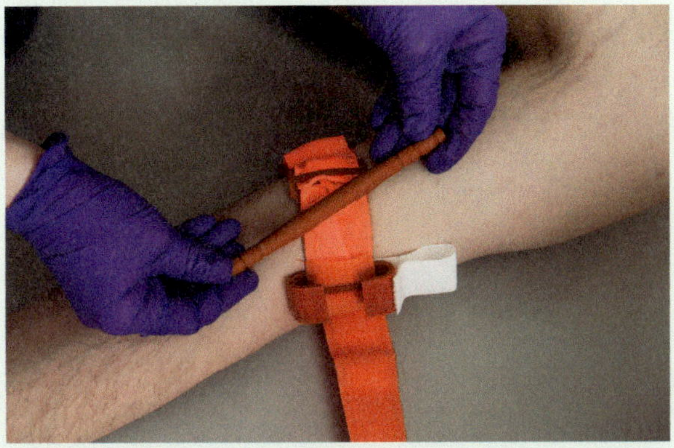	Some oozing may still occur from the bone end, but all other bleeding should cease.
6.	Once bleeding has ceased, keep turning the rod until it can be clipped into the holder. 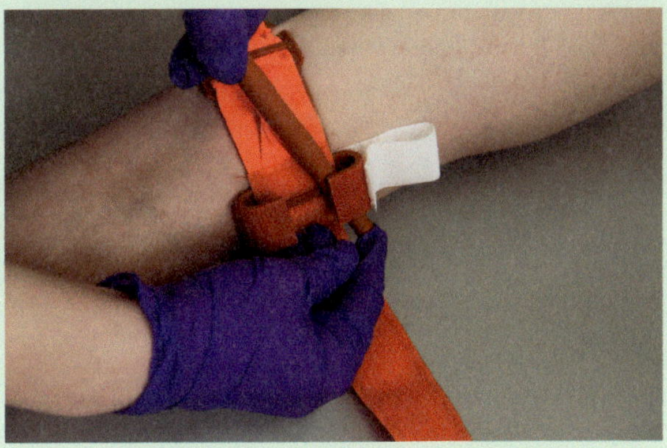	The rod must continue to be tightened until it can be clipped in to ensure bleeding does not restart.
7.	Wrap the remaining strap between the clips and then place the time strap over the top to secure the rod. 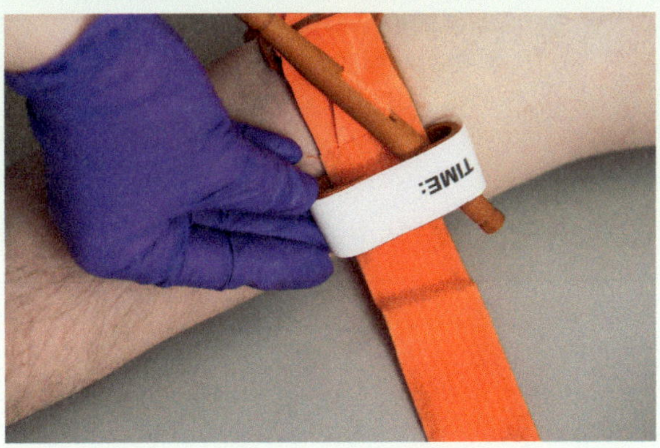	Place these straps appropriately to take up excess length and to secure the rod to prevent it from accidentally being released during movement etc.

Action		Rationale
8.	Document the procedure, including the time it was undertaken and any complications.	It is important to know how long the tourniquet has been applied for, as this will be used by senior clinicians to determine when to release it. You must keep full, clear and accurate records for everyone you care for, treat, or provide other services to (7).
9.	Continually reassess the tourniquet. If necessary, re-tighten it or add another tourniquet proximal to the first.	It is easy for a tourniquet to move during transfer, so this needs to be carefully observed for. As the patient is treated and blood pressure increases, bleeding may restart, in which case consider applying a second tourniquet.

References

1. Teixeira PGR, Brown CVR, Emigh B et al. Civilian prehospital tourniquet use is associated with improved survival in patients with peripheral vascular injury. *Journal of the American College of Surgeons*. 2018 May;226(5):769–776.e1.
2. Greaves I, Porter K, Wright C. *Trauma Care Pre-hospital Manual*. London: CRC Press; 2019.
3. Faculty of Pre-hospital Care. Position statement on the application of tourniquets [Internet]. 2017 [cited 2021 Dec 6]. Available from: https://fphc.rcsed.ac.uk/media/2398/position-statement-on-the-application-of-tourniquets-july-2017.pdf.
4. North American Rescue. Combat Application Tourniquet [Internet]. 2021 [cited 2021 Dec 6]. Available from: https://www.narescue.com/downloadable/download/sample/sample_id/791/.
5. Queensland Ambulance Service. Clinical practice procedure: trauma/arterial torniquet [Internet]. 2018 [cited 2022 Jan 2]. Available from: https://www.ambulance.qld.gov.au/docs/clinical/cpp/CPP_Arterial%20tourniquet.pdf.
6. British Medical Association. Ethics – general information [Internet]. 2018 [cited 2019 Dec 29]. Available from: https://www.bma.org.uk/advice/employment/ethics/consent/consent-tool-kit/2-general-information.
7. Health and Care Professions Council. Standards of conduct, performance and ethics [Internet]. 2016 [cited 2022 Jul 16]. Available from: https://www.hcpc-uk.org/standards/standards-of-conduct-performance-and-ethics/.
8. NHS England. Standard infection control precautions: national hand hygiene and personal protective equipment policy [Internet]. 2019 [cited 2022 Feb 13]. Available from: https://www.england.nhs.uk/publication/standard-infection-control-precautions-national-hand-hygiene-and-personal-protective-equipment-policy/.

Arterial Tourniquets (SOF®)

Indications

- Life-threatening limb haemorrhage unable to be controlled by simple techniques alone.

Contraindications

- Absence of bone inside the limb in cases of extreme trauma (tourniquets require a bone to compress against).

Advantages

- Can be rapidly applied.
- Improves survival from peripheral vascular injury when applied early (1).

Disadvantages

- Causes significant pain; strong analgesia likely to be required (2).
- Can worsen bleeding if applied incorrectly (increases venous bleeding if not applied tightly enough) (3).
- Can cause soft-tissue injury around the site of application.

Procedure – SOF® Tourniquet Application

Take the following steps to apply a SOF® Tourniquet (SOF-T) (3–5):

Action		Rationale
1.	Explain the procedure to the patient (including that the procedure may be painful) and obtain consent if appropriate to do so. If possible, arrange for analgesia to be administered.	You must make sure that you have valid consent from service users or other appropriate authority before you provide care, treatment or other services (6,7). Application of tourniquets can be extremely painful and analgesia should be given.
2.	Don appropriate personal protective equipment (PPE), and undertake appropriate hand hygiene.	This reduces the risk of cross-infection (8).

Action		Rationale
3.	Place the tourniquet around the limb, around 5–8 cm above the site of bleeding directly on to the skin. This can be on a single- or double-bone limb but should not be immediately over a joint. 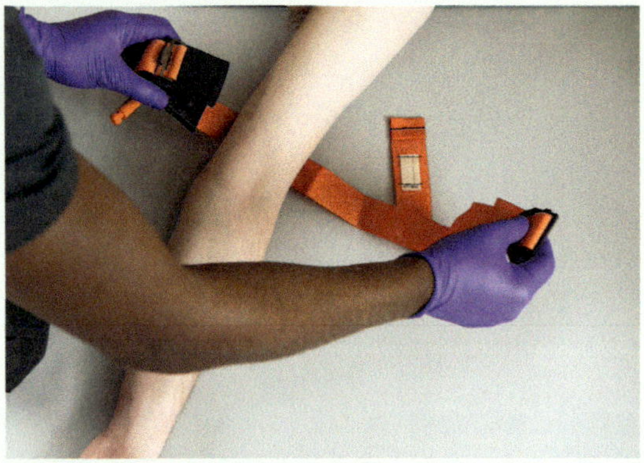	Clothing etc. should not be trapped under the tourniquet as it may reduce the tourniquet's efficacy and potentially cause more soft-tissue damage. Tourniquets can be effective over single- or double-bone limbs (3).
4.	Clip the buckle on the strap to the body of the tourniquet. Ensure it is properly clipped into place. 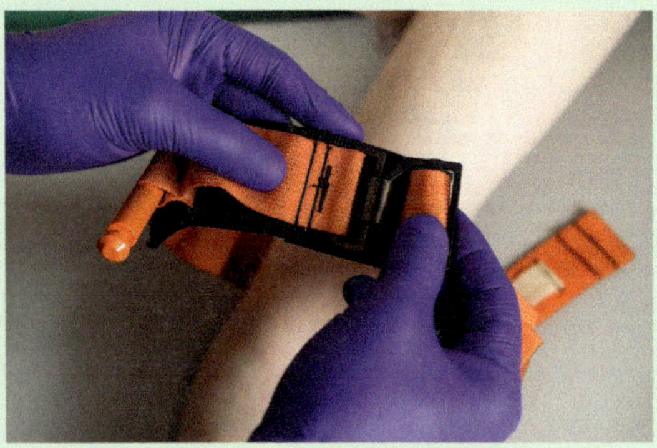	Failing to ensure the buckle is secure may result in the tourniquet not working.

Action		Rationale
5.	While stabilising the body of the tourniquet with one hand, pull the strap until the slack has been taken out. The band should be tight enough that three fingers cannot be slid between the band and the limb. 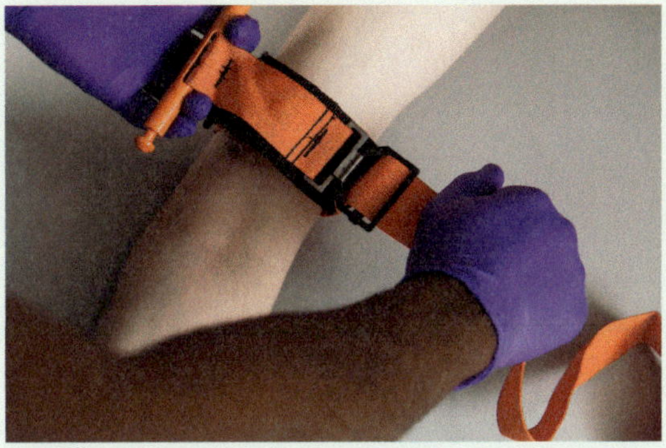	If the tourniquet is loose before tension is applied, it may not tighten enough to stop the bleeding.
6.	Turn the windlass rod until the bleeding stops. 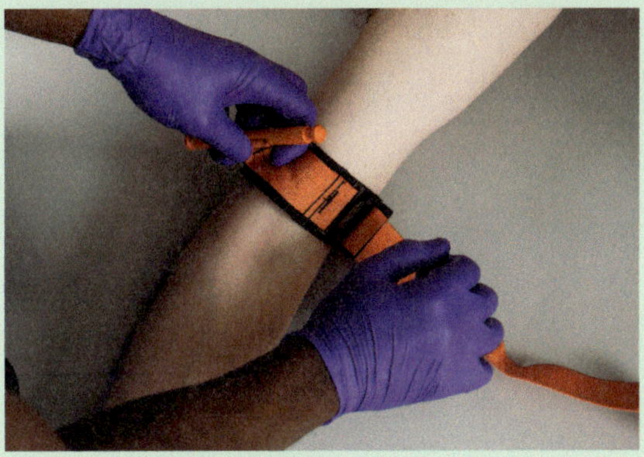	Some oozing may still occur from the bone end, but all other bleeding should cease.
7.	Once bleeding has ceased, keep turning the windlass until it can be clipped into the holder. 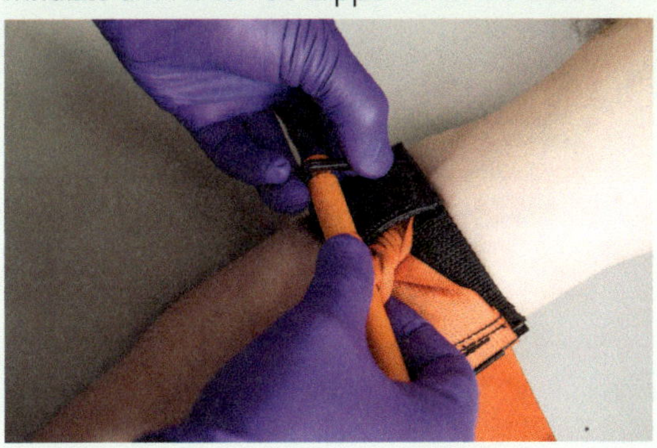	The rod must continue to be tightened until it can be clipped in to ensure bleeding does not restart.

Action		Rationale
8.	Wrap the remaining strap neatly round the windlass.	Excess strap can be caught during movement, displacing the tourniquet.
9.	Document the procedure, including the time it was undertaken and any complications. 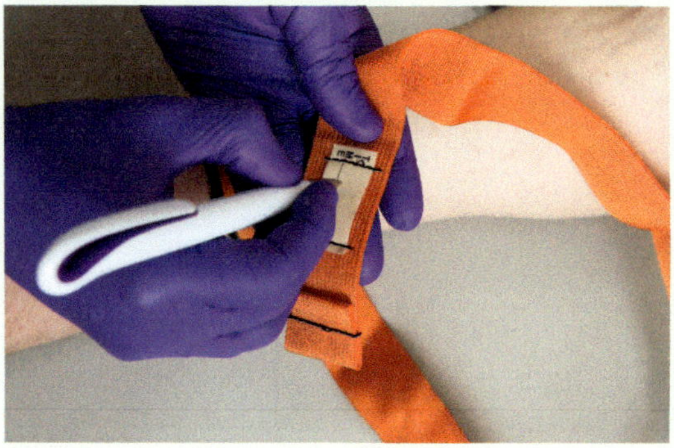	It is important to know how long the tourniquet has been applied for as this will be used by senior clinicians to determine when to release it. You must keep full, clear and accurate records for everyone you care for, treat, or provide other services to (7).
10.	Continually reassess the tourniquet. If necessary, re-tighten it or add another tourniquet proximal to the first.	It is easy for a tourniquet to move during transfer, so this needs to be carefully observed. As the patient is treated and blood pressure increases, bleeding may restart, in which case consider applying a second tourniquet.

References

1. Teixeira PGR, Brown CVR, Emigh B, et al. Civilian prehospital tourniquet use is associated with improved survival in patients with peripheral vascular injury. *Journal of the American College of Surgeons*. 2018 May;226(5):769–776.e1.
2. Greaves I, Porter K, Wright C. *Trauma Care Pre-hospital Manual*. London: CRC Press; 2019.
3. Faculty of Pre-hospital Care. Position statement on the application of tourniquets [Internet]. 2017 [cited 2021 Dec 6]. Available from: https://fphc.rcsed.ac.uk/media/2398/position-statement-on-the-application-of-tourniquets-july-2017.pdf.
4. Walters TJ, Wenke JC, Kauvar DS, et al. Effectiveness of self-applied tourniquets in human volunteers. *Prehospital Emergency Care*. 2005 Jan 2;9(4):416–422.
5. Queensland Ambulance Service. Clinical practice procedure: trauma/arterial torniquet [Internet]. 2018 [cited 2022 Jan 2]. Available from: https://www.ambulance.qld.gov.au/docs/clinical/cpp/CPP_Arterial%20tourniquet.pdf.
6. British Medical Association. Ethics – general information [Internet]. 2018 [cited 2019 Dec 29]. Available from: https://www.bma.org.uk/advice/employment/ethics/consent/consent-tool-kit/2-general-information.
7. Health and Care Professions Council. Standards of conduct, performance and ethics [Internet]. 2016 [cited 2022 Jul 16]. Available from: https://www.hcpc-uk.org/standards/standards-of-conduct-performance-and-ethics/.
8. NHS England. Standard infection control precautions: national hand hygiene and personal protective equipment policy [Internet]. 2019 [cited 2022 Feb 13]. Available from: https://www.england.nhs.uk/publication/standard-infection-control-precautions-national-hand-hygiene-and-personal-protective-equipment-policy/.

Intravenous Cannulation

Indications

- The immediate administration of drugs or fluid.
- Clinically unstable patients where drugs or fluids are likely to be required imminently.

Contraindications

- Patients unlikely to require intravenous (IV) drugs or fluids.
- You should not place a cannula in an arteriovenous fistula.
- You should not place a cannula in:*
  - Areas where lymphatic drainage has been affected.
  - Presence of injury (including burns), inflammation or infection.

*Note: These contraindications are relative to the clinical need and while they should be avoided, these sites could be utilised in a true emergency. For example, if a patient is in cardiac arrest and the only viable vein is in an arm where lymphatic drainage has been affected, then it may be acceptable. Alternatively, consider intraosseous access.

Advantages

- Effective route for fluid and drug administration.

Disadvantages

- Can be painful.
- Can damage nerves and tendons.
- Can inadvertently lead to arterial cannulation.
- Can cause bruising/haematoma (especially common for patients with clotting disorders or on anticoagulants).
- If not sited properly, drugs/fluids can cause extravasation injury.
- Infection (both locally and systemically from blood-borne pathogens).

Procedure – Intravenous Cannulation

Take the following steps to undertake intravenous cannulation (1,2):

Action		Rationale
1.	If the patient is conscious, explain the procedure and obtain consent if appropriate to do so.	You must make sure that you have valid consent from service users or other appropriate authority before you provide care, treatment or other services (3,4).
2.	Don appropriate personal protective equipment (PPE), and undertake appropriate hand hygiene.	This reduces the risk of cross-infection (5).

Action		Rationale
3.	Identify an appropriate site. To assist with this you may need to briefly apply a tourniquet to help identify suitable veins. Factors to consider include: • Size: For a small drug bolus, a small cannula and therefore a small vein may be appropriate. For larger fluid administrations, a larger cannula and vein is preferable. • Location: Typically look first at the dorsum of the hands and work up the arms to the antecubital fossa. Where more than one option exists, you should use the most appropriate distal site. • Pain: Consider sites that are less painful for the patient. For example: the dorsum of the hand is less painful than the palmar surface of the forearm. • Shape: Ideally, select a vein that runs in a straight line for approximately 5 cm from the insertion point. • Bifurcation: Try to avoid inserting where two veins join, as there are often valves in these areas. • Joint surfaces: Try to avoid placing a cannula directly over a joint surface (for example the wrist) as it can become more easily dislodged. • Feel: A full vein (when a tourniquet is applied) should feel 'springy' when palpated. If a vein either cannot be palpated or feels hard, cannulation is less likely to be successful and should be avoided if possible. Ultimately, any vein on the body can be used in an emergency, but always consider the points above. In a less urgent situation where identification of an appropriate site is proving challenging, consider if cannulation is required or if it could be delayed until arrival at hospital. If a tourniquet was applied to help identify a suitable vein, it should be removed while you prepare your equipment. A tourniquet for peripheral access should not be applied for longer than two minutes where possible.	Take time to consider the most appropriate site as this can increase the likelihood of your attempt being successful.

<table>
<tr><th colspan="2">Action</th><th>Rationale</th></tr>
<tr><td>4.</td><td>
Choose an appropriately sized cannula.
Cannulas come in multiple sizes, which determine their flow rate (1):
<table>
<tr><th>Size</th><th>Colour</th><th>Flow rate (ml/min)</th></tr>
<tr><td>22 ga</td><td>Blue</td><td>36</td></tr>
<tr><td>20 ga</td><td>Pink</td><td>60</td></tr>
<tr><td>18 ga</td><td>Green</td><td>90</td></tr>
<tr><td>16 ga</td><td>Grey</td><td>180</td></tr>
<tr><td>14 ga</td><td>Orange</td><td>270</td></tr>
</table>
Where only small boluses of drugs are going to be required, a 20 ga is likely to be sufficient. When multiple drugs and fluids are required, a larger cannula should be selected if it can be confidently placed.
It is more important to get a cannula placed successfully than it is to get a big cannula placed. Also consider that larger cannulas are more painful to insert.
</td><td>You should not place a cannula larger than is required, but do factor ongoing care. For example, if you take a patient with diabetic ketoacidosis to the emergency department, you may not need to administer much fluid initially, but in hospital it is likely they will receive a large infusion of fluids. If you have placed a 22 ga in the only viable vein when it could have easily accommodated a 16 ga, this may slow down onward care.</td></tr>
<tr><td>5.</td><td>
Prepare the remainder of your equipment:
<ul>
<li>Tourniquet</li>
<li>Appropriate skin preparation wipe (as per local policy)</li>
<li>Your selected size cannula and a size smaller</li>
<li>A 10 ml syringe, filled with 0.9% saline (or a pre-filled 0.9% saline syringe)</li>
<li>A sharps bin (not shown)</li>
<li>A cannula dressing</li>
<li>A dressing or gauze in case the attempt is unsuccessful.</li>
</ul>
Consider infection prevention.
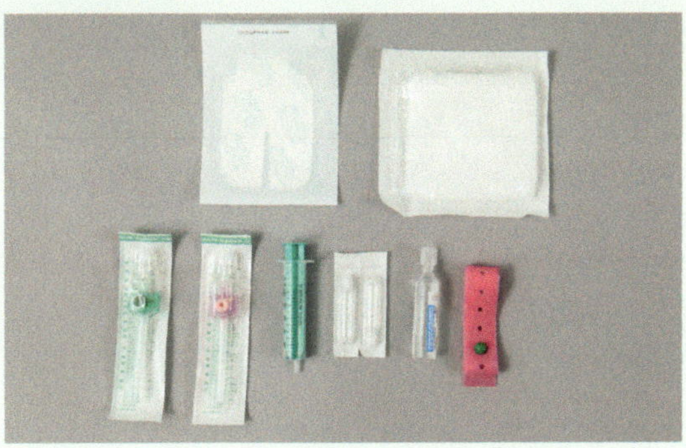
</td><td>Laying your equipment out neatly and in the order in which it is likely to be used will help ensure a smooth transition through the procedure.</td></tr>
</table>

Action		Rationale
6.	Apply the tourniquet above the site you previously identified as being appropriate for cannulation. Asking the patient to let the limb hang with gravity and pump their hand may help to make the vein more prominent quickly. Identify the target vessel and make a note of where and how you are going approach.	
7.	Thoroughly clean the site by using an appropriate skin-cleansing wipe (must contain 2% chlorhexidine in 70% isopropyl alcohol (6)). You should start in the centre where you plan to cannulate and then move outwards in increasing circles, avoiding going back over areas you have already cleaned. Allow the residue from the wipe to dry before continuing. You must not touch the target vessel again once it has been cleaned. If you need to re-palpate the vein, you must clean again afterwards or use sterile gloves. 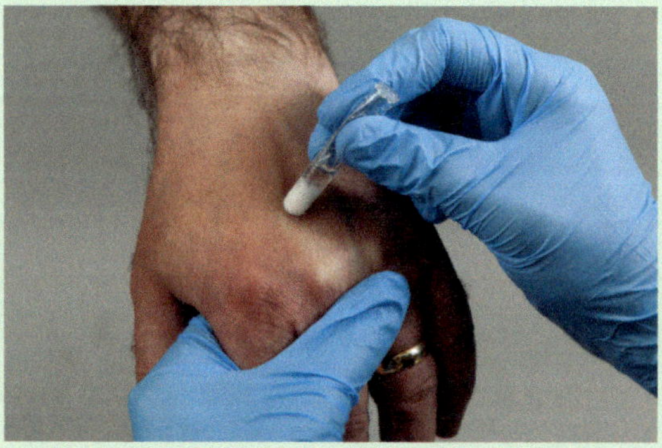	To reduce the risk of infection caused by insertion, national guidelines recommend use of single packaged wipes containing chlorhexidine (6). By moving in a continually outward motion, dirt and debris are always being carried away from the intended site of cannulation.

<table>
<tr><th></th><th>Action</th><th>Rationale</th></tr>
<tr><td>8.</td><td>Open the cannula packet and remove the cannula. Remove the protective cover over the sharp, taking care not to touch any part of the cannula that will go into the patient's vein.

With the cannula in your dominant hand, anchor the skin around the insertion site with your non-dominant hand, taking care not to touch the actual site of insertion. Placing the thumb of your non-dominant hand around 5–8 cm below the insertion site can help here.</td><td>

Anchoring the skin will make it less likely to move once you insert the cannula tip.</td></tr>
<tr><td>9.</td><td>Insert the cannula through the skin and towards the vein, running in line with it, at an angle of approximately 30°. Gently and slowly, keep advancing while observing the chamber in the back of the cannula for flashback.

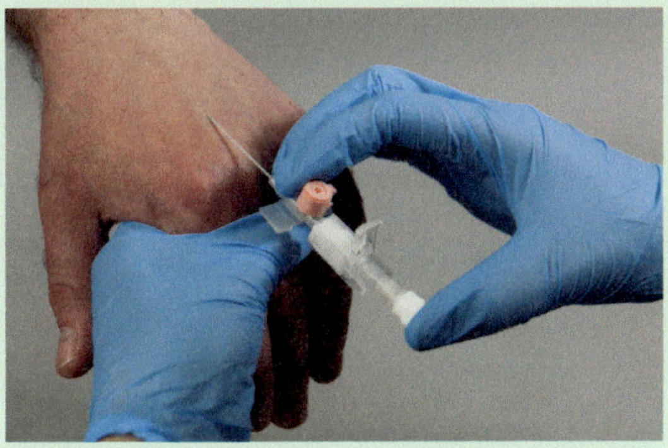</td><td>Once you see flashback, this indicates you are in the vein.

If you think you have inserted the cannula deep enough and have not got a flashback, you have probably gone to the side of the vessel. Withdraw until the tip of the cannula is only just under the skin, then change the angle slightly and try advancing again.</td></tr>
<tr><td>10.</td><td>Once you have flashback, flatten the cannula so it is nearly level with the skin and advance the whole device forwards by another 3–5 mm.

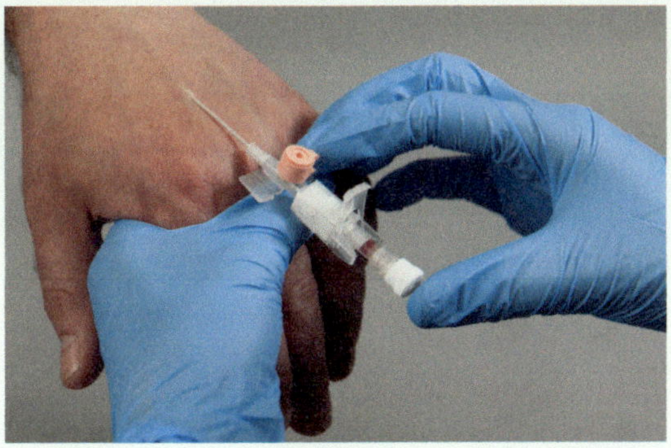</td><td>When you get flashback, it is likely that only the tip of the needle and not the cannula will be in the vein. Advancing slightly will ensure the cannula as well as the needle is within the vessel.

Flattening helps to reduce the risk of you poking the needle out through the back of the vein while advancing.</td></tr>
</table>

	Action	Rationale
11.	Release your non-dominant hand and grip the body of the cannula (around the injection port). Then use your dominant hand to gently pull the needle back slightly. You can now advance the plastic cannula forwards while holding the needle still until the entire plastic cannula is in the vein. 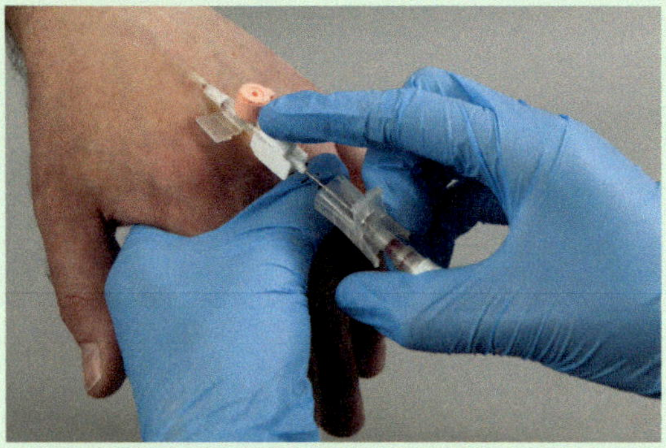	The entire cannula should be securely in the vein before being secured in place.
12.	Remove the tourniquet. 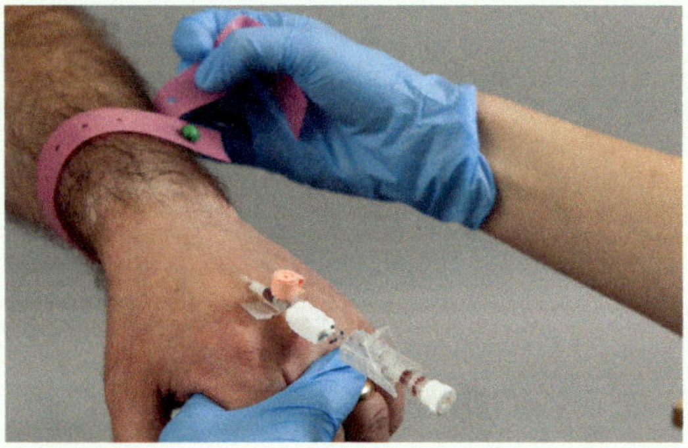	This is no longer required and should be removed to relieve pressure and prevent unnecessary bleeding when the needle is removed from the back of the cannula.

Action		Rationale
14.	With your non-dominant hand, anchor the cannula to the skin and occlude the tip by placing your finger firmly over the end of the plastic inside the vein. Remove the sharp and immediately screw the cap on to the back of the cannula. Dispose of the sharp in a sharps bin. 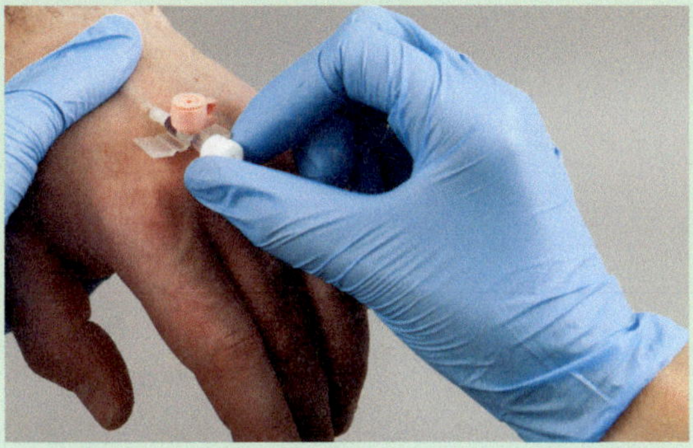	This occludes the tip of the cannula and prevents bleeding while the needle is removed.
15.	Depending on the dressing you have available, it may have two strips that go over the wings of the cannula. If these are present, apply them now. 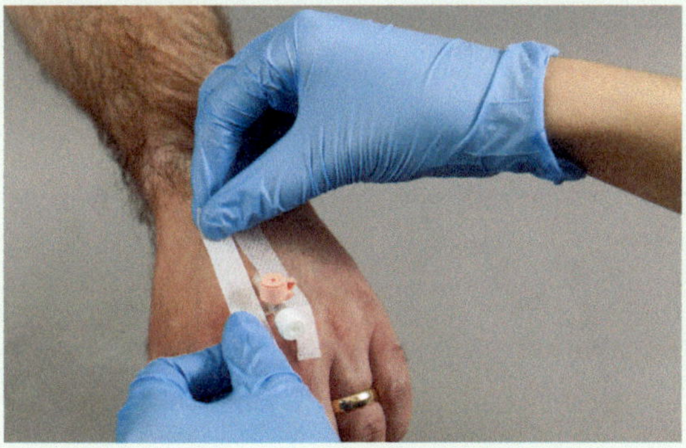	Apply the strips to anchor the cannula securely before you flush.

Action		Rationale
16.	Using the 10 ml syringe (or pre-filled syringe) of 0.9% saline you prepared earlier, flush the cannula. 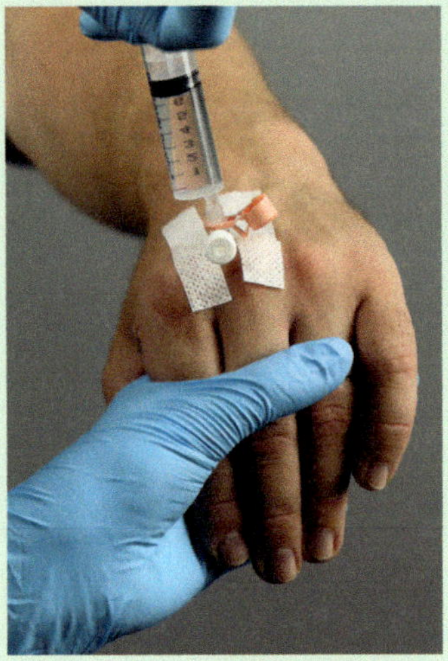	Fluid should run in freely, the flush should not be painful and there should be no swelling around the tip of the cannula in the vein. If it does not run freely or there is swelling, it is likely the cannula is misplaced and it should be removed.
17.	Once you have confirmed placement by flushing, fix the cannula down with the remainder of the dressing. This should include a label that details the date and time it was inserted. 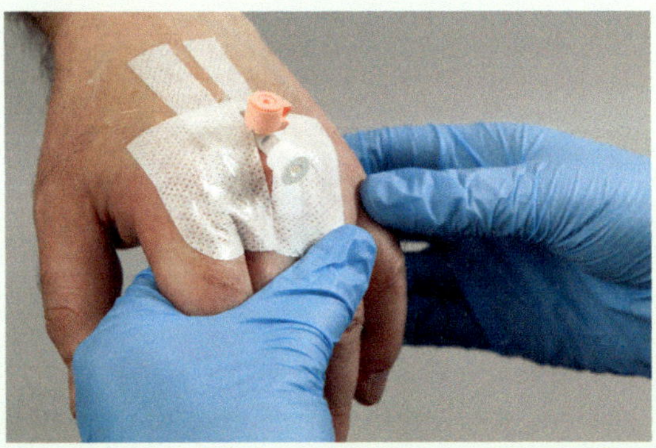	The cannula should be dressed to keep it secure and clean.
18.	Document the procedure.	You must keep full, clear and accurate records for everyone you care for, treat, or provide other services to (4).

References

1. Vygon. Biovalve safe: a guide to peripheral IV cannulation [Internet]. 2016 [cited 2022 Jul 16]. Available from: https://vygon.co.uk/wp-content/uploads/2019/01/BiovalveSafe-V2.pdf.
2. Porter L. Intravenous cannulation: OSCE guide [Internet]. Geeky Medics. 2021 [cited 2022 Jul 16]. Available from: https://geekymedics.com/how-to-perform-cannulation-osce-guide/.

3. British Medical Association. Ethics – general information [Internet]. 2018 [cited 2019 Dec 29]. Available from: www.bma.org.uk/advice/employment/ethics/consent/consent-tool-kit/2-general-information.
4. Health and Care Professions Council. Standards of conduct, performance and ethics [Internet]. 2016 [cited 2022 Jul 16]. Available from: www.hcpc-uk.org/standards/standards-of-conduct-performance-and-ethics/.
5. NHS England. Standard infection control precautions: national hand hygiene and personal protective equipment policy [Internet]. 2019 [cited 2022 Feb 13]. Available from: www.england.nhs.uk/publication/standard-infection-control-precautions-national-hand-hygiene-and-personal-protective-equipment-policy/.
6. National Institute for Health and Care Excellence. Healthcare-associated infections: prevention and control in primary and community care [Internet]. Clinical Guideline CG139. 2017 [cited 2022 Jul 16]. Available from: www.nice.org.uk/guidance/cg139/chapter/1-guidance.

External Jugular Vein Cannulation

Indications

- The emergency administration of drugs or fluids in adults.

Contraindications

- Patients unlikely to require intravenous (IV) drugs or fluids.
- Other suitable sites are available.

Advantages

- Effective route for fluid and drug administration.
- Large vein, which allows for placement of a wide-bore cannula and therefore rapid administration of a significant volume of fluid.
- In some patients the external jugular vein can be identified even when other veins are not visible.

Disadvantages

- Can be painful.
- Can lead to inadvertent artery or internal jugular vein cannulation.
- Can cause a pneumothorax if technique is incorrect.
- Can cause bruising or haematoma (especially common for patients with clotting disorders or on anticoagulants).
- If not sited properly, drugs or fluids can cause extravasation injury.
- Infection (both locally and systemically from blood-borne pathogens).
- Has a higher failure rate than other techniques (1).
- Valves in the external jugular vein may hinder attempt (2).

Procedure – External Jugular Vein Cannulation

Take the following steps to undertake external jugular vein cannulation (3,4):

Action		Rationale
1.	If the patient is conscious, explain the procedure and obtain consent if appropriate to do so.	You must make sure that you have valid consent from service users or other appropriate authority before you provide care, treatment or other services (5,6).
2.	Don appropriate personal protective equipment (PPE), and undertake appropriate hand hygiene.	This reduces the risk of cross-infection (7).

<table>
<tr><th></th><th>Action</th><th>Rationale</th></tr>
<tr><td>3.</td><td>Lay the patient flat or, if safe, slightly head down.

Identify the external jugular vein by asking the patient to turn their head, or turn it yourself if the patient is unable to. They should turn their head away from the side you intend to cannulate (contralateral).

The external jugular vein runs from just behind the angle of the mandible at the base of the jaw to the mid-clavicular area. Observe for a vein running in this location.

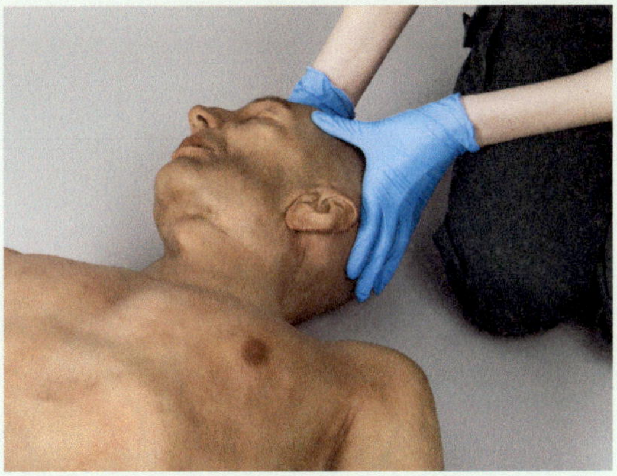</td><td>Turning the head to the contralateral side of where you intend to insert the cannula will make identification of the external jugular vein easier.</td></tr>
<tr><td>4.</td><td>Once you have identified the external jugular vein, choose an appropriately sized cannula.

Cannulas come in multiple sizes, which determine their flow rate (3):

<table><tr><th>Size</th><th>Colour</th><th>Flow rate (ml/min)</th></tr><tr><td>22 ga</td><td>Blue</td><td>36</td></tr><tr><td>20 ga</td><td>Pink</td><td>60</td></tr><tr><td>18 ga</td><td>Green</td><td>90</td></tr><tr><td>16 ga</td><td>Grey</td><td>180</td></tr><tr><td>14 ga</td><td>Orange</td><td>270</td></tr></table>
External jugular vein cannulation is more commonly performed in the context of requiring large volumes of fluid, in which case the largest cannula that can confidently be placed should be selected.</td><td>You should use a cannula suitable for the reason it is being placed, but consider what might come after you hand the patient over at hospital. Once the external jugular vein has been cannulated by a prehospital team, the hospital cannot insert another cannula in the same vein anytime soon, so it is likely the cannula you have placed is the one the patient will be keeping for some time.</td></tr>
</table>

Action		Rationale
5.	Prepare the remainder of your equipment: • Appropriate skin preparation wipe (as per local policy) • Your selected size cannula and a size smaller • A 10 ml syringe, filled with 0.9% saline or a pre-filled syringe • A sharps bin • A cannula dressing • A dressing or gauze in case the attempt is unsuccessful. Consider infection prevention.	Laying your equipment out neatly and in the order it is likely to be used will help ensure a smooth transition through the procedure.
6.	Thoroughly clean the site by using an appropriate skin-cleansing wipe (containing 2% chlorhexidine in 70% isopropyl alcohol). You should start in the centre where you plan to cannulate and then move outwards in increasing circles, avoiding going back over areas you have already cleaned. Allow the residue from the wipe to dry before continuing. You must not touch the target vessel again once it has been cleaned. If you need to re-palpate the vein, you must clean again afterwards or use sterile gloves. 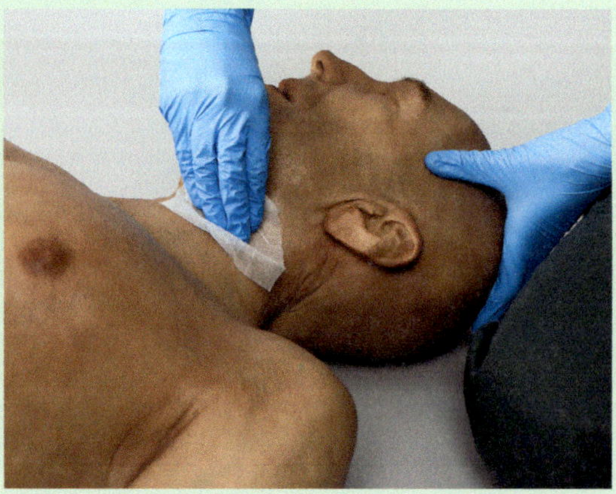	To reduce risk of infection caused by insertion, national guidelines recommend use of single packaged wipes containing chlorhexidine (8). By moving in a continually outward motion, dirt and debris are always being carried away from the intended site of cannulation.

	Action	Rationale
7.	Open the cannula packet and remove the cannula. Remove the protective cover over the sharp, taking care not to touch any part of the cannula that will go into the patient's vein. With the cannula in your dominant hand, anchor the skin around the insertion site with your non-dominant hand, taking care not to touch the actual site of insertion. Placing the thumb of your non-dominant hand around 5–8 cm above the site of insertion can help here. 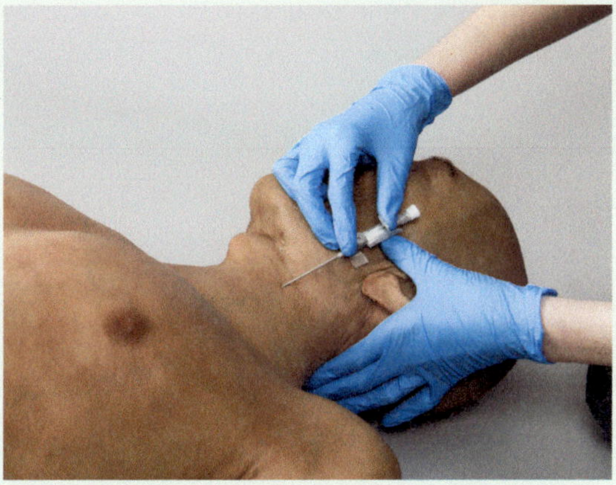	Anchoring the skin will make it less likely to move once you insert the cannula tip.
8.	Insert the cannula through the skin and towards the vein, running in line with it, at an angle of approximately 30°. Gently and slowly, keep advancing while observing the chamber in the back of the cannula for flashback.	Once you see flashback, this indicates you are in the vein. If you think you have inserted the cannula deep enough and not got a flashback, you have probably gone to the side of the vessel. Withdraw until the tip of the cannula is only just under the skin, then change angle slightly and try advancing again. Do not advance too far as doing so risks damaging other underlying structures including the carotid artery and lungs.

Action		Rationale
9.	Once you have flashback, flatten the cannula so it is nearly level with the skin and advance the whole device forwards by another 3–5 mm. 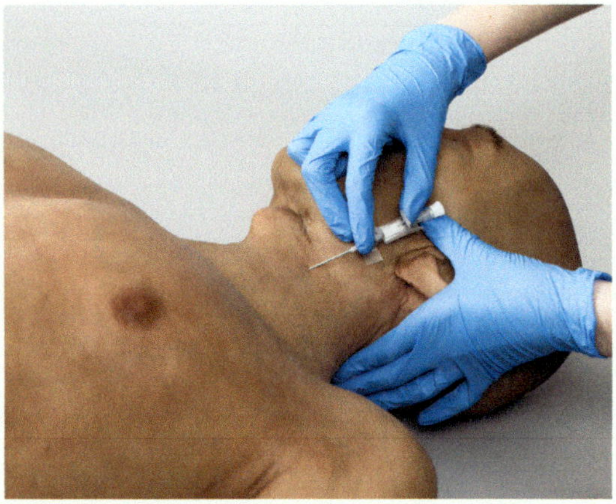	When you get flashback, it is likely that only the tip of the needle and not the cannula will be in the vein. Advancing slightly will ensure the cannula as well as the needle is within the vessel. Flattening helps to reduce the risk of poking the needle out through the back of the vein while advancing.
10.	Release your non-dominant hand and grip the body of the cannula (around the injection port). Then use your dominant hand to gently pull the needle back slightly. You can now advance the plastic cannula forwards while holding the needle still until the entire plastic cannula is in the vein. 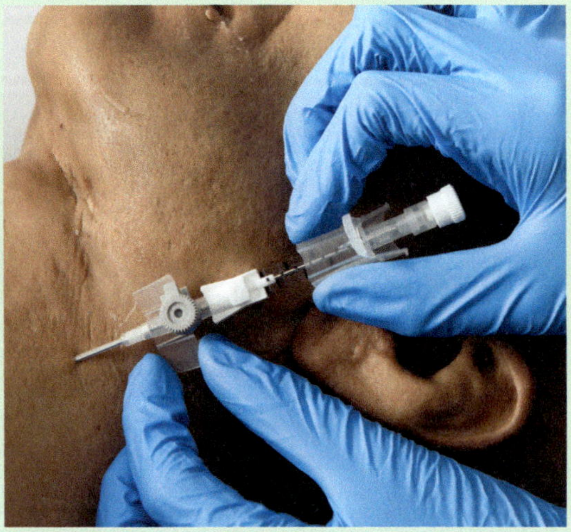	The entire cannula should be securely in the vein before being secured in place.

Action		Rationale
11.	With your non-dominant hand, anchor the cannula to the skin and occlude the tip by placing your finger firmly over the end of the plastic inside the vein. Remove the sharp and immediately screw the cap on to the back of the cannula. Dispose of the sharp in a sharps bin. 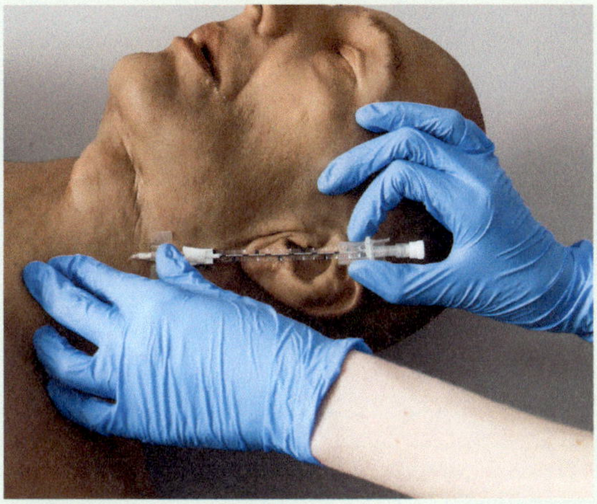	This occludes the tip of the cannula and prevents bleeding while the needle is removed. Beware not to leave the back of the cannula exposed without a cap once the needle is removed, as this could potentially cause air to be drawn in during the respiratory cycle, which can itself cause a pulmonary embolism.
12.	Apply a cannula dressing. 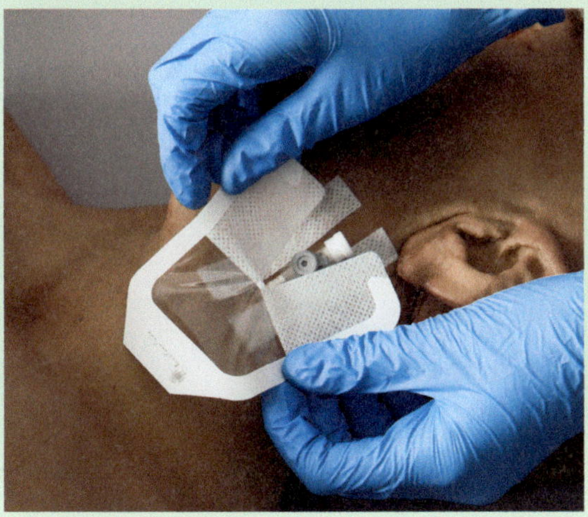	External jugular vein cannulas are easily displaced, but applying a dressing will keep it secure. This needs to be performed quickly though as the cannula needs to be flushed. If for any reason the application of the dressing cannot be completed quickly, consider moving on to the next step and coming back to put on a dressing afterwards.

	Action	Rationale
13.	Using the 10 ml syringe of 0.9% saline (or pre-filled syringe) you prepared earlier, flush the cannula. 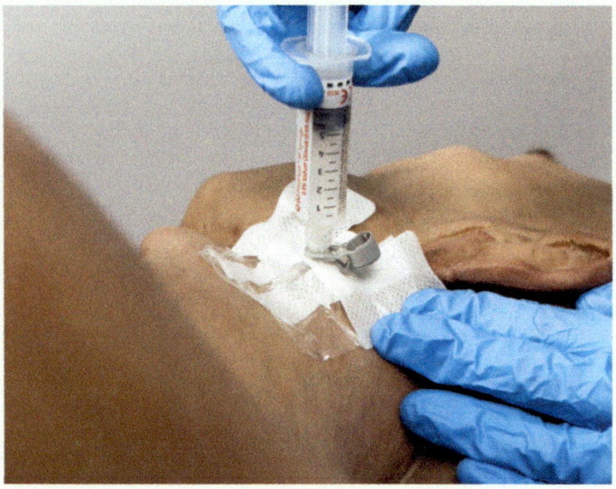	Fluid should run in freely, the flush should not be painful and there should be no swelling around the tip of the cannula in the vein. If it does not run freely or there is swelling, it is likely the cannula is misplaced and it should be removed.
14.	Once you have confirmed placement by flushing, ensure that the dressing is secure. This should include a label that details the date and time it was inserted.	The cannula should be dressed to keep it secure and clean.
15.	Document the procedure.	You must keep full, clear and accurate records for everyone you care for, treat, or provide other services to (6).

References

1. Lahtinen P, Musialowicz T, Hyppölä H, et al. Is external jugular vein cannulation feasible in emergency care? A randomised study in open heart surgery patients. *Resuscitation*. 2009;80(12).
2. Anaesthesia UK. Cannulation of the external jugular vein [Internet]. 2004 [cited 2022 Jul 17]. Available from: www.frca.co.uk/article.aspx?articleid=100033.
3. Vygon. Biovalve Safe: A guide to peripheral IV cannulation [Internet]. 2016 [cited 2022 Jul 16]. Available from: https://vygon.co.uk/wp-content/uploads/2019/01/BiovalveSafe-V2.pdf.
4. Porter L. Intravenous cannulation: OSCE guide [Internet]. Geeky Medics. 2021 [cited 2022 Jul 16]. Available from: https://geekymedics.com/how-to-perform-cannulation-osce-guide/.
5. British Medical Association. Ethics – general information [Internet]. 2018 [cited 2019 Dec 29]. Available from: www.bma.org.uk/advice/employment/ethics/consent/consent-tool-kit/2-general-information.
6. Health and Care Professions Council. Standards of conduct, performance and ethics [Internet]. 2016 [cited 2022 Jul 16]. Available from: www.hcpc-uk.org/standards/standards-of-conduct-performance-and-ethics/.
7. NHS England. Standard infection control precautions: national hand hygiene and personal protective equipment policy [Internet]. 2019 [cited 2022 Feb 13]. Available from: www.england.nhs.uk/publication/standard-infection-control-precautions-national-hand-hygiene-and-personal-protective-equipment-policy/.
8. National Institute for Health and Care Excellence. Healthcare-associated infections: prevention and control in primary and community care [Internet]. Clinical Guideline CG139. 2017 [cited 2022 Jul 16]. Available from: www.nice.org.uk/guidance/cg139/chapter/1-guidance.

Intraosseous Access

Indications

- Requirement for immediate vascular access to administer medication, fluids or blood products, where peripheral access has either been attempted and failed, or is considered highly unlikely to be successful in a suitable timeframe.

Contraindications

- Fracture in target bone.
- Excessive tissue or absence of adequate landmarks.
- Infection at the area of insertion.
- Previous significant orthopaedic procedure at the site.
- Prosthetic limb or joint.
- Intraosseous (IO) access in target bone within the last 48 hours.

Caution

- A conscious patient who cannot be given local anaesthetic. Careful consideration should be given to whether the procedure is appropriate to perform without the availability of local anaesthetic.

Advantages

- Rapid and simple procedure.
- Suitable for all age ranges.
- Comparable peak drug administration to intravenous (IV) access.
- All drugs and fluids typically found in prehospital practice can be administered via the IO route.

Disadvantages

- Very expensive in comparison to peripheral IV cannulation.
- IO infusions can be very painful.
- Drugs and fluids typically need to be administered under pressure: they will not normally flow under the pressure of gravity as they will when being administered via an IV route.
- Much more challenging with higher failure rates when inserting in infants and neonates.

Procedure – Intraosseous Access (EZ-IO®)

Take the following steps to obtain intraosseous access with an EZ-IO® needle (1):

Note: For this procedure, the proximal tibia is being demonstrated. Other sites require different landmarking to identify the correct insertion point.

Action		Rationale
1.	If the patient is conscious, explain the procedure and obtain consent if appropriate to do so.	You must make sure that you have valid consent from service users or other appropriate authority before you provide care, treatment or other services (2,3).
2.	Don appropriate personal protective equipment (PPE), and undertake appropriate hand hygiene.	This reduces the risk of cross-infection (4).

Action		Rationale
3.	Consider which site would be most suitable. In adults the possible sites are: • Proximal humerus • Proximal tibia • Distal tibia. The preferred site for adult EZ-IO® insertion is the proximal humerus. For paediatrics, sites are the same as in adults, but with the addition of the distal femur (5).	Choosing the correct site is important to ensure maximum flow and that drugs and fluids get to the target sites quickly. The proximal humerus has better flow rates than other sites – it takes only three seconds for medication to get to the heart – and it has lower insertion and infusion pain than other sites (6).
4.	Gather the required equipment and prime the infusion line with sodium chloride 0.9%. Equipment you will require is: • A skin-cleansing wipe • An appropriately sized needle • The insertion driver • Primed connecting line • 10 ml syringe with sodium chloride for flushing the line • Lidocaine (if conscious) • An appropriate dressing • Sharps bin (not shown). 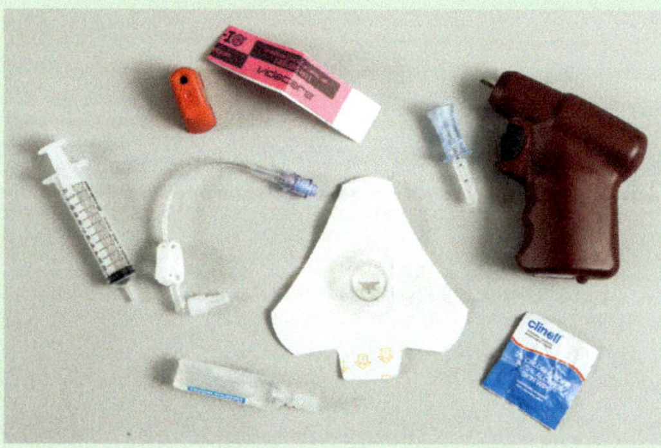	To prevent complications, ensure all the required equipment is present prior to commencing the procedure.

	Action	Rationale
5.	Identify the site (here the tibial tuberosity is being demonstrated). Locate the inferior edge of the patella, measure down two finger breadths and move slightly medially. You should be able to clearly palpate a large, relatively flat surface of bone shallow to the surface. 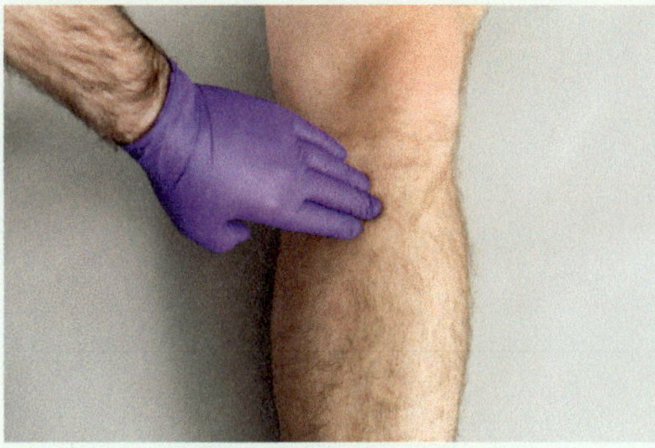	The tibial tuberosity is the site recommended by the manufacturer for proximal tibial access.
6.	Choose an appropriately sized needle. Three needles are available depending on the site and the size of the patient. All of the needles have the same diameter (15 ga), but come in different lengths (**Figure 4.1**): • Pink = 15 mm needle • Blue = 25 mm needle • Yellow = 45 mm needle. Typically the pink needle is used in infants and small children. The blue needle is used for adult proximal or distal tibia sites, while the yellow needle is used for the adult humeral head.	If the incorrect needle size is chosen, the procedure is unlikely to be successful as the tip of the device will not be placed in the intramedullary space. The actual needle used should be selected based on the chosen site and the amount of overlying tissue.
7.	Clean the site with an appropriate skin preparation. 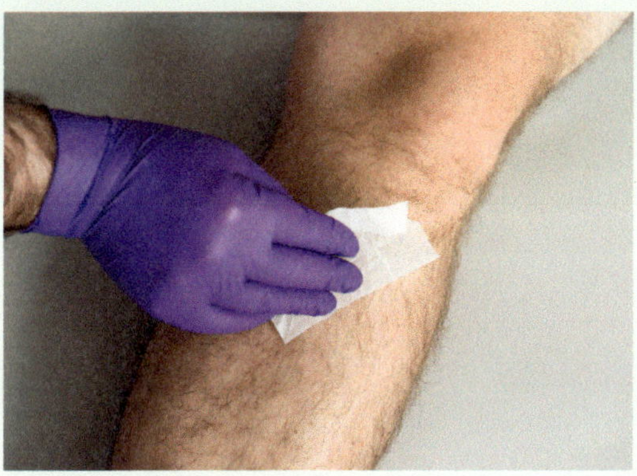	This reduces the risk of infection caused by insertion.

Action		Rationale
8.	Quickly test the driver by pulling the trigger. Attach the needle to the end of the driver and ensure it is being held firm by the magnetic lock. Remove the protective cover from the needle. 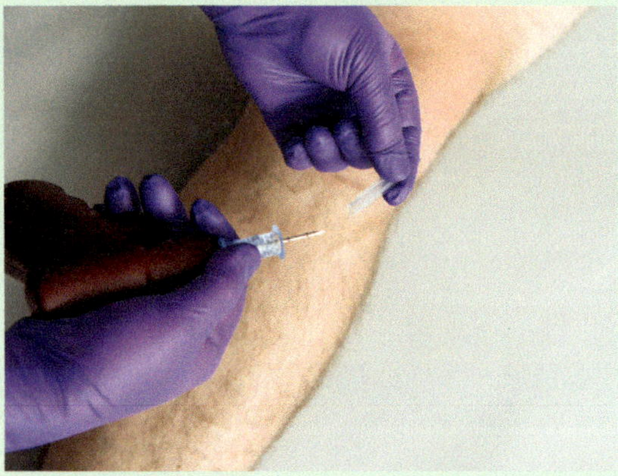	If the light-emitting diode (LED) on the back of the device shines red, the battery is running low. If possible, use another driver to reduce the risk of failure during insertion.
9.	Stabilise the extremity. Aim the needle set at a 90° angle to the centre of the bone 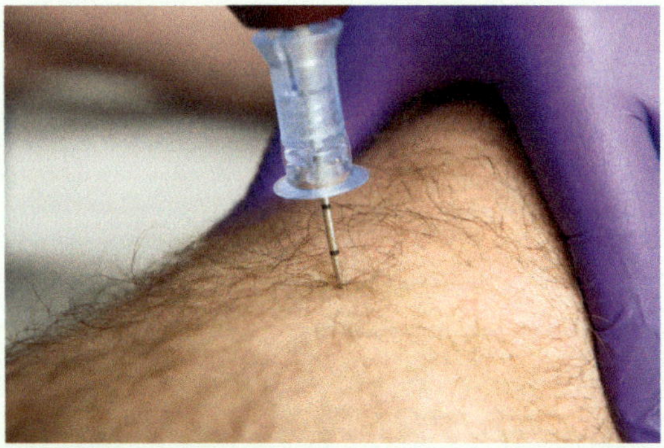	Limb movement during insertion could damage the needle.
10.	**Without** pulling the trigger, insert the needle through the skin at the insertion site. Advance the needle until contact is made with bone.	The needle is sharp enough to penetrate the skin and underlying tissue without activating the drilling mechanism.

Action		**Rationale**
11.	Once in contact with bone, check that the angle of the drill appears appropriate to penetrating the underlying bone. Check that at least one 5 mm black marker is visible above the skin on the needle (**Figure 4.2**). 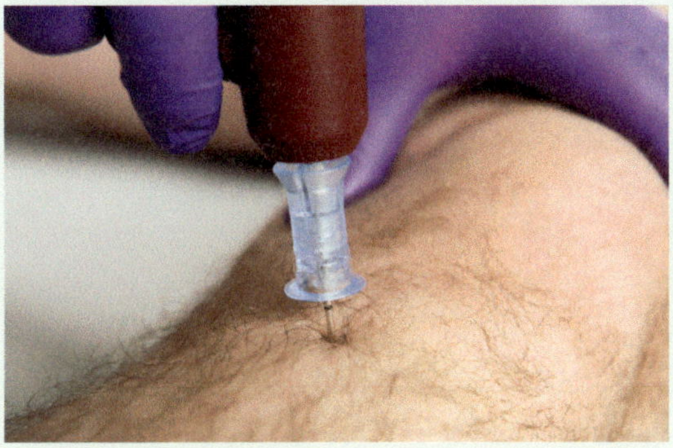	Checking alignment may help to prevent the needle accidentally passing through the side of a bone. One marker must be visible, otherwise the needle is unlikely to penetrate deep enough into the target bone.
12.	Pull the trigger while applying light pressure to the device. Keep the trigger squeezed until the needle is pulled into the bone, at which point release the trigger. If the driver fails during insertion, disconnect it from the needle and finish the insertion by gripping the needle in your hand and rotating it with gentle downward pressure. 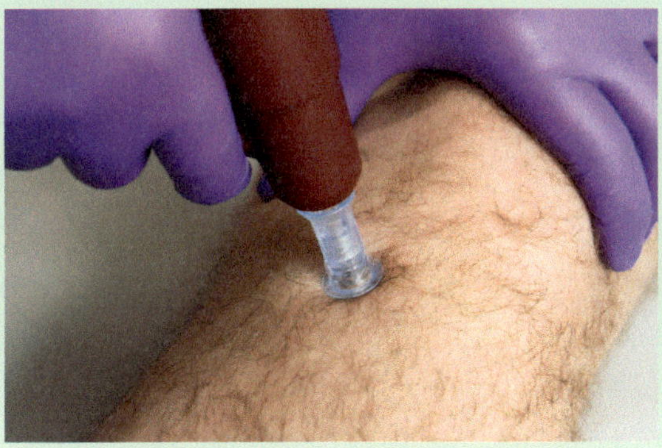	A common mistake with the EZ-IO® is to apply too much pressure to the drill, causing it to stall. Light pressure to keep the needle in firm contact with the bone is all that is required.

<table>
<tr><th colspan="2">Action</th><th>Rationale</th></tr>
<tr><td>13.</td><td>Once the needle is in the bone, the driver can be disconnected.
Using your non-dominant hand to stabilise the needle, unscrew and remove the stylet, and place it in an appropriate sharps container.
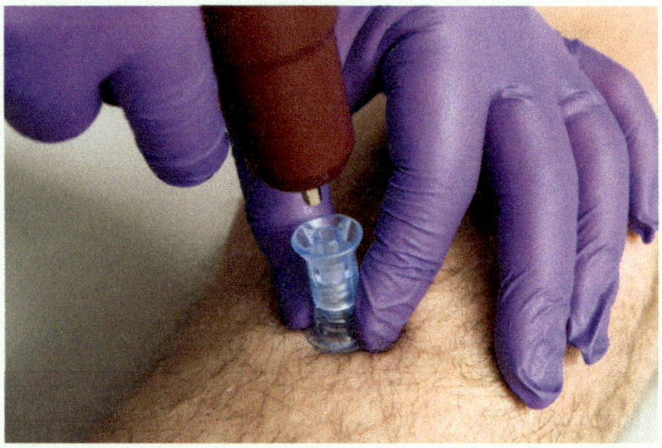</td><td>The stylet can now be removed and safely disposed of, leaving space for the drug administration circuit to be connected.</td></tr>
<tr><td>14.</td><td>Place the stabiliser dressing over the needle</td><td>The stabiliser must be applied now as the administration set is connected through the gap in the dressing.</td></tr>
<tr><td>15.</td><td>Attach the administration set and rapidly flush with 5–10 ml of normal saline (2–5 ml in paediatrics).
This can be extremely painful, and in conscious patients local anaesthetic should be considered in line with local policy.
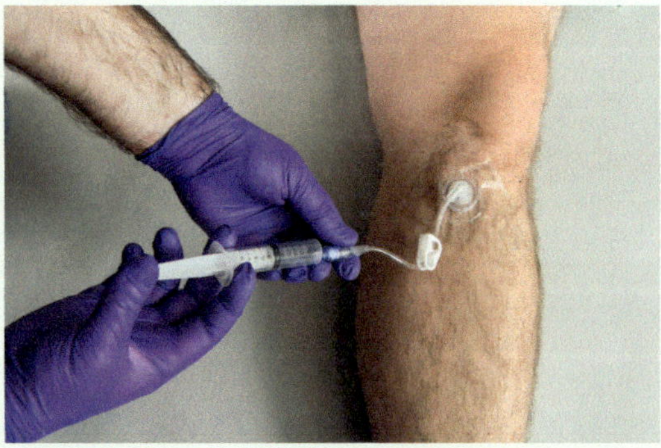</td><td>A firm flush helps to create a potential space for drugs and fluids to be infused into.</td></tr>
<tr><td>16.</td><td>If not already completed, peel the covers off the back of the stabiliser dressing and fix down.</td><td>The stabiliser dressing will help to keep the needle securely in place.</td></tr>
</table>

Action		Rationale
17.	Apply the wrist band that came in the needle pack to the patient with the site and time of insertion recorded. Make sure the insertion of an IO is clearly communicated as part of the handover at hospital. 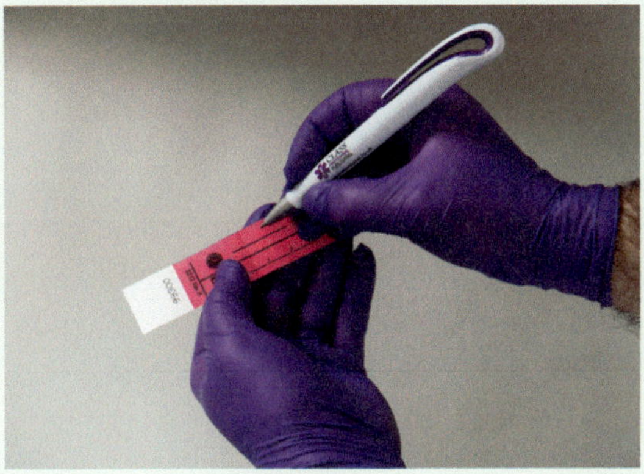	It is important that the hospital team are aware of the insertion of an IO needle for ongoing management and timely removal.
18.	Document the procedure.	You must keep full, clear and accurate records for everyone you care for, treat, or provide other services to (3).

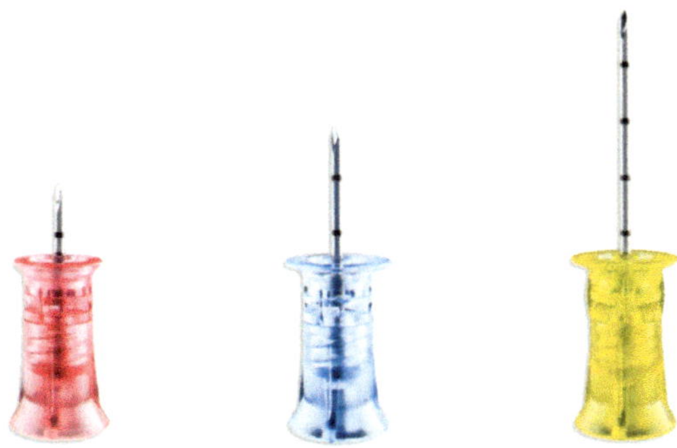
15 mm
15 gauge
Indicated for patients weighing 3–39kg
25 mm
15 gauge
Indicated for patients weighing 3 kg or over
45 mm
15 gauge
Indicated for patients weighing 40 kg or over excessive tissue depth

Figure 4.1 EZ-IO® needles.

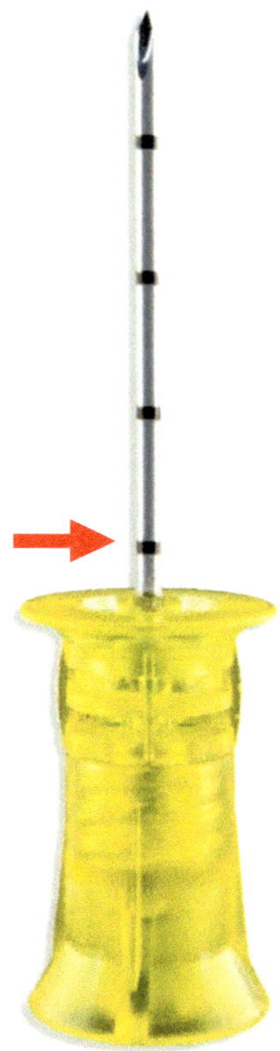

Figure 4.2 5 mm-mark closest to the needle hub.

References

1. Teleflex. 2017 The science and fundamentals of intraosseous vascular access [Internet]. 2017 [cited 2021 Apr 11]. Available from: www.teleflex.com/usa/en/clinical-resources/ez-io/documents/EZ-IO_Science_Fundamentals_MC-003266-Rev1-1.pdf.
2. British Medical Association. Ethics – general information [Internet]. 2018 [cited 2019 Dec 29]. Available from: www.bma.org.uk/advice/employment/ethics/consent/consent-tool-kit/2-general-information.
3. Health and Care Professions Council. Standards of conduct, performance and ethics [Internet]. 2016 [cited 2022 Jul 16]. Available from: www.hcpc-uk.org/standards/standards-of-conduct-performance-and-ethics/.
4. NHS England. Standard infection control precautions: national hand hygiene and personal protective equipment policy [Internet]. 2019 [cited 2022 Feb 13]. Available from: www.england.nhs.uk/publication/standard-infection-control-precautions-national-hand-hygiene-and-personal-protective-equipment-policy/.
5. Teleflex. EZ-IO intraosseous vascular access system pocket guide [Internet]. 2016 [cited 2021 Jun 13]. Available from: www.teleflex.com/usa/en/product-areas/emergency-medicine/intraosseous-access/arrow-ez-io-system/literature/VA_IOS_EZ-IO_Pocket_Guide.pdf.
6. Teleflex. Clinical resources: proximal humerus [Internet]. 2021 [cited 2022 Jul 16]. Available from: https://p.widencdn.net/hbbcp7/MCI-2019-0085_IN_DS_Arrow-EZ-IO-Proximal-Humerus-Clinical-Resource_EN_1905_LR.

Chapter

5 Drug Administration

The administration of medications forms an important component of providing emergency care, and will be a common aspect of any prehospital clinician's role. Knowing how to prepare and administer medication safely and effectively are core skills that should be developed and maintained to a high standard.

Despite the frequency with which clinicians have to handle and administrate medications, it is still a common area of preventable errors in healthcare. It is estimated that more than 237 million medication errors are made annually in England, the avoidable consequences of which cost the NHS upwards of £98 million and result in more than 1,700 lives lost (1). In prehospital practice medication errors are common, especially during time-sensitive emergencies, when dealing with complex patients or responding to incidents during the early hours of the morning (2).

Avoiding harm remains the first priority of prehospital care and maintaining high standards in the preparation and administration of medications will help to ensure you avoid making medication errors. In addition, adopting some form of mandatory check immediately prior to administering a medicine is another effective technique for reducing error.

As a practitioner you should develop and maintain high standards in preparing and administering medication. Even when familiar with administering medication, it may be of some benefit to revisit these pages and ensure that your ongoing practice remains in line with best practice around safe and secure handling of medicines.

References

1. Elliott RA, Camacho E, Jankovic D, et al. Economic analysis of the prevalence and clinical and economic burden of medication error in England. *BMJ Quality and Safety*. 2021;30(2):95–105.
2. Ramadanov N, Klein R, Schumann U, et al. Factors, influencing medication errors in prehospital care: A retrospective observational study. *Medicine* (United States). 2019;98(49):e18200.

Penthrox® (Methoxyflurane)

Indications

- Refer to guidelines used by your organisation for indications.

Contraindications

- Refer to guidelines used by your organisation for contraindications.

Cautions

- Refer to guidelines used by your organisation for cautions.

Advantages

- Can be administered by non-registered clinicians following a robust protocol.
- Provides a more rapid analgesia effect than inhaled Entonox (1).
- Effective analgesia for use in the prehospital setting (1).

Disadvantages

- Exhaled methoxyflurane can pose an occupational exposure hazard as it can be inhaled by clinicians caring for a patient (2). To reduce this risk, Penthrox® should only be used in well-ventilated environments, following local policy on reducing risks of occupational exposure.

Procedure – Penthrox® (Methoxyflurane) Administration

Take the following steps to prepare and administer Penthrox® (methoxyflurane) (3,4):

Action		Rationale
1.	Explain the procedure and obtain consent if appropriate to do so.	You must make sure that you have valid consent from service users or other appropriate authority before you provide care, treatment or other services (5,6). As Penthrox® is self-administered, the patient must be conscious and able to comply with instructions.
2.	Don appropriate personal protective equipment (PPE), and undertake appropriate hand hygiene.	This reduces the risk of cross-infection (7).

Action		Rationale
3.	Open the package. Ensure all components are present and the vial containing the medication is intact and securely sealed. 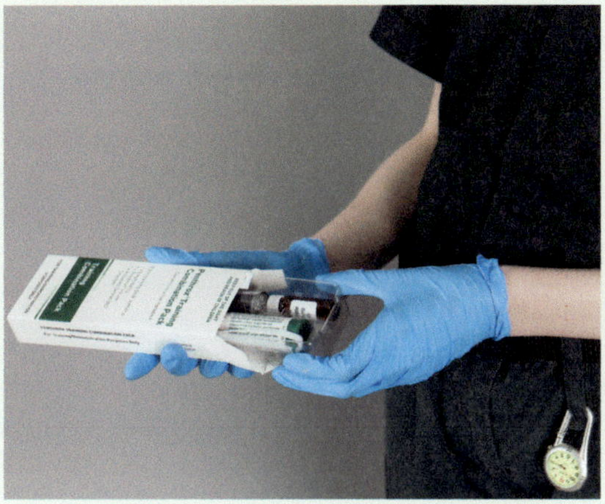	If any part of the device or vial is damaged, or if the security seal on the drug ampoule has been compromised, the set should not be used.
4.	Attach the activated carbon filter to the body of the Penthrox® inhaler by pushing it into the top of the device. 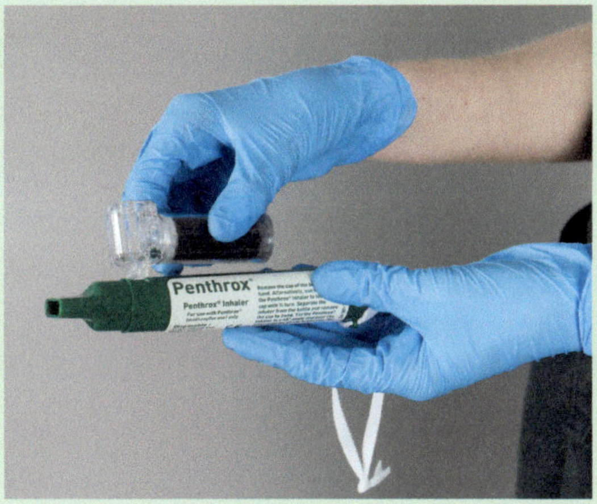	The activated charcoal filter absorbs the active drug as the patient exhales, reducing the risk of occupational exposure (8).

	Action	Rationale
5.	Open the vial containing the methoxyflurane medication, either by hand or by inserting it into the end of the inhaler as pictured and then twisting to release the cap. 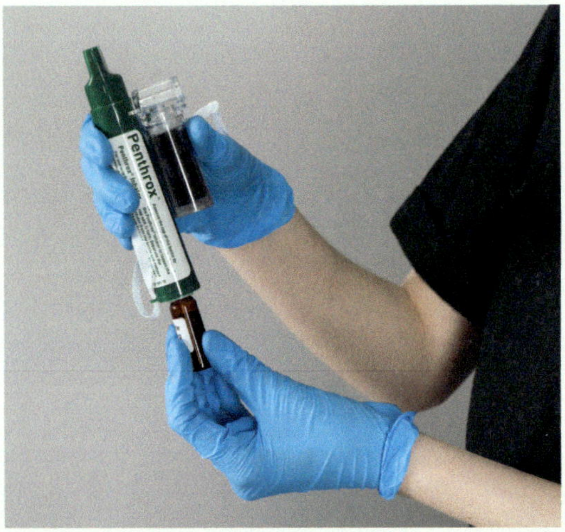	
6.	Tilt the inhaler to a 45° angle with the mouthpiece pointing down. Pour the methoxyflurane into the back of the device while continually rotating it. 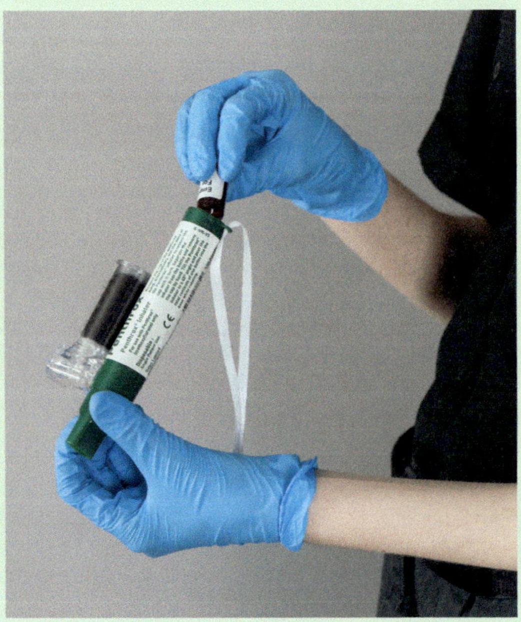	Inside the inhaler is a material which absorbs the liquid. Holding the device at 45° and rotating it will ensure that the methoxyflurane is evenly distributed across the material.

<table>
<tr><th colspan="2">Action</th><th>Rationale</th></tr>
<tr><td>7.</td><td>Place the wrist loop over the patient's wrist.
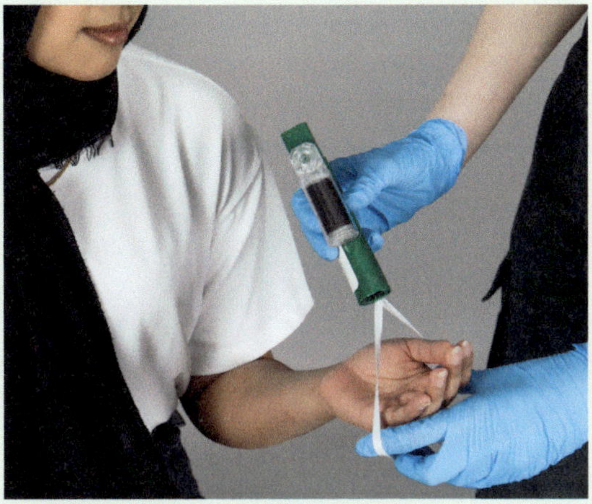</td><td>Penthrox is self-administered. The loop ensures that if the patient drops the device, it doesn't fall to the floor and become contaminated or lost.</td></tr>
<tr><td>8.</td><td>Instruct the patient to breathe through the inhaler. The first few breaths should be gentle, then normal breaths can be resumed.
Patients should inhale and exhale through the device.
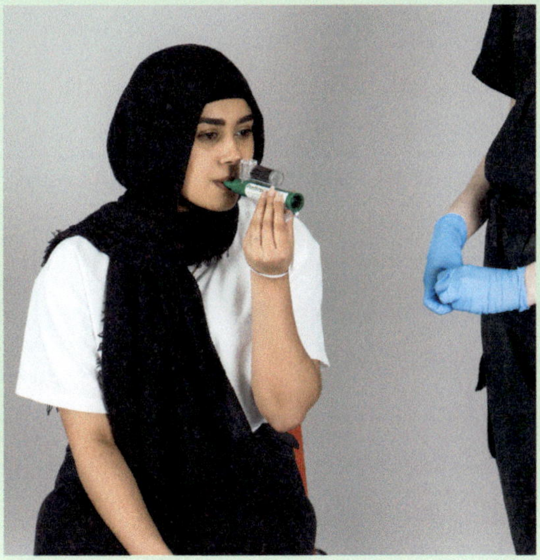</td><td>This will help patients get used to the sweet taste and odour of the methoxyflurane, which some may find unpleasant (9).
It is important to exhale through the device to ensure that exhaled methoxyflurane is captured in the activated charcoal filter.</td></tr>
</table>

Action		Rationale
9.	Patients should be instructed to inhale intermittently as the need for pain relief dictates, and not continuously.	Patients can adjust the amount of medication they receive (and therefore the amount of analgesia) by taking breaks from the inhaler.
10.	For maximum analgesic effect the patient can cover the dilutor hole at the top of the filter device. 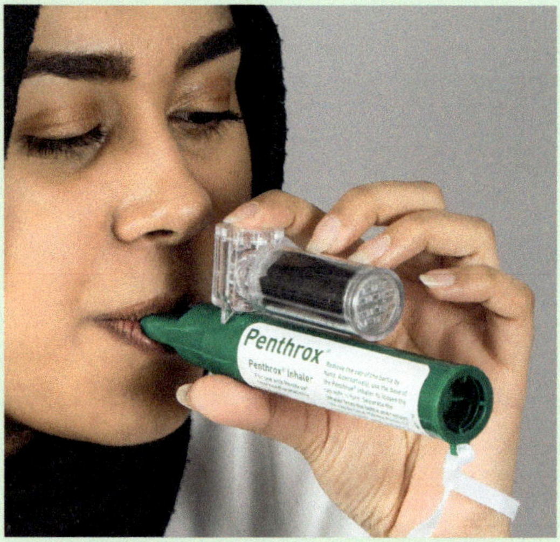	This will increase the concentration of inhaled methoxyflurane.
11.	If further analgesia is required, a second bottle of methoxyflurane can be added to the inhaler.	A Penthrox® inhaler will provide analgesia for approximately 20 minutes. Follow your organisation's policy on repeat dosing.
12.	Once you have finished using the device, place it into the plastic bag provided as part of the Penthrox® kit, seal, and dispose of it in line with your organisation's policy.	
13.	Document the procedure.	You must keep full, clear and accurate records for everyone you care for, treat, or provide other services to (6).

References

1. Siriwardena AN, Smith MD, Rowan E, et al. Clinical effectiveness and costs of pre-hospital inhaled methoxyflurane for acute pain in trauma in adults: non-randomised control group study. *British Paramedic Journal*. 2021;5(4):66–67.
2. Allison SJ, Docherty PD, Pons D, et al. Frequency and duration of ambulance officer exposure to nitrous oxide and methoxyflurane in New Zealand. *International Archives of Occupational and Environmental Health*. 2021;94(8):1773–1782.
3. Galen. Penthrox methoxyflurane [Internet]. 2022 [cited 2022 Aug 5]. Available from: https://penthrox.co.uk/wp-content/uploads/2022/06/MAT-PEN-UK-000523-Where-to-Poster-A4-PI-Price-Increase-May-22.pdf.
4. Electronic Medicines Compendium. PENTHROX 99.9%, 3 ml inhalation vapour, liquid [Internet]. 2021 [cited 2022 Aug 5]. Available from: www.medicines.org.uk/emc/product/1939/smpc#CONTRAINDICATIONS.
5. British Medical Association. Ethics – General information [Internet]. 2018 [cited 2019 Dec 29]. Available from: www.bma.org.uk/advice/employment/ethics/consent/consent-tool-kit/2-general-information.
6. Health and Care Professions Council. Standards of conduct, performance and ethics [Internet]. 2016 [cited 2022 Jul 16]. Available from: www.hcpc-uk.org/standards/standards-of-conduct-performance-and-ethics/.
7. NHS England. Standard infection control precautions: National hand hygiene and personal protective equipment policy [Internet]. 2019 [cited 2022 Feb 13]. Available from: www.england.nhs.uk/publication/standard-infection-control-precautions-national-hand-hygiene-and-personal-protective-equipment-policy/.
8. Griffiths E. Efficacy and safety of methoxyflurane: Managing trauma associated pain in UK SAR helicopter paramedic practice [Internet]. *Journal of Paramedic Practice*. 2017;9(3) [cited 2022 Aug 5]. Available from: https://www.paramedicpractice.com/features/article/efficacy-and-safety-of-methoxyflurane-managing-trauma-associated-pain-in-uk-sar-helicopter-paramedic-practice.
9. Trimmel H, Egger A, Doppler R, et al. Usability and effectiveness of inhaled methoxyflurane for prehospital analgesia – A prospective, observational study [Internet]. *BMC Emergency Medicine*. 2022;22(8) [cited 2022 Oct 31]. Available from: https://doi.org/10.1186/s12873-021-00565-6.

Spacer Device

Indications
- To be used with pressurised metred dose inhalers (pMDIs).

Contraindications
- Device is damaged or in some other way defective.

Advantages (1)
- Reduces oropharyngeal deposition of a drug.
- Improves lung deposition of a drug.

Disadvantages
- Requires regular cleaning to remain effective.
- Due to its size, can be inconvenient for patients to keep with them constantly.

Procedure – Spacer Device

Take the following steps to use a spacer device with a pMDI (2):

Action		Rationale
1.	Explain the procedure and obtain consent if appropriate to do so.	You must make sure that you have valid consent from service users or other appropriate authority before you provide care, treatment or other services (3,4).
2.	Don appropriate personal protective equipment (PPE), and undertake appropriate hand hygiene.	This reduces the risk of cross-infection (5).
3.	Carefully examine the spacer for any damage, missing parts or foreign bodies within the chamber of the device. 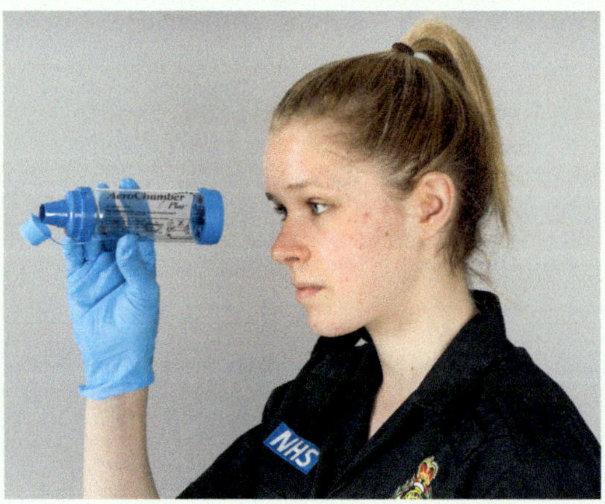	The device should not be used if there are any damaged or missing components. If any foreign bodies are seen, they should be removed prior to use.

Action		Rationale
4.	Remove the cap from the pMDI and shake. Then insert into the back of the chamber. 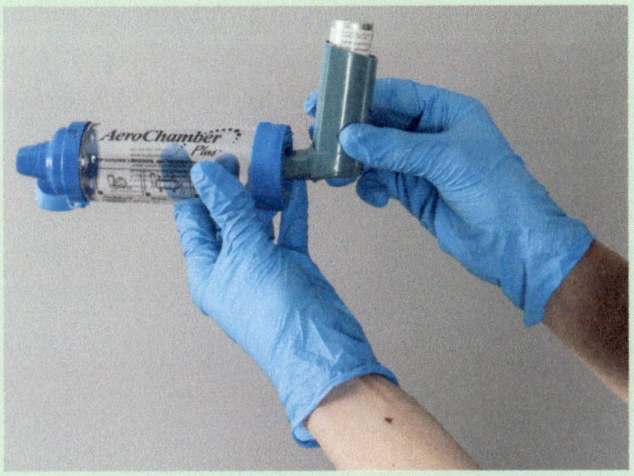 	Ensure the pMDI has been firmly inserted so that a good seal is created.
5.	Explain to the patient the technique they need to follow in advance. 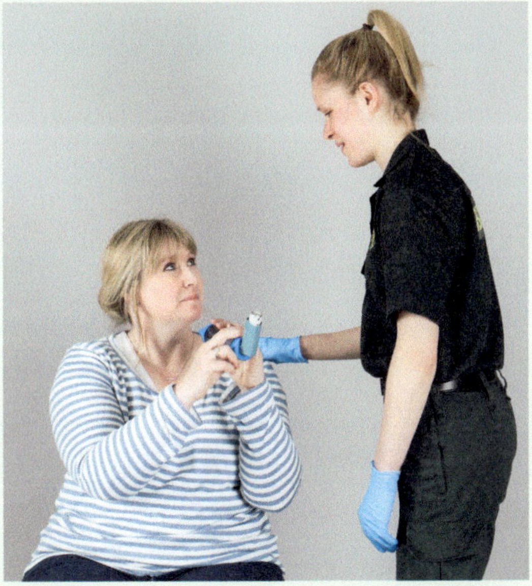	Patients need to coordinate breathing and administering a dose of the pMDI at the right time for maximum drug delivery.
6.	Instruct the patient to make a seal around the mouthpiece with their lips and to take gentle breaths. Some devices have an inbuilt whistle. If the whistle sounds, the patient is inhaling too quickly and should be instructed to slow their breathing.	Optimum drug delivery occurs during gentle deep respiration.

Action		Rationale
	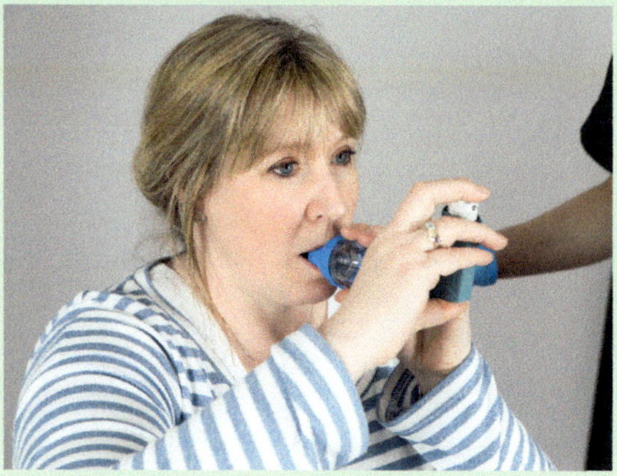	
7.	At the end of gentle expiration, the patient should deliver a single dose of medication from the pMDI. This should coincide with the start of inspiration.	
8.	The patient should take a deep full breath and hold it for 5–10 seconds if possible.	Holding their breath will aid in drug absorption. If this is not possible, the patient should keep their lips firmly sealed around the chamber and take two to three further breaths through the device.
9.	Repeat steps 6–8 to deliver additional doses as directed on the pMDI instructions or as prescribed.	
10.	Document the procedure.	You must keep full, clear and accurate records for everyone you care for, treat, or provide other services to (4).

References

1. Vincken W, Levy ML, Scullion J, et al. Spacer devices for inhaled therapy: Why use them, and how? *ERJ Open Research*. 2018;4:00065–2018.
2. AeroChamber. Learning how to use your AeroChamber Plus® Flow-Vu® [Internet]. 2022 [cited 2022 Aug 7]. Available from: www.aerochambervhc.com/instructions-for-use.
3. British Medical Association. Ethics – General information [Internet]. 2018 [cited 2019 Dec 29]. Available from: www.bma.org.uk/advice/employment/ethics/consent/consent-tool-kit/2-general-information.
4. Health and Care Professions Council. Standards of conduct, performance and ethics [Internet]. 2016 [cited 2022 Jul 16]. Available from: www.hcpc-uk.org/standards/standards-of-conduct-performance-and-ethics/.
5. NHS England. Standard infection control precautions: National hand hygiene and personal protective equipment policy [Internet]. 2019 [cited 2022 Feb 13]. Available from: www.england.nhs.uk/publication/standard-infection-control-precautions-national-hand-hygiene-and-personal-protective-equipment-policy/.

Inhalers

Indications

- To deliver inhaled medications.

Contraindications

- Device is damaged or in some other way defective.
- Medication is past its expiry date.
- Other forms of drug delivery, for example a nebuliser, are available and more clinically appropriate.

Advantages

- Does not require any other equipment.

Disadvantages

- Technique has a significant impact on efficacy of drug delivery and is often poor, especially in children. Where possible, a spacer device should be used to improve drug delivery (1).

Procedure – Inhaler

Take the following steps to use a metered dose inhaler (2,3):

Action		Rationale
1.	Explain the procedure and obtain consent if appropriate to do so.	You must make sure that you have valid consent from service users or other appropriate authority before you provide care, treatment or other services (4,5).
2.	Don appropriate personal protective equipment (PPE), and undertake appropriate hand hygiene.	This reduces the risk of cross-infection (6).
3.	Inspect the inhaler for any damage and note the date on the metal canister to ensure it is in date. 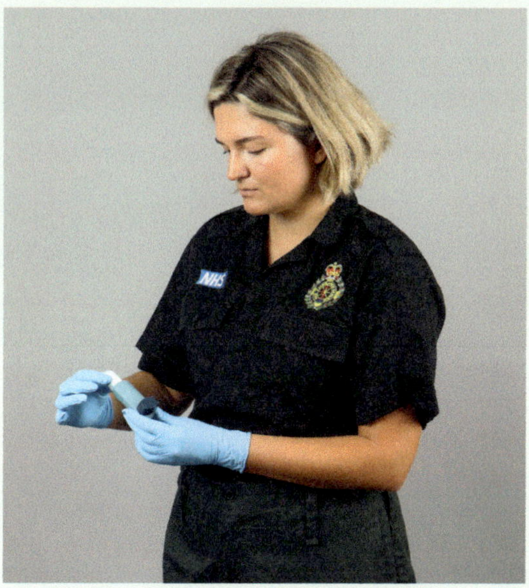	The inhaler should not be used if it is damaged or the medication has expired.

Action		Rationale
4.	Remove the cap from the end of the inhaler and inspect the inside of the device to ensure there is no foreign body present. 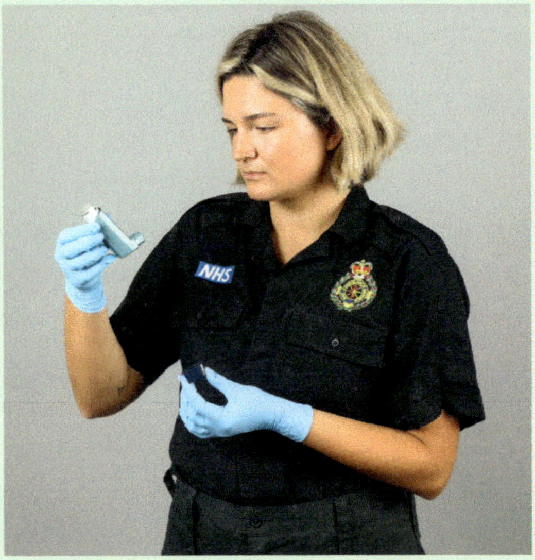	Any debris inside the inhaler could be inhaled during use if not removed.
5.	Shake the inhaler well, typically four to five times prior to use.	This ensures all the medication is correctly mixed and distributed inside the canister prior to administration.
6.	With the patient in the sitting position, instruct them to grasp the inhaler so their thumb is under the base of the device and their index finger is on the top of the canister, ready to push it down. 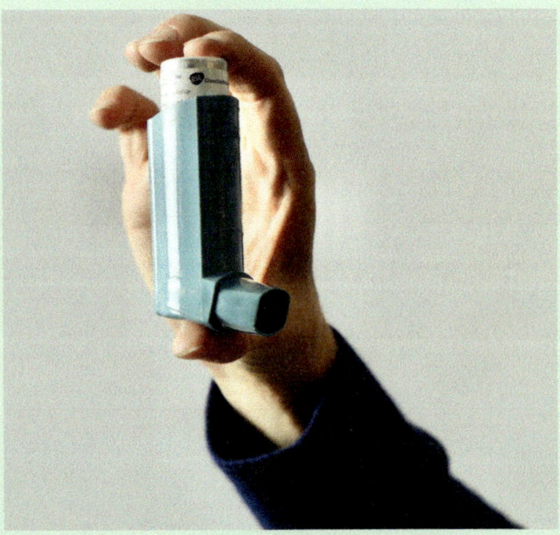	
7.	Instruct the patient to breathe fully out, without the inhaler in their mouth, until their lungs feel empty.	By fully exhaling, the patient will be able to take a deeper inhalation, which may make drug delivery more effective.

Action		Rationale
8.	Instruct the patient to insert the inhaler into their mouth and make a seal around the mouthpiece with their lips. Then instruct them to start slowly taking a deep breath in.	
9.	Once the patient has started to breathe in, they should smoothly and firmly press on the canister until one dose is released. Once the dose has been released, the patient should continue to inhale until their lungs feel full. 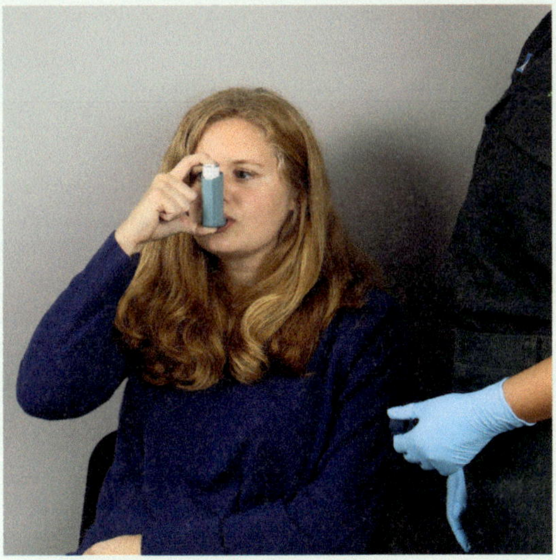	
10.	The patient can now remove the inhaler from their mouth and seal their lips. They should hold their breath for 10 seconds.	Holding one's breath optimises drug delivery.
11.	At the end of the 10 seconds instruct the patient to gently exhale.	
12.	If further doses are required, repeat steps 6–11 after 30–60 seconds.	
13.	When the patient is finished with the inhaler, they should replace the cap and store safely.	
14.	Document the procedure.	You must keep full, clear and accurate records for everyone you care for, treat, or provide other services to (5).

References

1. Gillette C, Rockich-Winston N, Kuhn JBA, et al. Inhaler technique in children with asthma: A systematic review. *Academic Pediatrics*. 2016;16(7):605–615.
2. Asthma and Lung UK. Using your inhalers [Internet]. 2021 [cited 2022 Aug 22]. Available from: www.asthma.org.uk/advice/inhalers-medicines-treatments/using-inhalers/.
3. Geeky Medics. Inhaler technique – OSCE guide [Internet]. 2022 [cited 2022 Aug 22]. Available from: https://geekymedics.com/inhaler-technique-osce-guide/.
4. British Medical Association. Ethics – General information [Internet]. 2018 [cited 2019 Dec 29]. Available from: www.bma.org.uk/advice/employment/ethics/consent/consent-tool-kit/2-general-information.
5. Health and Care Professions Council. Standards of conduct, performance and ethics [Internet]. 2016 [cited 2022 Jul 16]. Available from: www.hcpc-uk.org/standards/standards-of-conduct-performance-and-ethics/.
6. NHS England. Standard infection control precautions: National hand hygiene and personal protective equipment policy [Internet]. 2019 [cited 2022 Feb 13]. Available from: www.england.nhs.uk/publication/standard-infection-control-precautions-national-hand-hygiene-and-personal-protective-equipment-policy/.

Infusion

Indications

- To prepare infusion medications for administration.

Contraindications

- None.

Advantages

- Since preparation takes time, can be undertaken concurrently with obtaining intravenous access, (assuming sufficient personnel available), minimising subsequent delay to the administration of fluids.

Disadvantages

- Takes time to correctly prepare.
- If not prepared correctly, dangerous complications such as air in the line can result.

Procedure – Preparing an Infusion

Take the following steps to prepare an infusion:

Action		Rationale
1.	Don appropriate personal protective equipment (PPE), and undertake appropriate hand hygiene.	This reduces the risk of cross-infection (1).
2.	Prepare required equipment. You will need: • The fluid for administration • A giving set. 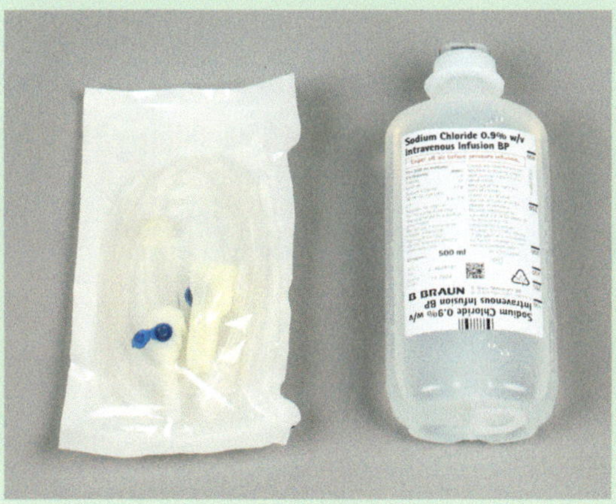	Preparing all equipment in advance will help ensure the process is completed without unnecessary interruption.
3.	Check the packaging of the giving set to ensure it is intact and in date. Examine the fluid and ensure: • It is the fluid intended for preparation • The packaging is intact • The fluid is in date • The fluid inside the bag appears as expected (it is clear, without floating debris).	If there are any concerns about the medication or the giving set, it should be discarded and a new item prepared.

Action		Rationale
4.	Remove the protective packaging and hang up the bag of fluid. In an ambulance, ceiling-mounted hooks are normally provided for this. In other locations you may need to hang it from a handy item or ask a bystander to hold the fluid. Do not place any part of the giving set on the floor or other contaminated surfaces.	Fluid infusions typically rely on gravity to facilitate administration.
5.	Twist and remove the foil covering or rubber pigtail of the outlet channel at the base of the fluid bag. Fluid will not flow out until the bag is spiked with a giving set. 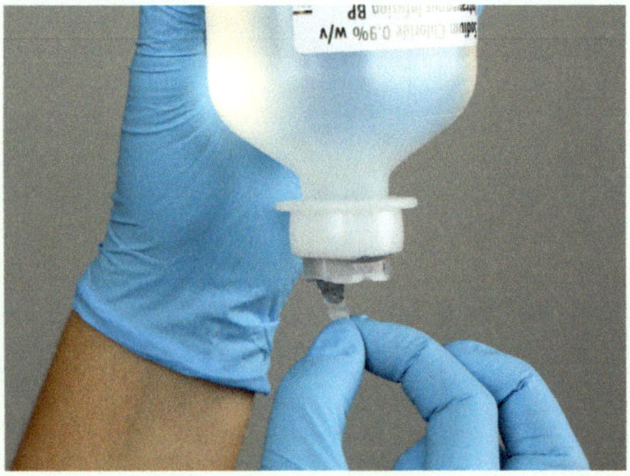	
6.	Open the package of the giving set. Close the roller clamp by rolling the clamp until it is tight on the fluid line. 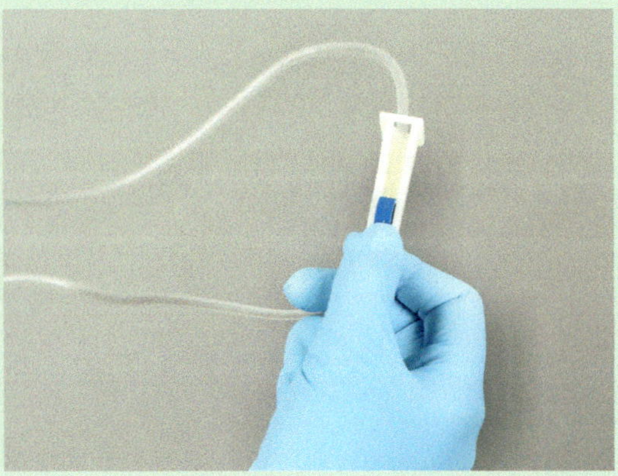	Closing the clamp at this stage will prevent fluid flowing into the line when the bag is spiked. This should also prevent air being drawn into the line prior to it being correctly primed.

Action		Rationale
7.	Remove the protective cap from the end of the spike. Do not touch the spike. 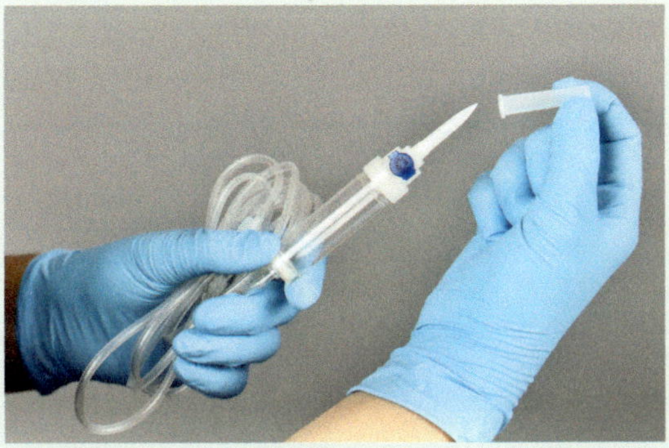	The spike is sharp and sterile. Touching the spike can cause a sharps injury and will contaminate the spike. If you do inadvertently touch the spike, discard the giving set and replace with a new set.
8.	Push the spike straight into the fluid outlet channel (where you have just removed the foil covering or rubber pigtail). If using a bag of fluid, grip the fluid channel on the bag with one hand, and push the spike into the bag with the other hand. For rigid containers, use the technique shown in the photograph below. It may help to use a twisting motion to push the spike into the outlet channel. Once fluid starts to enter the drip chamber, the spike has been inserted far enough. 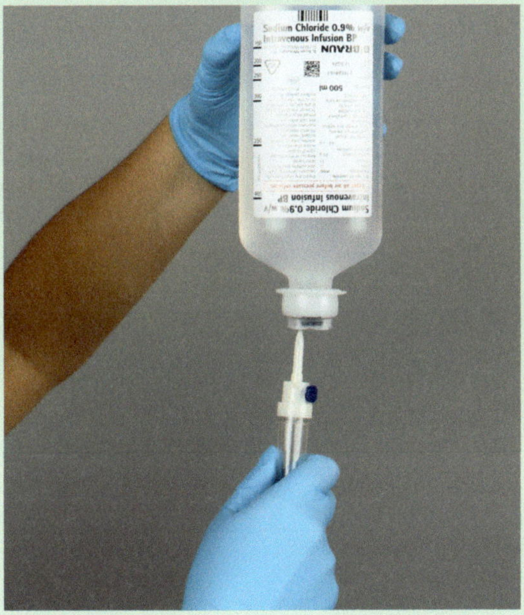	Be careful to push the spike in straight. If pushed in at an angle, it can inadvertently push back out through the side of the bag, causing a leak. Pushing the spike into the bag will break a seal allowing fluid to flow into the chamber.

Action		Rationale
9.	Prime the drip chamber by squeezing it between your thumb and forefinger. Repeat this until the drip chamber is half full of fluid. 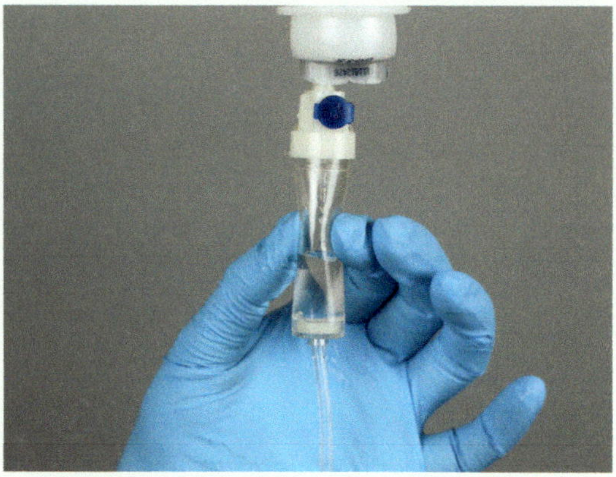	Priming the chamber will enable the line to be easily primed with fluid and prevent air from entering the line.
10.	Gently open the roller clamp until fluid starts to slowly flow through the line. Allow fluid to continue to slowly flow until it reaches the distal end of the line, then close the roller clamp again. 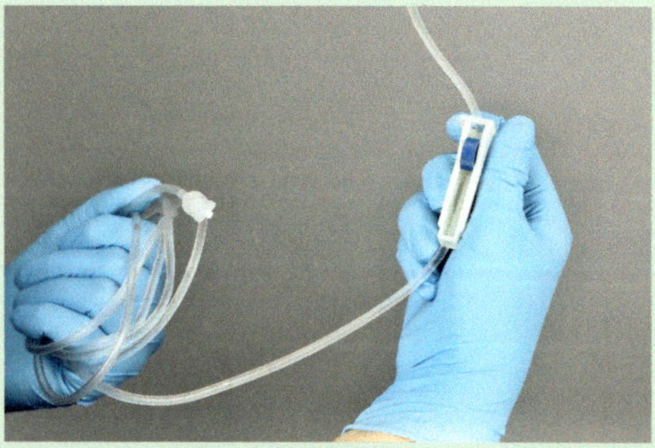	Controlling the rate of fluid flow through the giving-set line will reduce the likelihood of air being inadvertently drawn into the line along with the fluid.

	Action	Rationale
11.	Inspect the line for any air bubbles. If bubbles are present immediately prior to connecting the infusion to the patient, discard the cap from the end of the infusion line and open the roller clamp. This will allow fluid to flow out of the giving set until all the air has been removed. Discard the fluid into a vomit bowl, clinical waste bag or similar. 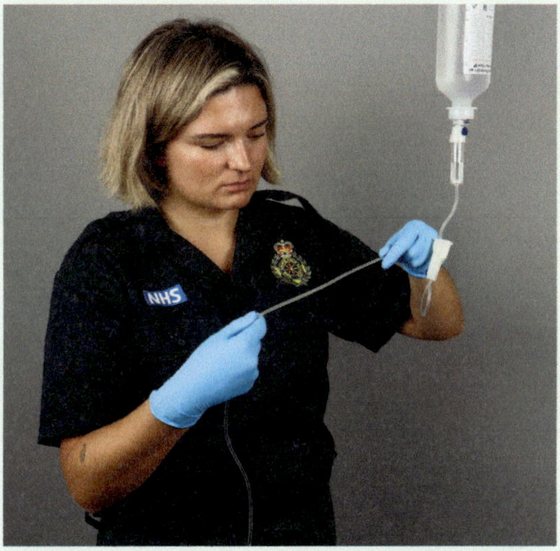	Air bubbles must not be administered to a patient. Air can gather within the circulation and in larger quantities can result in a fatal air embolus.
12.	Inspect the drip chamber. If the fluid level has dropped below half, then re-pinch the chamber until it is half full again.	The chamber must have a fluid level within it to prevent air from entering the line.
13.	Document the procedure.	You must keep full, clear and accurate records for everyone you care for, treat, or provide other services to (2).

References

1. NHS England. Standard infection control precautions: National hand hygiene and personal protective equipment policy [Internet]. 2019 [cited 2022 Feb 13]. Available from: www.england.nhs.uk/publication/standard-infection-control-precautions-national-hand-hygiene-and-personal-protective-equipment-policy/.
2. Health and Care Professions Council. Standards of conduct, performance and ethics [Internet]. 2016 [cited 2022 Jul 16]. Available from: www.hcpc-uk.org/standards/standards-of-conduct-performance-and-ethics/.

Drawing Up an Ampoule

Indications

- To prepare a drug for administration.

Contraindications

- If a pre-filled syringe of the same medication is available and the clinical urgency means its use would be more appropriate, then this should be used instead of drawing up an ampoule.

Advantages

- Due to the size of ampoules, multiple drugs can be carried in a compact manner.

Disadvantages

- Takes time to draw up.
- Ampoules can break if not opened correctly, rendering the medication unusable, and causing sharps injury in some cases.

Procedure – Drawing Up an Ampoule

Take the following steps to draw up an ampoule:

Action		Rationale
1.	Don appropriate personal protective equipment (PPE), and undertake appropriate hand hygiene.	This reduces the risk of cross-infection (1).
2.	Prepare the required equipment. You will need: • The ampoule of medication • An appropriately sized syringe • Ampoule breakers • Drawing-up needle • Syringe bung • Drug label (if appropriate) • Sharps bin.	Preparing all equipment in advance will help ensure the process is completed without unnecessary interruptions.

<table>
<tr><th colspan="2">Action</th><th>Rationale</th></tr>
<tr><td>3.</td><td>Check the following:
• Integrity of the ampoule
• The medication is the correct drug and dose
• The contents appear as expected
• The expiry date is clearly visible and the ampoule is within date.
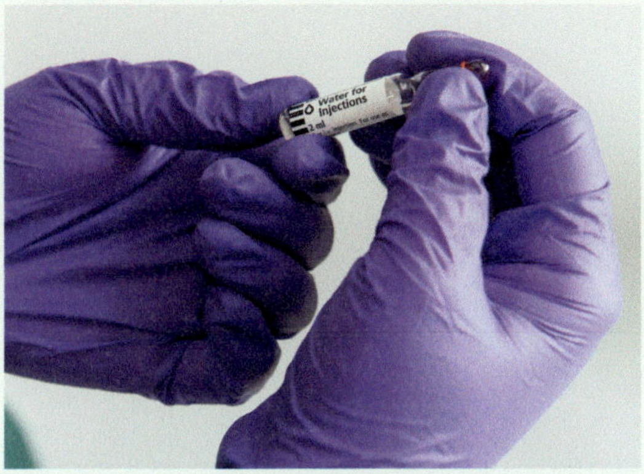
</td><td>If there are any concerns about the medication, it should be discarded.</td></tr>
<tr><td>4.</td><td>Ensure all the liquid is in the main body of the ampoule and not in the neck. If fluid is in the neck, grip the ampoule by the tip and gently rotate in your hand, being careful not to drop the ampoule.</td><td>The centrifugal effect from gentle rotation will move the fluid from the neck into the body of the ampoule.</td></tr>
<tr><td>5.</td><td>Place a disposable ampoule breaker over the tip and slide down until it sits on the neck of the ampoule.
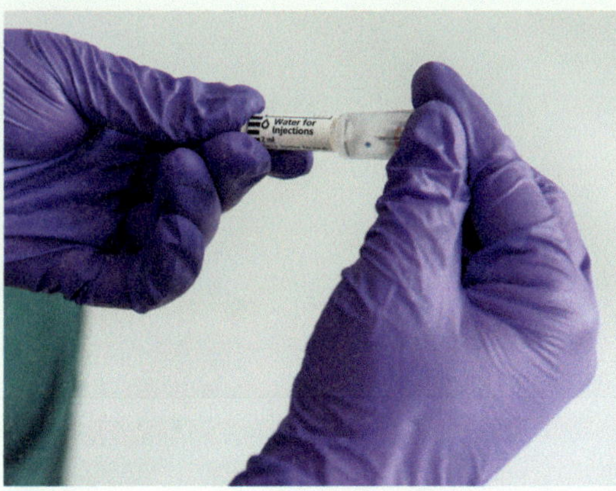
</td><td>Ampoules can break when opened, resulting in sharps injuries. Using an ampoule breaker will ensure no sharps injuries occur if the ampoule does break when opened.</td></tr>
</table>

Action		Rationale
6.	With the dot on the neck of the ampoule facing away from you, snap the top off the ampoule and dispose of it in a sharps bin. 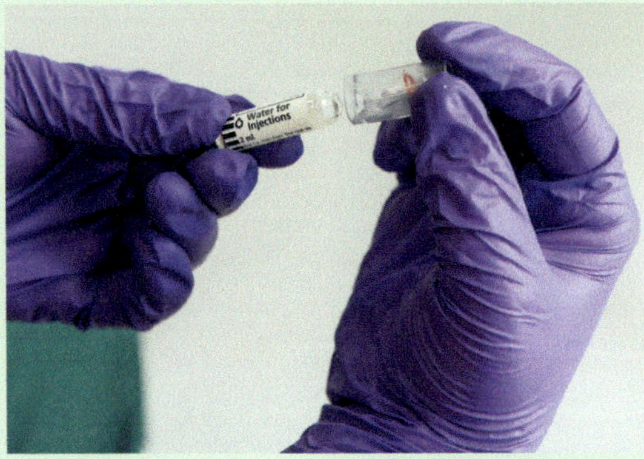	The dot identifies an area of the ampoule that has been scored, so is weaker. If no dot is present, the ampoule has been scored all around so can be snapped in any direction.
7.	Inspect the contents of the ampoule for any evidence of glass fragments.	If any glass fragments are seen, the ampoule and contents should be discarded.
8.	Attach a blunt filter needle (drawing-up needle) to the syringe. 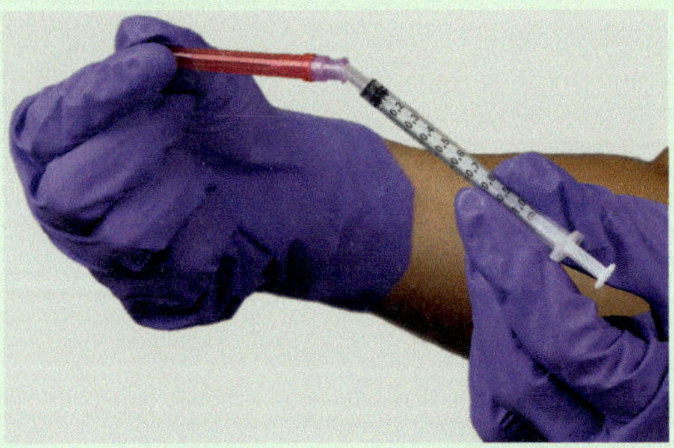	The use of a filter needle will ensure that any glass particles released when opening the ampoule are not inadvertently administered to the patient as part of the medication. They should be used routinely when drawing up medications (2).

Action		Rationale
9.	Without touching the sharp edges, take hold of the ampoule. Insert the syringe with the drawing-up needle and pull back on the plunger to aspirate the fluid into the syringe. 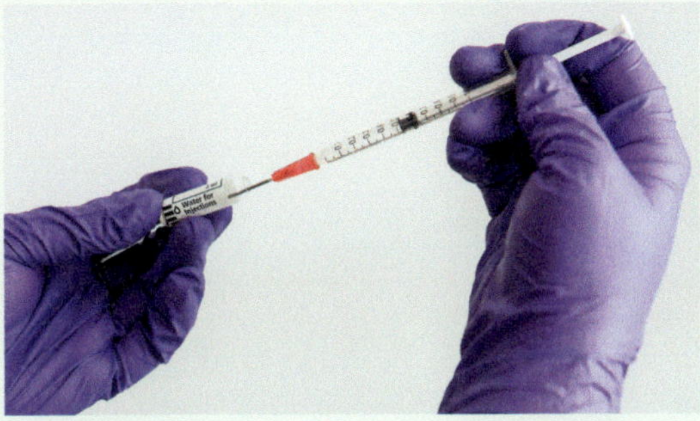	Tilting the ampoule and placing the tip of the needle into the lowest part of the ampoule will help to reduce air being accidentally aspirated as part of drawing up.
10.	If any air is inadvertently drawn up, hold the syringe by the body with the needle pointing up and gently tap the air bubbles until they travel to the top of the syringe. They can then be expelled by gently pushing on the syringe plunger. 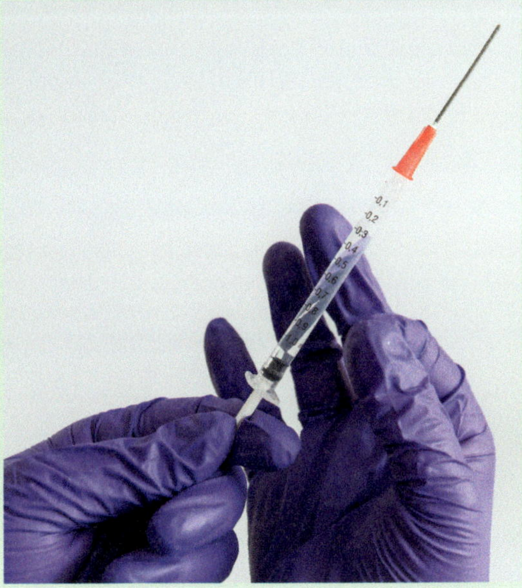	Air can cause an embolism if administered directly into a vein, so care should be taken to remove all air prior to administration.

Action		Rationale
11.	Remove the drawing-up needle and dispose of it safely. 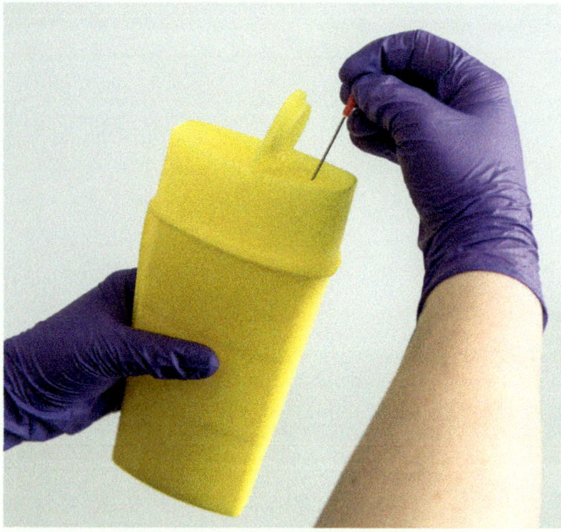	
12.	If the medication is not going to be administered immediately, it should be labelled and a syringe bung placed on the end.	All medication should be labelled to prevent drug errors.
13.	Document the procedure.	You must keep full, clear and accurate records for everyone you care for, treat, or provide other services to (3).

References

1. NHS England. Standard infection control precautions: National hand hygiene and personal protective equipment policy [Internet]. 2019 [cited 2022 Feb 13]. Available from: https://www.england.nhs.uk/publication/standard-infection-control-precautions-national-hand-hygiene-and-personal-protective-equipment-policy/.
2. NHS Business Service Authority. Clinical review: Blunt drawing up devices with and without filter [Internet]. 2016 [cited 2022 Aug 7]. Available from: https://www.nhsbsa.nhs.uk/sites/default/files/2017-04/Clinical%20review%20blunt%20drawing%20up%20devices%20with%20and%20without%20filter%20-%20Final%20%28V1.0%29%2012%202016.pdf.
3. Health and Care Professions Council. Standards of conduct, performance and ethics [Internet]. 2016 [cited 2022 Jul 16]. Available from: https://www.hcpc-uk.org/standards/standards-of-conduct-performance-and-ethics/.

Oral Administration

Indications

- Administration of drugs given via the oral route.

Contraindications

- Patient's level of consciousness is decreased such that they cannot safely take oral medication.
- Unable to swallow safely.

Cautions

- Active vomiting (as will reduce absorption).

Advantages

- Simple technique.
- Non-invasive.

Disadvantages

- Some patients, especially children, struggle to swallow tablets.

Procedure – Oral Administration

Take the following steps to administer drugs via the oral route:

Action		Rationale
1.	Explain the procedure and obtain consent if appropriate to do so.	You must make sure that you have valid consent from service users or other appropriate authority before you provide care, treatment or other services (1,2).
2.	Don appropriate personal protective equipment (PPE), and undertake appropriate hand hygiene.	This reduces the risk of cross-infection (3)
3.	Check the package of the medication to be administered to ensure: • Integrity of all packaging • The medication is the correct drug and dose • The expiry date is visible and the drug is within date. 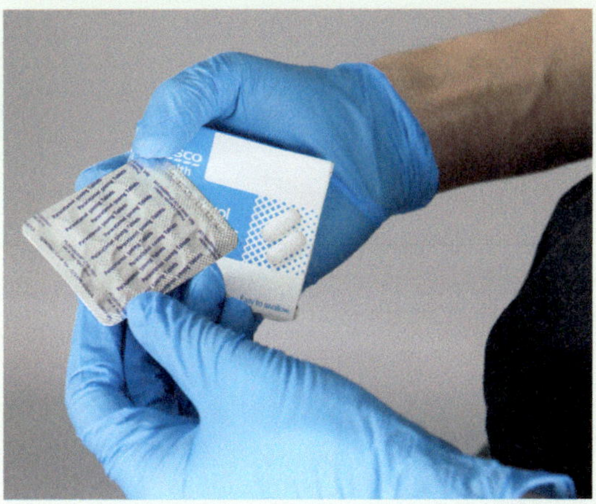	Tablets are easily confused, so carefully check you have the correct medication.

Action		Rationale
4.	Prior to administration, complete a med-check process. Your organisation may have a dedicated procedure for this, but if not, confirm the following with a colleague: • The drug to be administered • The reason for administration • The dose (and how this was calculated if relevant, for example, JRCALC Page for Age) • The route • Patient allergy status.	Drug errors are a common form of clinical error, especially in emergency situations. Taking a moment to check with a colleague can help to identify and potentially reduce drug administration errors.
5.	Present the medication to the patient with clear instructions, depending on the route of administration. **Oral tablets**, such as paracetamol, can be swallowed with a small amount of water (provide a small amount of water if appropriate). The common exception to this in ambulance practice is aspirin, which should be chewed. **Sublingual tablets**, such as glyceryl trinitrate (GTN), are placed under the tongue and allowed to slowly dissolve. **Buccal tablets**, such as prochlorperazine, are placed between the gum and cheek and allowed to be absorbed slowly through the buccal mucosa. 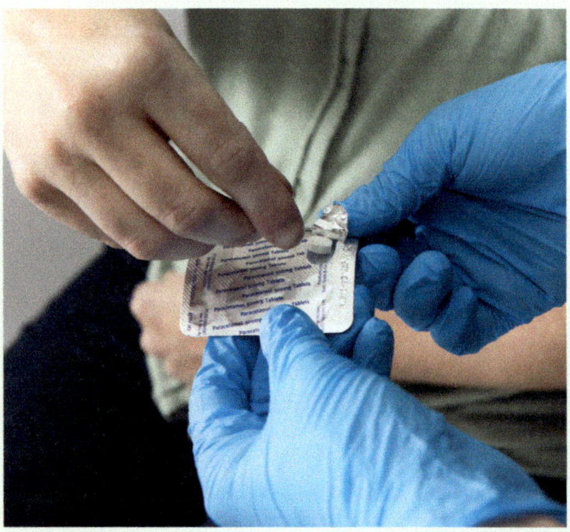	Different routes will have different absorption speeds and other impacts on pharmacokinetics. Manufacturers choose the appropriate route of administration based on a range of characteristics of the medication and speed of onset. Make sure the patient is aware of how they should self-administer the medication for maximum efficacy.

Action		Rationale
6.	If a patient is not able to administer the medication themselves, due to an arm injury, for example, it is acceptable to place the tablet into their mouth and provide a small sip of water if appropriate. Ensure you are wearing gloves in this case. Do not place a tablet into the mouth of a patient unless you are confident they can swallow effectively.	Tablets can cause an airway obstruction, so they should not be administered to an unconscious patient or one who does not have an effective swallow.
7.	Document the procedure.	You must keep full, clear and accurate records for everyone you care for, treat, or provide other services to (2).

References

1. British Medical Association. Ethics – General information [Internet]. 2018 [cited 2019 Dec 29]. Available from: https://www.bma.org.uk/advice/employment/ethics/consent/consent-tool-kit/2-general-information.
2. Health and Care Professions Council. Standards of conduct, performance and ethics [Internet]. 2016 [cited 2022 Jul 16]. Available from: https://www.hcpc-uk.org/standards/standards-of-conduct-performance-and-ethics/.
3. NHS England. Standard infection control precautions: National hand hygiene and personal protective equipment policy [Internet]. 2019 [cited 2022 Feb 13]. Available from: https://www.england.nhs.uk/publication/standard-infection-control-precautions-national-hand-hygiene-and-personal-protective-equipment-policy/.

Nebulising Medication

Indications
- To administer drugs given via nebulisation.

Contraindications
- None.

Advantages
- Non-invasive.

Disadvantages
- The patient needs to be able to sit up for a nebuliser mask to work effectively.

Procedure – Nebulising Medication

Take the following steps to administer nebulised medication (1):

Action		Rationale
1.	Explain the procedure and obtain consent if appropriate to do so.	You must make sure that you have valid consent from service users or other appropriate authority before you provide care, treatment or other services (2,3).
2.	Don appropriate personal protective equipment (PPE) and undertake appropriate hand hygiene.	This reduces the risk of cross-infection (4).
3.	Open the packaging of the nebuliser mask. Depending on the manufacturer of the nebuliser device, you may need to dismantle the chamber prior to adding the medication. 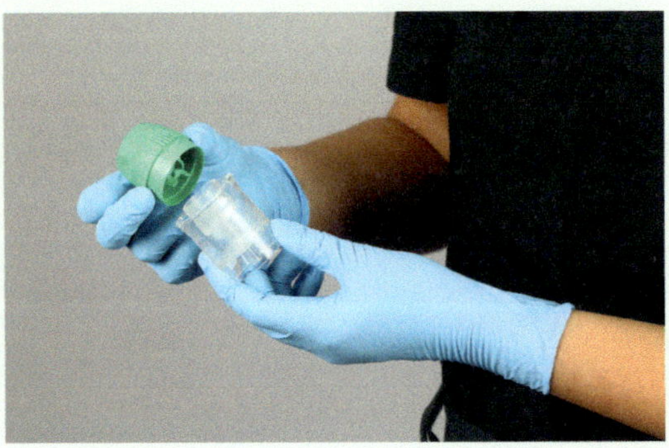	Different manufacturers' nebulisers are prepared differently. Here a device which has to be unscrewed before medication is added has been shown.

Action		Rationale
4.	Add medication to the nebuliser chamber and reassemble the chamber if necessary. 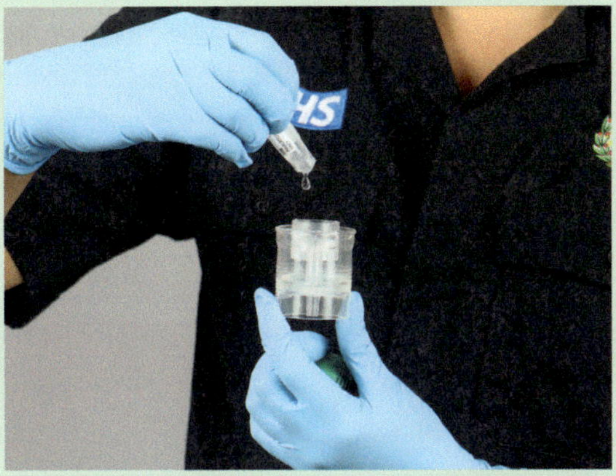	
5.	Connect gas tubing to the chamber and correctly seat the mask on the patient's face. 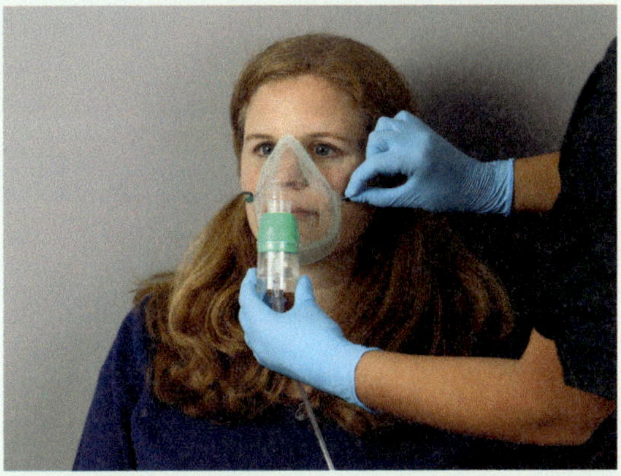	Positioning the mask correctly should ensure a good seal between the mask and the patient's face. This may help to improve the delivery of medication to the patient's lungs.
6.	Turn on the gas flow to 8 litres per minute. 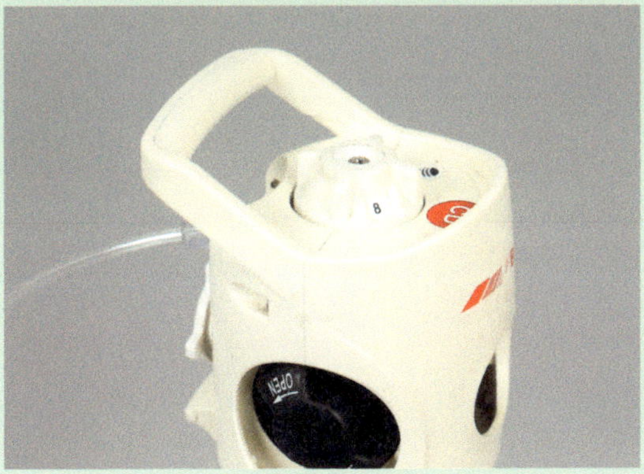	The gas must be at the correct flow rate to ensure the medication is nebulised to the correct droplet size, which in turn aids delivery of the medication to the lungs. Ensure you check the manufacturer's guidelines regarding the correct gas flow rate for the mask you are using. The type shown here requires 8 litres per minute (5).

Action		Rationale
7.	Prior to administration, complete a med-check process. Your organisation may have a dedicated procedure for this, but if not, confirm the following with a colleague: • The drug to be administered • The reason for administration • The dose (and how this was calculated if relevant, for example, JRCALC Page for Age) • The route.	Drug errors are a common form of clinical error, especially in emergency situations. Taking a moment to check with a colleague can help to identify and potentially reduce drug administration errors.
8.	Coach the patient's breathing, encouraging them to take deep breaths and briefly hold their breath for two to three seconds before exhaling. 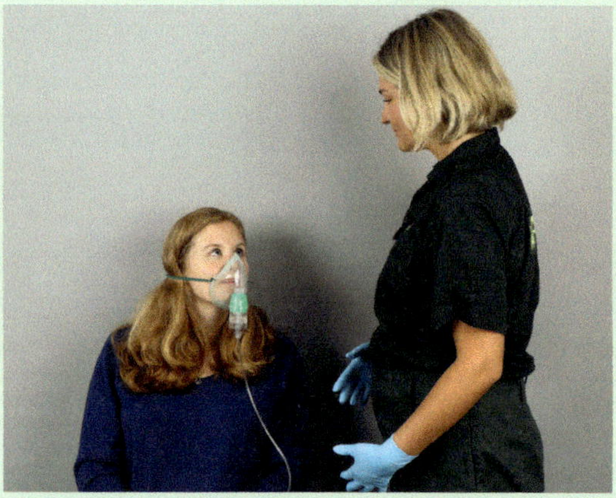	This may help drug absorption within the lungs.
9.	Monitor the administration of nebulised medication by observing the fine mist being created. Ensure the patient remains upright, and once the medication within the chamber has all been nebulised, remove the chamber.	If the chamber is not upright, nebulisation may not occur.
10.	Document the procedure.	You must keep full, clear and accurate records for everyone you care for, treat, or provide other services to (3).

References

1. Queensland Ambulance Service. Drug administration /Nebulisation [Internet]. 2022 [cited 2022 Aug 21]. Available from: www.ambulance.qld.gov.au/docs/clinical/cpp/CPP_Nebulisation.pdf.
2. British Medical Association. Ethics – General information [Internet]. 2018 [cited 2019 Dec 29]. Available from: www.bma.org.uk/advice/employment/ethics/consent/consent-tool-kit/2-general-information.
3. Health and Care Professions Council. Standards of conduct, performance and ethics [Internet]. 2016 [cited 2022 Jul 16]. Available from: www.hcpc-uk.org/standards/standards-of-conduct-performance-and-ethics/.
4. NHS England. Standard infection control precautions: National hand hygiene and personal protective equipment policy [Internet]. 2019 [cited 2022 Feb 13]. Available from: www.england.nhs.uk/publication/standard-infection-control-precautions-national-hand-hygiene-and-personal-protective-equipment-policy/.
5. Intersurgical. Cirrus 2 [Internet]. 2012 [cited 2022 Aug 21]. Available from: www.intersurgical.com/content/files/65259/-1507526261.

Reconstituting Medications

Indications

- To prepare powdered medications for administration.

Contraindications

- None.

Advantages

- Non-invasive.

Disadvantages

- Reconstituting can be slow and challenging.

Procedure – Reconstituting Medication

Take the following steps to reconstitute medication:

Action		Rationale
1.	Explain the procedure and obtain consent if appropriate to do so.	You must make sure that you have valid consent from service users or other appropriate authority before you provide care, treatment or other services (1,2).
2.	Don appropriate personal protective equipment (PPE), and undertake appropriate hand hygiene.	This reduces the risk of cross-infection (3).
3.	Prepare the required equipment: • The ampoule of medication to be prepared • Required quantity of base fluid, typically 0.9% sodium chloride or water for injection (as directed by the drug manufacturer) • Appropriately sized syringe • Blunt filter needle • Sharps bin.	Ensure you have the required equipment prepared in advance.
4.	Before commencing, confirm: • The medication • The dose • The type of base fluid to use (sodium chloride 0.9% or water for injection).	Reconstituting drugs is a common opportunity for a drug error to occur. Check the medication and method of reconstitution carefully. Where possible, cross-check your decisions with a suitably qualified colleague.

Action		Rationale
5.	Draw up the correct amount of base fluid (sodium chloride 0.9% or water for injection) into a syringe. 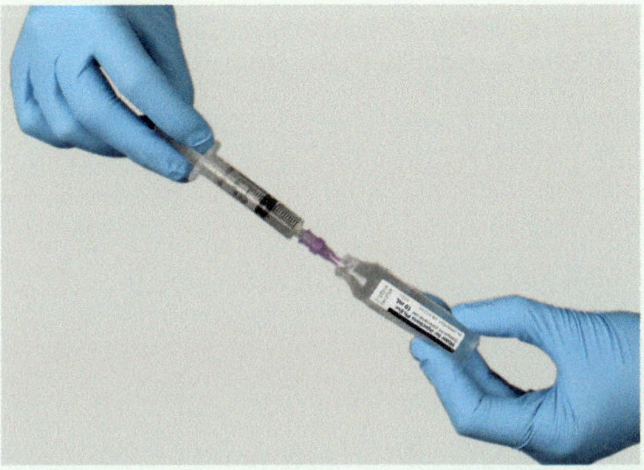	Drawing up the correct amount of fluid into the syringe will ensure the correct concentration of medication once reconstituted.
6.	Take the cap off the vial for reconstitution. Place the blunt needle through the rubber seal and inject the base fluid into the ampoule. 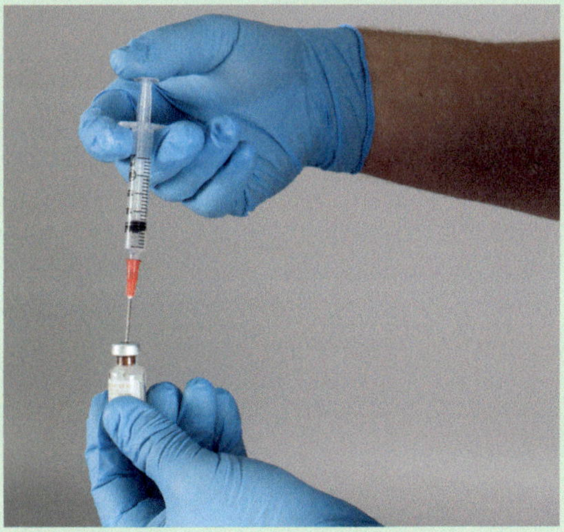	If the cap from the top of the vial is missing, it should not be used. Discard and replace with a new vial.

Action		Rationale
7.	Without removing the needle or syringe, gently roll the bottle in your hand so that the fluid and drug mix together. Keep doing this until no powder medication can be seen. 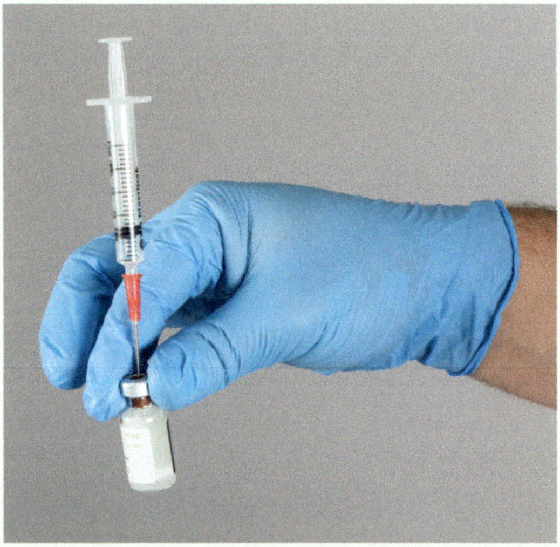	Gently rolling the medication will help the product to dissolve more quickly.
8.	Invert the vial, then aspirate the contents into the syringe. Ensure the full contents of the vial are aspirated. 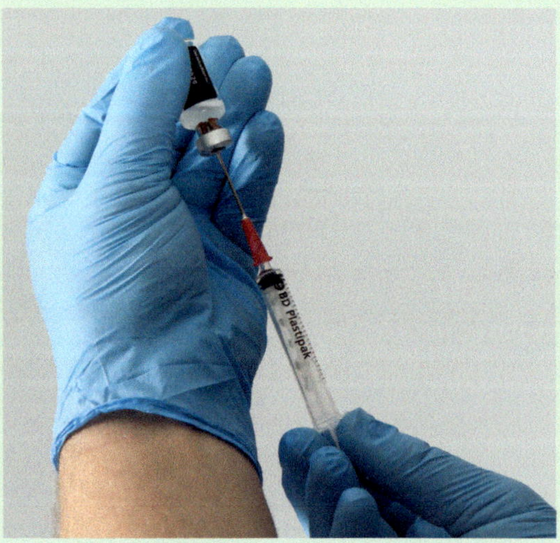	Due to the design of the bottles, inverting the vial will help to ensure the full volume is aspirated back into the syringe.

	Action	Rationale
9.	Once aspirated, inspect the contents of the syringe for: • Volume: Ensure that the volume aspirated into the syringe is the same as the amount calculated and injected into the vial for reconstitution. • Appearance: The fluid should have no particles visible within it, although sometimes the colour of the fluid will change slightly, such as with co-amoxiclav, which may transiently appear pink (4).	Ensure the medication appears appropriate prior to administration. If there are any concerns about the appearance following reconstitution, the medication should be discarded and a new medication prepared.
10.	Prior to administration, complete a med-check process. Your organisation may have a dedicated procedure for this, but if not, confirm the following with a colleague: • The drug to be administered • The reason for administration • The dose (and how this was calculated if relevant, for example, JRCALC Page for Age) • The route.	Drug errors are a common form of clinical error, especially in emergency situations. Taking a moment to check with a colleague can help to identify and potentially reduce drug administration errors. This should be completed separately to the calculations for reconstitution.
11.	Dispose of the ampoule and drawing-up needle securely. 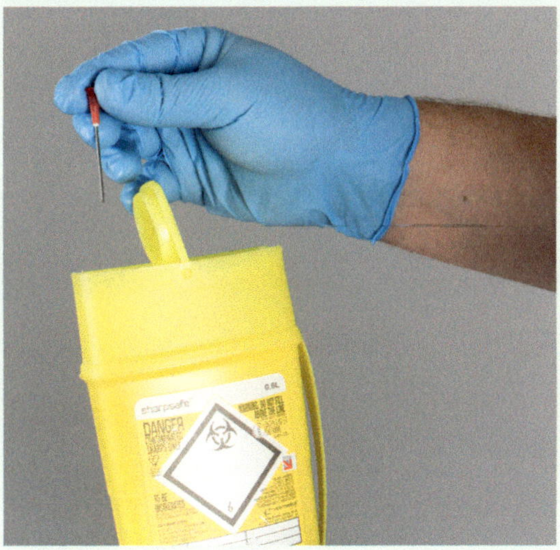	Follow your organisation's policy on safe disposal.
12.	Document the procedure.	You must keep full, clear and accurate records for everyone you care for, treat, or provide other services to (2).

References

1. British Medical Association. Ethics – General information [Internet]. 2018 [cited 2019 Dec 29]. Available from: www.bma.org.uk/advice/employment/ethics/consent/consent-tool-kit/2-general-information.
2. Health and Care Professions Council. Standards of conduct, performance and ethics [Internet]. 2016 [cited 2022 Jul 16]. Available from: www.hcpc-uk.org/standards/standards-of-conduct-performance-and-ethics/.
3. NHS England. Standard infection control precautions: national hand hygiene and personal protective equipment policy [Internet]. 2019 [cited 2022 Feb 13]. Available from: www.england.nhs.uk/publication/standard-infection-control-precautions-national-hand-hygiene-and-personal-protective-equipment-policy/.
4. Electronic Medicines Compendium. Co-Amoxiclav 1000 mg/200 mg powder for solution for injection/infusion [Internet]. 2020 [cited 2022 Aug 21]. Available from: www.medicines.org.uk/emc/product/7211/smpc#USEHANDLING.

Intramuscular Administration

Indications

- Administration of drugs given via the intramuscular route.

Contraindications

- When other routes are more clinically appropriate.
- Infection at site.
- Patient in cardiac arrest.

Cautions

- The absorption of intramuscular drugs is impaired in patients who are cold, hypovolaemic or in a compromised haemodynamic state.

Advantages

- May be an appropriate route to administer medications in non-compliant patients.

Disadvantages

- Can be painful.
- Small risk of injuring underlying vessels or nerves.

Procedure – Intramuscular Administration

Take the following steps to administer drugs via the intramuscular route (1):

Action		Rationale
1.	Explain the procedure and obtain consent if appropriate to do so.	You must make sure that you have valid consent from service users or other appropriate authority before you provide care, treatment or other services (2,3).
2.	Don appropriate personal protective equipment (PPE), and undertake appropriate hand hygiene.	This reduces the risk of cross-infection (4).
3.	Prepare the required equipment, including: • The appropriate medication • An appropriately sized syringe, depending on the volume to be administered • A blunt filter drawing-up needle • Sharps bin • Disinfectant wipe • A syringe label (if appropriate) • Gauze	Preparing all equipment in advance will help ensure the process is completed without unnecessary interruption.

	Action	Rationale
	• Roll of medical tape • A needle for administering the medication, typically 25 mm long and 21–23 ga • Plaster. 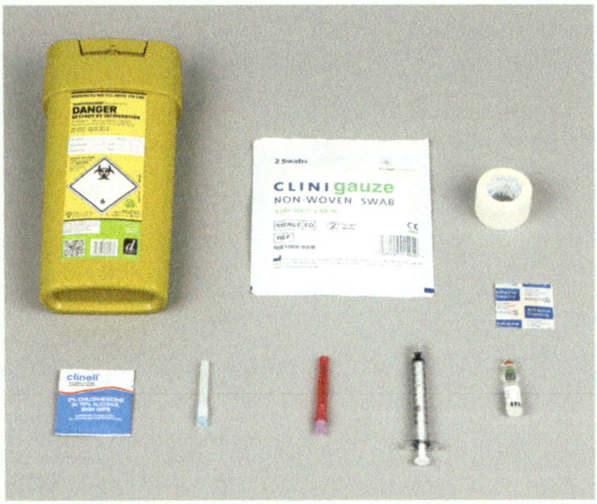	
4.	Follow the ampoule drawing-up procedure to prepare the medication in the syringe for administration.	
5.	Inspect the site for injection. In prehospital practice the most appropriate location is typically the vastus lateralis, which is easily identified as the antero-lateral aspect of the thigh. Alternate sites include the deltoid muscle or ventrogluteal region. Here the deltoid is shown. 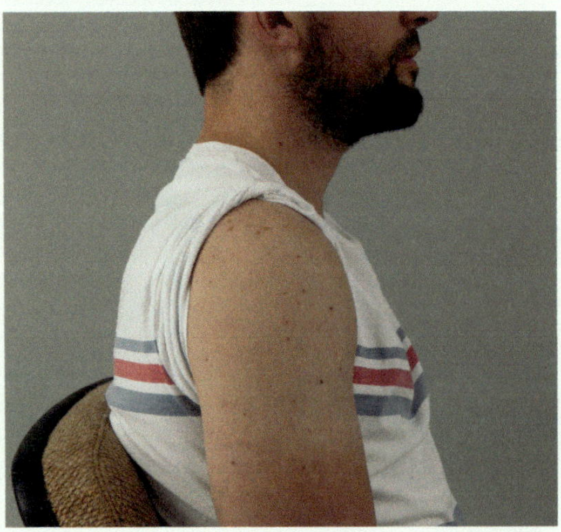	Site selection is based on identifying muscles with good vascular supplies but where the risk of causing neurovascular injury is low. The vastus lateralis is suitable for this, though in cases where this may not be possible (bilateral amputee or trauma, for example) you should be aware of the alternate sites.

Action		Rationale
6.	Thoroughly clean the site by using an appropriate skin-cleansing wipe (must contain 2% chlorhexidine in 70% isopropyl alcohol). 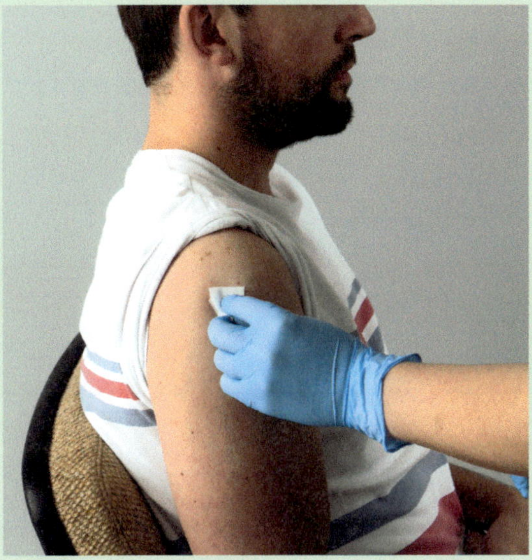	May reduce the risk of infection, although there is some debate as to whether this is necessary if the skin is not visibly dirty (5). Follow local guidance.
7.	Prior to administration, complete a med-check process. Your organisation may have a dedicated procedure for this, but if not, confirm the following with a colleague: • The drug to be administered • The reason for administration • The dose (and how this was calculated if relevant, for example, JRCALC Page for Age) • The route.	Drug errors are a common form of clinical error, especially in emergency situations. Taking a moment to check with a colleague can help to identify and potentially reduce drug administration errors.
8.	Firmly attach the needle to the syringe and remove the cap.	Ensure the needle is firmly attached so it does not accidentally become dislodged during the procedure.

Action		Rationale
9.	Using your non-dominant hand, apply gentle traction to the site where the injection will occur. 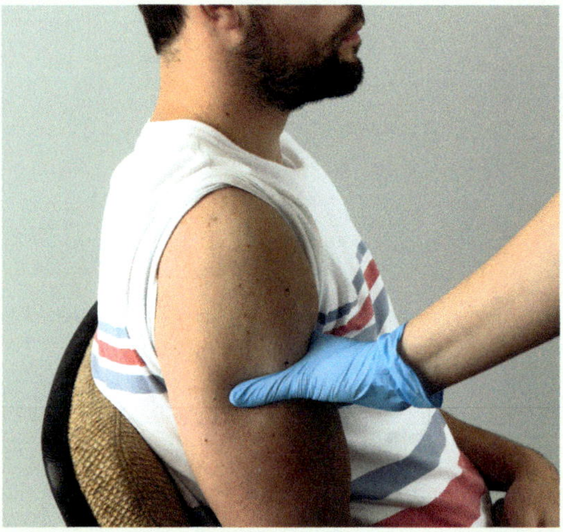	Applying traction is the first part of the 'Z-track technique' which helps to keep injected fluid in the muscle when the needle is removed. Once applied, maintain traction until the needle is withdrawn (6).
10.	Warn the patient of a sharp scratch. Holding the syringe in your dominant hand like a dart, insert the needle at a 90° angle to the skin. Insert quickly with the bevel of the needle facing upwards. 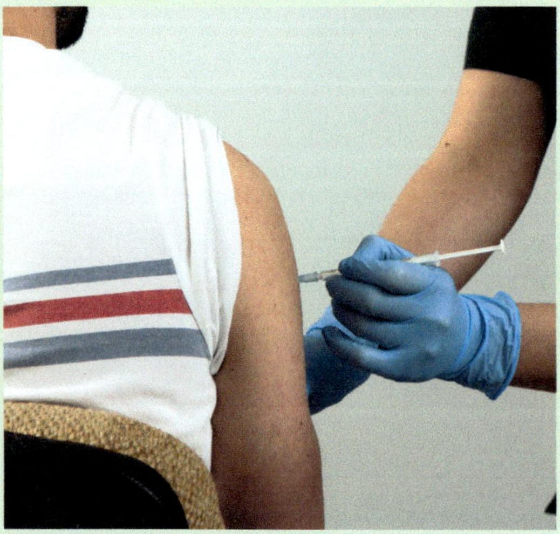	The depth of the muscle under the surface will vary, and consideration should be given to this based on a visual assessment of the patient's body habitus. Adjust the depth of insertion as appropriate.

Action		Rationale
11.	Aspirate the syringe and observe for blood. If blood is seen, remove the needle, prepare a fresh syringe and try again in a different location. 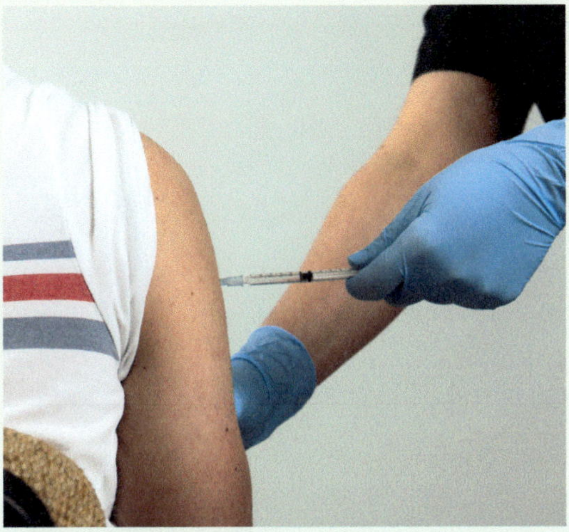	This will ensure the tip of the needle is not placed within a vessel.
12.	Inject the fluid at a rate of approximately 1 ml every 10 seconds. Once all the fluid has been injected, leave the needle in situ for a further 10 seconds before removing. 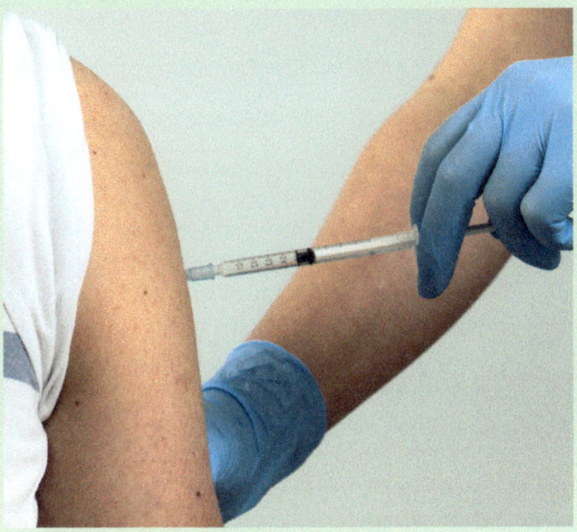	This rate is less painful than a faster injection and allows time for the fluid to be distributed into the muscle.
13.	Remove the needle and immediately place into a sharps bin.	This reduces the risk of an inadvertent sharps injury.

	Action	Rationale
14.	Release traction on the skin and apply pressure with a small patch of gauze for a few seconds. 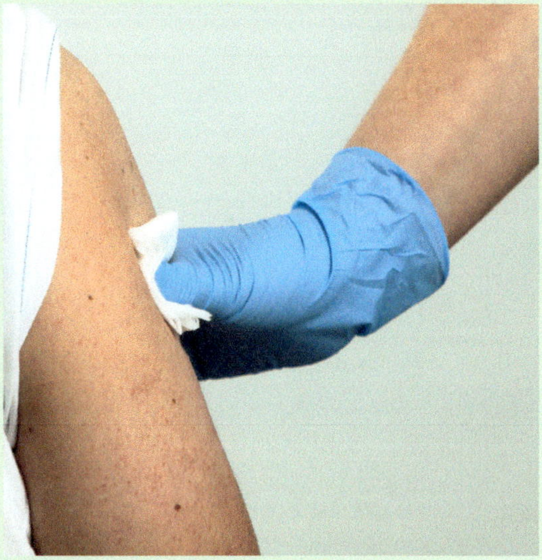	
15.	Replace the gauze with a small plaster.	This ensures the site is covered and kept clean after the injection has been administered.
16.	Document the procedure.	You must keep full, clear and accurate records for everyone you care for, treat, or provide other services to (3).

References

1. Geeky Medics. Intramuscular injection (IM) – OSCE guide [Internet]. 2021 [cited 2022 Aug 21]. Available from: https://geekymedics.com/intramuscular-injection-im-osce-guide/.
2. British Medical Association. Ethics – General information [Internet]. 2018 [cited 2019 Dec 29]. Available from: www.bma.org.uk/advice/employment/ethics/consent/consent-tool-kit/2-general-information.
3. Health and Care Professions Council. Standards of conduct, performance and ethics [Internet]. 2016 [cited 2022 Jul 16]. Available from: www.hcpc-uk.org/standards/standards-of-conduct-performance-and-ethics/.
4. NHS England. Standard infection control precautions: National hand hygiene and personal protective equipment policy [Internet]. 2019 [cited 2022 Feb 13]. Available from: www.england.nhs.uk/publication/standard-infection-control-precautions-national-hand-hygiene-and-personal-protective-equipment-policy/.
5. UK Health Security Agency. Immunisation procedures: The green book, chapter 4 [Internet]. 2013 [cited 2022 Oct 31] Available from: https://www.gov.uk/government/publications/immunisation-procedures-the-green-book-chapter-4.
6. Nicoll LH, Hesby A. Intramuscular injection: An integrative research review and guideline for evidence-based practice. *Applied Nursing Research*. 2002;15(3):149–162.

Rectal Administration

Indications

- To administer appropriate drugs rectally, for example rectal diazepam.

Contraindications

- Drugs not intended for rectal administration.
- Other, more appropriate routes are available.
- Anal or peri-anal trauma or recent surgery.

Advantages

- Can be used in the full range of ages when other routes are not available or not safe, for example during seizures, when intravenous access may not be possible.

Disadvantages

- Passing stool or diarrhoea around the time of administration will reduce efficacy of absorption.
- Low level of patient acceptance of procedure.
- Can trigger an episode of autonomic dysreflexia in patients with spinal cord injury.

Procedure – Rectal Administration

Take the following steps to administer drugs via the rectal (PR) route (1,2):

Action		Rationale
1.	Explain the procedure and obtain consent if appropriate to do so.	You must make sure that you have valid consent from service users or other appropriate authority before you provide care, treatment or other services (3,4).
2.	Don appropriate personal protective equipment (PPE), and undertake appropriate hand hygiene.	This reduces the risk of cross-infection (5).
3.	Due to the intimate nature of the procedure, you should always have a chaperone present. Follow your organisation's chaperone policy.	
4.	Position the patient appropriately: • For adults and large children: Position them on their side. • For smaller children: Consider placing them on their front. 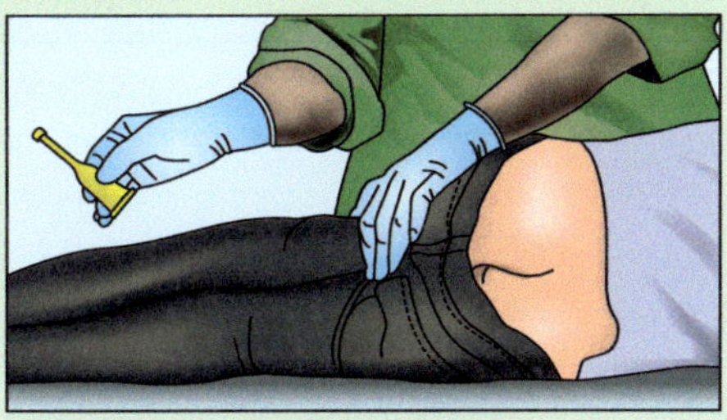	Appropriate positioning of the patient will make administration easier, though consider the overall patient condition. Placing a seizing child on their front may compromise their airway, so consider carefully the most appropriate position.

Action		Rationale
5.	Inspect the packaging: • Ensure the packaging is intact • Check the expiry date. If packaging is intact and in date, rip open the foil and remove the medication.	If packaging is damaged or the expiry date has passed, the medication must not be used.
6.	Remove the cap from the end of the rectal tube.	
7.	Prior to administration, complete a med-check process. Your organisation may have a dedicated procedure for this, but if not, confirm the following with a colleague: • The drug to be administered • The reason for administration • The dose (and how this was calculated if relevant, for example, JRCALC Page for Age) • The route.	Drug errors are a common form of clinical error, especially in emergency situations. Taking a moment to check with a colleague can help to identify and potentially reduce drug administration errors.
8.	Using one hand to lift the upper buttock (in a patient lying on their side) to reveal the anus, insert the nozzle completely into the rectum. For children under 15 kg insert the nozzle half-way. 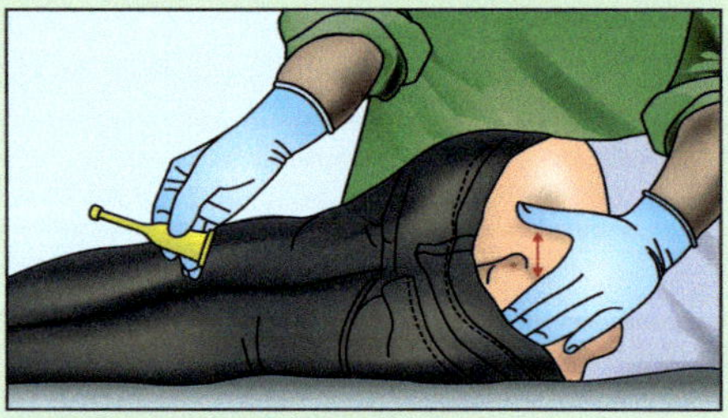	The nozzle should only be inserted half-way in small children due to the length of the rectum and a small increased risk of internal injury occurring.
9.	Empty the tube by firmly pressing the medication reservoir between the thumb and forefinger. 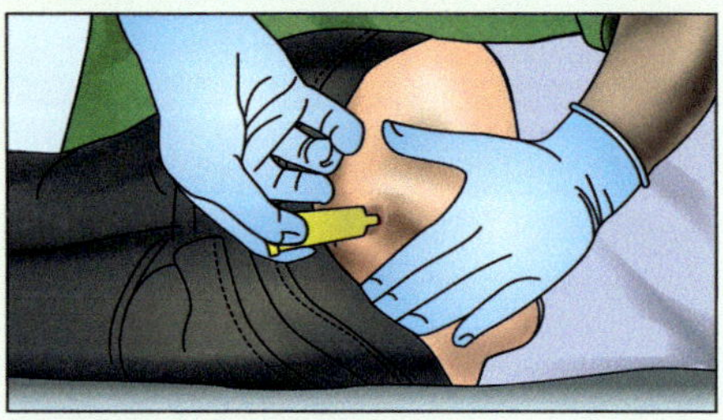	Keep the reservoir pressed until the rectal tube has been removed to prevent it from invertedly suctioning the medication out.

Action		Rationale
10.	Remove the tube and dispose of into a clinical waste bin.	
11.	If possible and safe, maintain the patient in the side or face-down position for a couple of minutes.	Maintaining position will help to improve drug absorption.
12.	Document the procedure.	You must keep full, clear and accurate records for everyone you care for, treat, or provide other services to (4).

References

1. Lowry M. Rectal drug administration in adults: How, when, why. *Nursing Times*. 2016;112(8):12–14.
2. Wockhardt. Diazepam RecTubes: Patient Leaflet [Internet]. 2019 [cited 2022 Aug 22]. Available from: www.medicines.org.uk/emc/files/pil.6799.pdf.
3. British Medical Association. Ethics – General Information [Internet]. 2018 [cited 2019 Dec 29]. Available from: www.bma.org.uk/advice/employment/ethics/consent/consent-tool-kit/2-general-information.
4. Health and Care Professions Council. Standards of conduct, performance and ethics [Internet]. 2016 [cited 2022 Jul 16]. Available from: www.hcpc-uk.org/standards/standards-of-conduct-performance-and-ethics/.
5. NHS England. Standard infection control precautions: National hand hygiene and personal protective equipment policy [Internet]. 2019 [cited 2022 Feb 13]. Available from: www.england.nhs.uk/publication/standard-infection-control-precautions-national-hand-hygiene-and-personal-protective-equipment-policy/.

Intranasal Administration

Indications

- Administration of drugs suitable for intranasal administration.

Contraindications

- When other routes are more clinically appropriate.
- Legal authority to administer drugs via intranasal route is absent (for example, a medication cannot be administered under a patient group direction (PGD) unless it has *intranasal* listed in approved routes of administration).

Cautions

- Changes to the nasal mucosal characteristics, including the presence of mucus and/or blood, that may impact on drug absorption.

Advantages

- Allows for medication to be administered without the need for sharps to be used.
- Less invasive than other routes.

Disadvantages

- Absorption is less predictable and slower than some other routes (intravenous or intramuscular) (1).

Procedure – Intranasal Administration

Take the following steps to administer drugs via the intranasal route (2):

Action		Rationale
1.	Explain the procedure and obtain consent if appropriate to do so.	You must make sure that you have valid consent from service users or other appropriate authority before you provide care, treatment or other services (3,4).
2.	Don appropriate personal protective equipment (PPE), and undertake appropriate hand hygiene.	This reduces the risk of cross-infection (5).

Action		Rationale
3.	Prepare the required equipment. For this procedure you will need: • The appropriate medication • An appropriately sized Luer Lock syringe (1 ml, 2 ml or 3 ml) depending on the volume to be administered • A blunt filter drawing-up needle • Sharps bin • A nasal atomiser device • A syringe label (if appropriate). 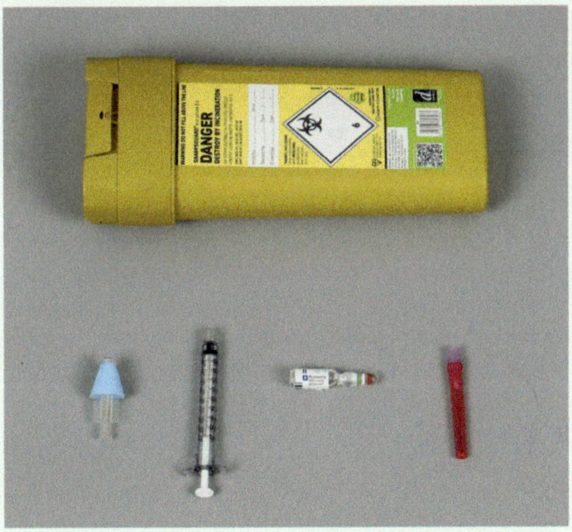	Preparing all equipment in advance will help ensure the process is completed without unnecessary interruptions.
4.	Follow the procedure for drawing up an ampoule to prepare the medication in the syringe. Only draw up the amount of medication to be administered, plus an additional 0.1 ml, as this accounts for the dead space inside the nasal atomiser device.	Drawing up only the required amount reduces the risk of inadvertently administering too much medication.

	Action	Rationale
5.	Connect the nasal atomiser device to the syringe by screwing it into the Luer Lock connector. 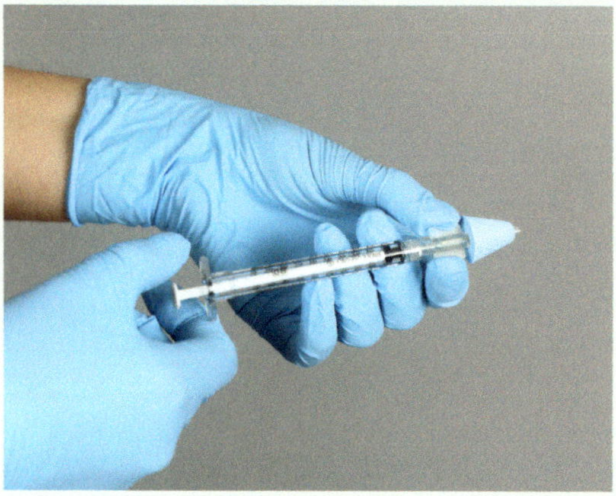	Luer Lock connectors are more secure than Luer Slip connectors. Using a Luer Lock will ensure the atomiser device does not become detached from the syringe or leak during administration.
6.	Prior to administration, complete a med-check process. Your organisation may have a dedicated procedure for this, but if not, confirm the following with a colleague: • The drug to be administered • The reason for administration • The dose (and how this was calculated if relevant, for example, JRCALC Age per Page). • The route.	Drug errors are a common form of clinical error, especially in emergency situations. Taking a moment to check with a colleague can help to identify and potentially reduce drug administration errors.
7.	Using your free hand to hold the occiput of the patient's head stable, place the tip of the nasal atomiser device snugly against the nostril, aiming slightly up and outward (towards the top of the ear). 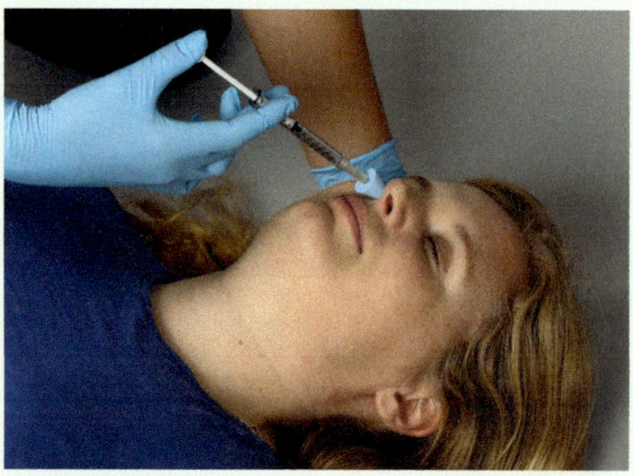	This direction will help to distribute the aerosolised medication across a greater surface area of nasal mucosa.

Action		Rationale
8.	Briskly depress the plunger and deliver half of the medication into one nostril.	In order for medication to be effectively delivered, it needs to be atomised, which is best achieved with a brisk push on the syringe. Pushing too slowly will result in fluid being released as droplets, which will be absorbed less effectively.
9.	Move the syringe and nasal atomiser device to the other nostril and repeat steps 7 and 8 to deliver the remaining 50% of the medication. 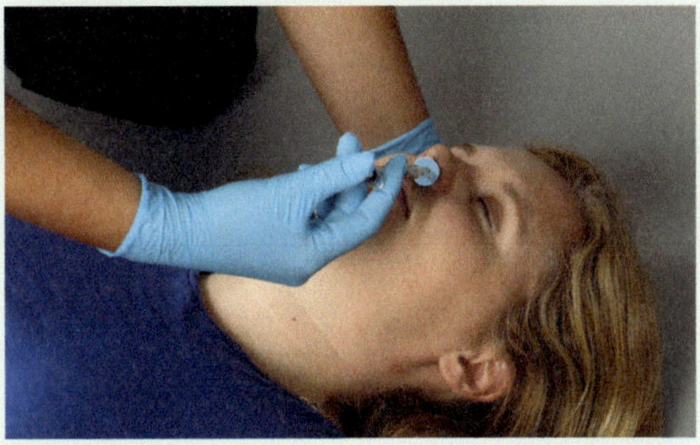	Switching nostrils will increase the total surface area over which the atomised drug is delivered. This should make absorption more effective.
10.	Document the procedure.	You must keep full, clear and accurate records for everyone you care for, treat, or provide other services to (4).

References

1. Dietze P, Jauncey M, Salmon A, et al. Effect of intranasal vs intramuscular naloxone on opioid overdose: A randomized clinical trial. *JAMA Network Open*. 2019;2(11):e1914977.
2. Teleflex. MAD Nasal™ intranasal mucosal atomization device [Internet]. 2017 [cited 2022 Aug 8]. Available from: www.teleflex.com/usa/en/product-areas/anesthesia/atomization/mad-nasal-device/AN_ATM_Anesthesia-MAD-Nasal-User-Guide_MC_MC-001925_Rev1.pdf.
3. British Medical Association. Ethics – General information [Internet]. 2018 [cited 2019 Dec 29]. Available from: www.bma.org.uk/advice/employment/ethics/consent/consent-tool-kit/2-general-information.
4. Health and Care Professions Council. Standards of conduct, performance and ethics [Internet]. 2016 [cited 2022 Jul 16]. Available from: www.hcpc-uk.org/standards/standards-of-conduct-performance-and-ethics/.
5. NHS England. Standard infection control precautions: National hand hygiene and personal protective equipment policy [Internet]. 2019 [cited 2022 Feb 13]. Available from: www.england.nhs.uk/publication/standard-infection-control-precautions-national-hand-hygiene-and-personal-protective-equipment-policy/.

Chapter

6 Trauma

Prehospital clinicians will frequently attend a wide variety of traumatic incidents, from the relatively minor injury through to life-threatening multi-system trauma. Major trauma remains a leading cause of death of young people in the UK (1) and many of these deaths may be prevented with early appropriate clinical intervention.

Due to the fact that some skills need to be performed on a more regular basis, you will rapidly become familiar with certain techniques, like spinal immobilisation. Opportunities to use other skills, such as femoral traction, are likely to occur less frequently, and regular practice or revision of the appropriate technique may be required to ensure that, when called upon, you can remember how to perform that intervention.

As with many aspects of medicine, a range of devices exist, and often there are even multiple devices available for the same intervention. An example here, which will be covered in more detail later in this chapter, is pelvic binders. Numerous binders exist, but there is no compelling evidence to suggest that one saves more lives than the others. What is clear from the literature is that despite the relative simplicity of these devices, they are often applied incorrectly and risk doing more damage than benefit, unless care is taken in ensuring their correct application.

It would not have been possible to cover all the devices available for prehospital trauma patients, so instead we have selected a number of the more common devices found in practice and described these. It is important that you are familiar with the equipment available in your service and the local guidelines and standard operating procedures governing their use.

While this chapter will cover in detail devices utilised when for caring for trauma patients, it cannot replace the benefits of hands-on practise. Seek out opportunities to develop expertise in the use of these pieces of equipment with the procedures in the following pages to help guide your practice.

References

1. Office for National Statistics. Leading causes of death, UK: 2001 to 2018. [Internet]. 2020 [cited 2022 Sep 16]. Available from: https://www.ons.gov.uk/peoplepopulationandcommunity/healthandsocialcare/causesofdeath/articles/leadingcausesofdeathuk/2001to2018.

Broad Arm Sling

Indications
- To provide support to an injury of the arm.

Contraindications
- None – though consider whether other forms of splinting or immobilisation may be more appropriate, for example, vacuum splint.

Advantages
- Simple to apply.
- Minimal equipment required.
- Can provide effective analgesia by supporting the weight of the limb.

Disadvantages
- Does not provide complete immobilisation of the limb.

Procedure – Broad Arm Sling

Take the following steps to apply a broad arm sling (1,2):

Action		Rationale
1.	Explain the procedure and obtain consent if appropriate to do so.	You must make sure that you have valid consent from service users or other appropriate authority before you provide care, treatment or other services (3,4).
2.	Don appropriate personal protective equipment (PPE), and undertake appropriate hand hygiene.	This reduces the risk of cross-infection (5).
3.	Ensure that all clothing is removed from the injured limb and a full neurovascular assessment has been completed. Any wounds should be dressed.	Injured limbs should be exposed so they can be fully assessed. A neurovascular assessment will help to determine the injury and appropriate management. This should be completed before deciding to apply a sling.
4.	Ensure the patient has adequate analgesia.	Moving the limb can be painful, so ensure appropriate analgesia has been administered.

Action		Rationale
5.	Ask the patient to support their injured arm with the uninjured arm and to flex the elbow to 90°. 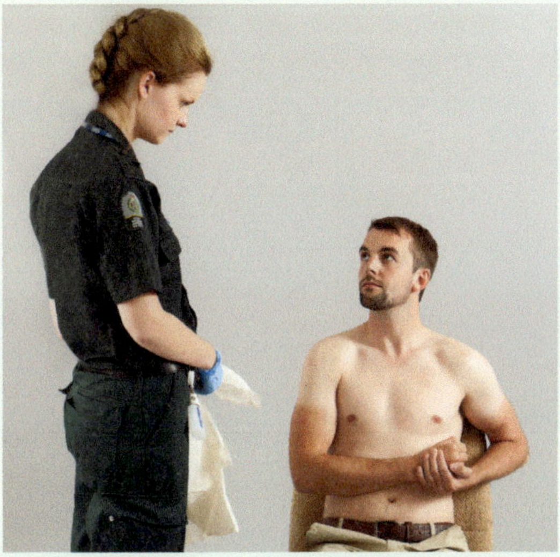	This will position the arm appropriately to give you space to introduce the triangular bandage.
6.	Open the triangular bandage and gently pass it under the injured arm with the point under the elbow of the injured arm. 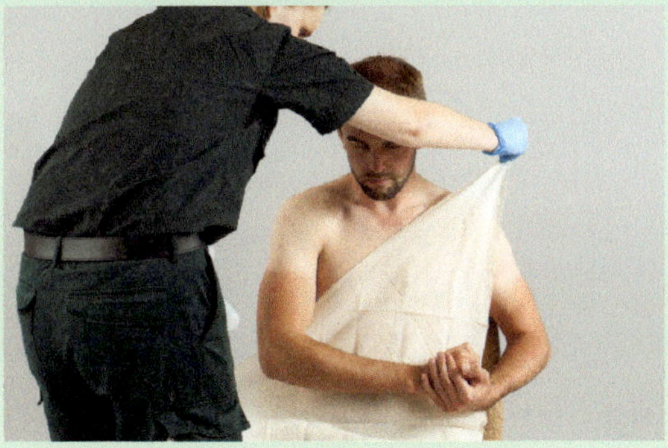	The widest part of the triangular bandage should be under the arm to provide maximum support.

Action		Rationale
7.	Slide the upper end of the triangular bandage around the back of the neck towards the shoulder on the injured side. 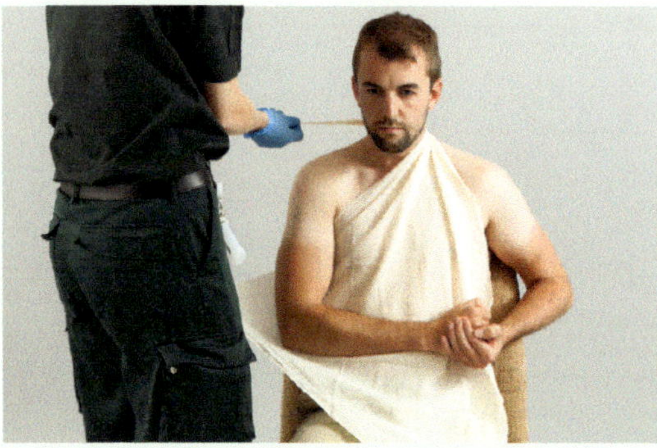	This is done in anticipation of being tied to the other end.
8.	Lift the other end of the triangular bandage up over the forearm. 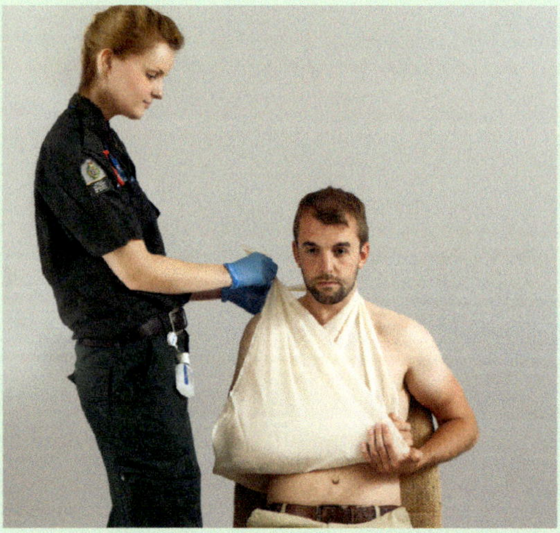	

Action		Rationale
9.	Tie the two ends together, preferably using a reef knot, to the side of the neck. Consider using a piece of gauze padding under the knot if it sits directly on skin. 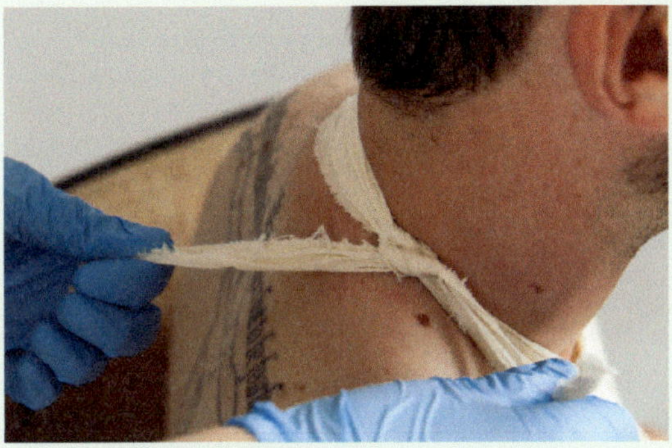	A reef knot will not slip when pressure is applied, and keeping the knot off the neck reduces the risk of pressure injury.
10.	Take hold of the point of the bandage beyond the elbow and twist until the fabric is snug to the elbow. Then fold the excess into the bandage or tape it to the outside. 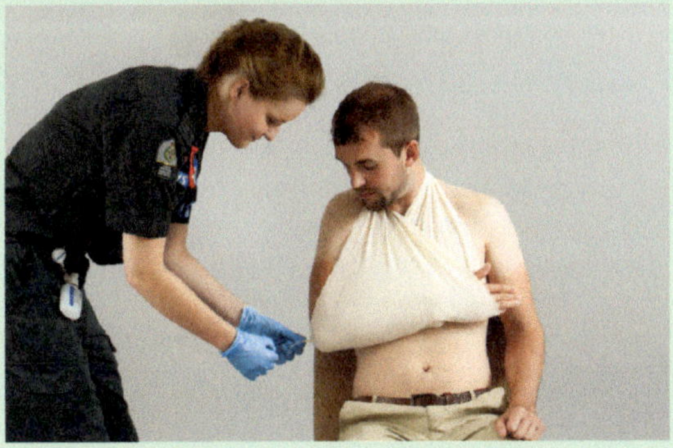	This keeps the sling in shape and stops the arm sliding out at the back.

Action		Rationale
11.	Recheck the limb distally for any change in neurovascular status. 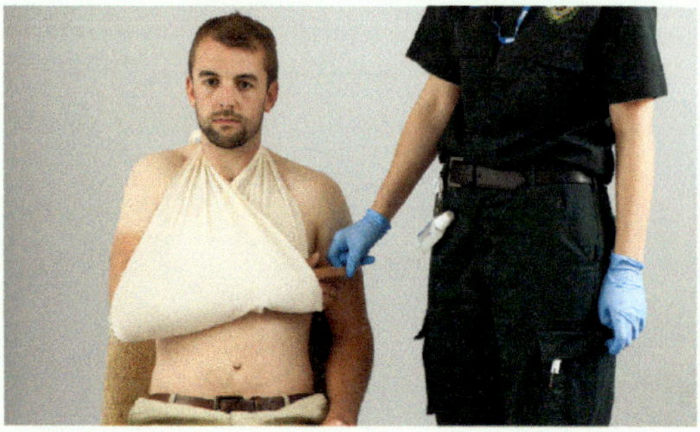	Neurovascular compromise can result in long-term injury to the limb or in the worst cases death of the limb tissue, rendering the limb unsalvageable.
12.	Document the procedure.	You must keep full, clear and accurate records for everyone you care for, treat, or provide other services to (4).

References

1. St John Ambulance. How to make an arm sling [Internet]. 2021 [cited 2022 Jul 25]. Available from: www.sja.org.uk/get-advice/first-aid-advice/how-to/how-to-make-an-arm-sling/.
2. Queensland Ambulance Service. Trauma/Bandaging – Simple bandaging and slings [Internet]. 2020 [cited 2022 Jul 25]. Available from: www.ambulance.qld.gov.au/docs/clinical/cpp/CPP_Bandaging_Simple%20bandaging.pdf.
3. British Medical Association. Ethics – General information [Internet]. 2018 [cited 2019 Dec 29]. Available from: www.bma.org.uk/advice/employment/ethics/consent/consent-tool-kit/2-general-information.
4. Health and Care Professions Council. Standards of conduct, performance and ethics [Internet]. 2016 [cited 2022 Jul 16]. Available from: www.hcpc-uk.org/standards/standards-of-conduct-performance-and-ethics/.
5. NHS England. Standard infection control precautions: National hand hygiene and personal protective equipment policy [Internet]. 2019 [cited 2022 Feb 13]. Available from: www.england.nhs.uk/publication/standard-infection-control-precautions-national-hand-hygiene-and-personal-protective-equipment-policy/.

Elevated Arm Sling

Indications

- To provide support to an injury of the arm.

Contraindications

- None – though consider whether other forms of splinting or immobilisation may be more appropriate, for example, vacuum splint.

Advantages

- Simple to apply.
- Minimal equipment required.
- Can provide effective analgesia by supporting the weight of the limb.
- Elevation may help to control bleeding or minimise swelling to hand.

Disadvantages

- Does not provide complete immobilisation of the limb.

Procedure – Elevated Arm Sling

Take the following steps to apply an elevated arm sling (1,2):

Action		Rationale
1.	If the patient is conscious, explain the procedure and obtain consent if appropriate to do so.	You must make sure that you have valid consent from service users or other appropriate authority before you provide care, treatment or other services (3,4).
2.	Don appropriate personal protective equipment (PPE), and undertake appropriate hand hygiene.	This reduces the risk of cross-infection (5).
3.	Ensure that all clothing is removed from the injured limb and a full neurovascular assessment has been completed. Any wounds should be dressed.	Injured limbs should be exposed so they can be fully assessed. A neurovascular assessment will help to determine the injury and appropriate management. This should be completed before deciding to apply a sling.
4.	Ensure the patient has adequate analgesia.	Moving the limb can be painful, so ensure appropriate analgesia has been administered.

Action		Rationale
5.	Ask the patient to support their injured arm with the uninjured arm. The injured arm should be placed across their chest with the fingers of the injured arm resting on the opposite shoulder. 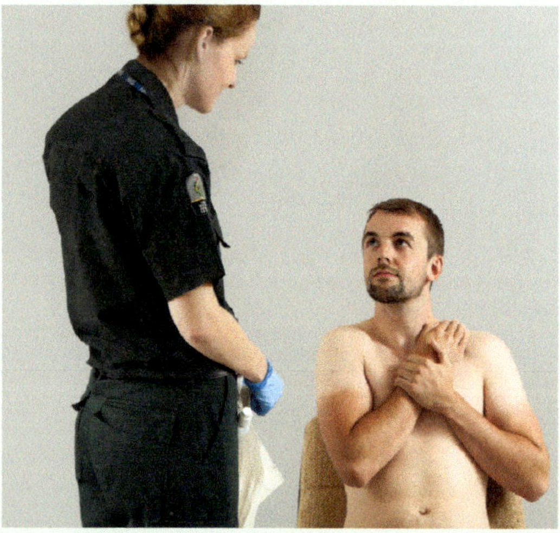	This will position the arm appropriately to give you space to introduce the triangular bandage.
6.	Place the triangular bandage over the injured arm with the point on the bandage just beyond the elbow of the injured arm. 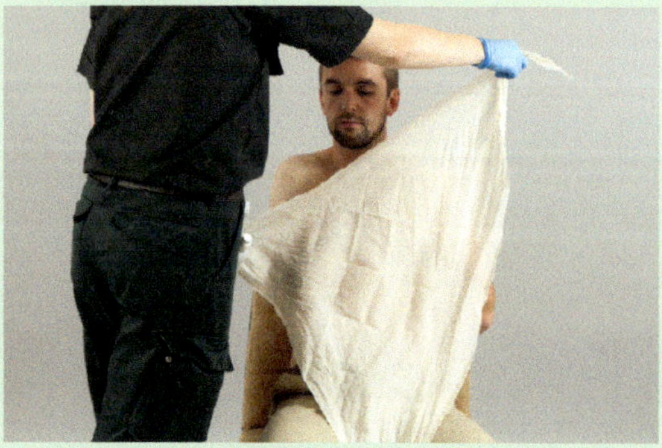	

Action		Rationale
7.	Ask the patient to let go of the injured arm and tuck the bandage under the injured arm and bring it around to their back. 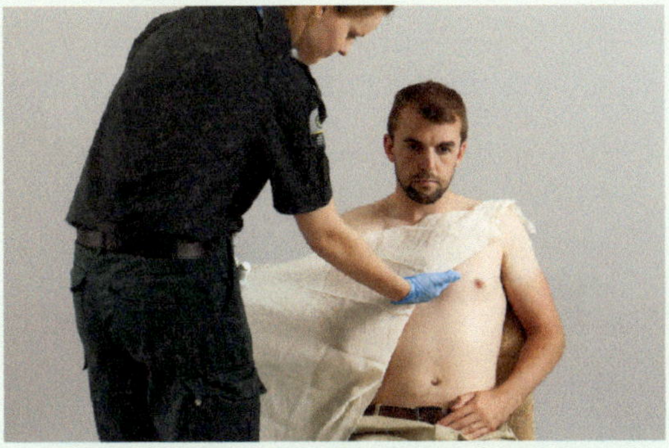	Tucking the bandage under the arm ensures it will support the injured arm once tied.
8.	Bring the bandage up across the patients back to meet the other end at the shoulder on the uninjured side. 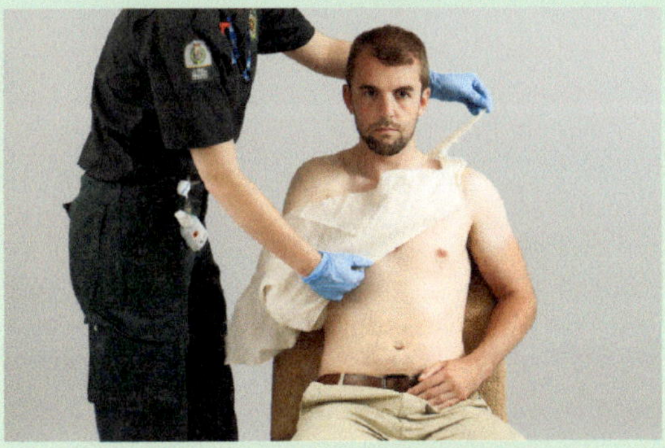	
9.	Tie the two ends together, preferably using a reef knot, to the side of the neck. Consider using a piece of gauze padding under the knot if it sits directly on skin. 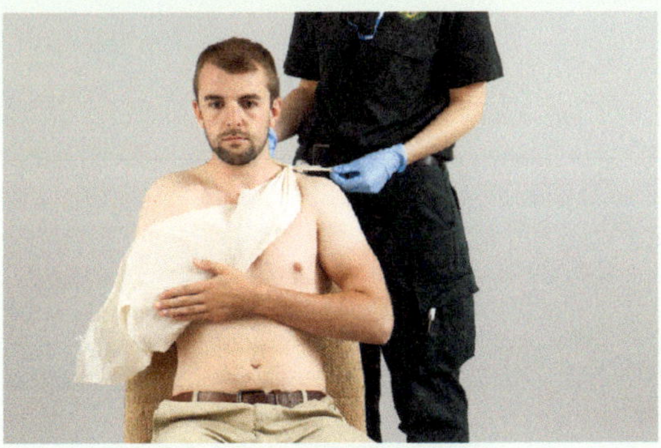	A reef knot will not slip when pressure is applied, and keeping the knot off the neck reduces the risk of pressure injury.

	Action	Rationale
10.	Take hold of the point of the bandage beyond the elbow and twist until the fabric is snug to the elbow. Then fold the excess into the bandage or tape it to the outside. 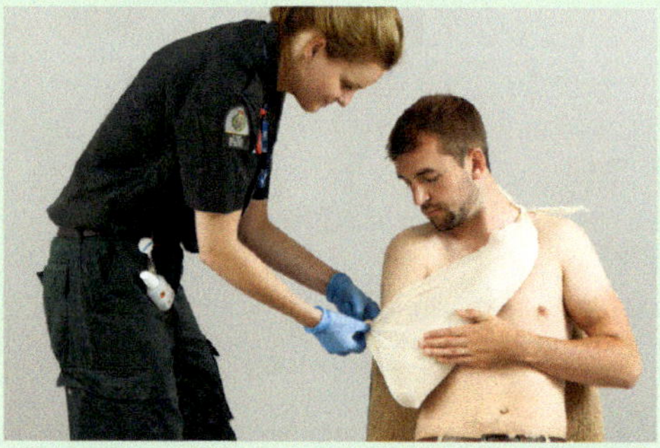	This keeps the sling in shape and stops the arm sliding out at the back.
11.	Recheck the limb distally for any change in neurovascular status. 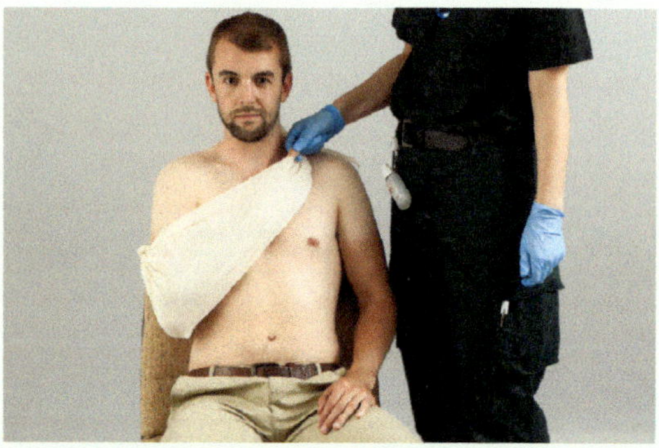	Neurovascular compromise can result in long-term injury to the limb or in the worst cases death of the limb tissue, rendering the limb unsalvageable.
12.	Document the procedure.	You must keep full, clear and accurate records for everyone you care for, treat, or provide other services to (4).

References

1. Queensland Ambulance Service. Trauma/Bandaging – Simple bandaging and slings [Internet]. 2020 [cited 2022 Jul 25]. Available from: www.ambulance.qld.gov.au/docs/clinical/cpp/CPP_Bandaging_Simple%20bandaging.pdf.
2. St John Ambulance. How to make an elevation sling [Internet]. 2021 [cited 2022 Jul 31]. Available from: www.sja.org.uk/get-advice/first-aid-advice/how-to/how-to-make-an-elevation-sling/.
3. British Medical Association. Ethics – General information [Internet]. 2018 [cited 2019 Dec 29]. Available from: www.bma.org.uk/advice/employment/ethics/consent/consent-tool-kit/2-general-information.
4. Health and Care Professions Council. Standards of conduct, performance and ethics [Internet]. 2016 [cited 2022 Jul 16]. Available from: www.hcpc-uk.org/standards/standards-of-conduct-performance-and-ethics/.
5. NHS England. Standard infection control precautions: National hand hygiene and personal protective equipment policy [Internet]. 2019 [cited 2022 Feb 13]. Available from: www.england.nhs.uk/publication/standard-infection-control-precautions-national-hand-hygiene-and-personal-protective-equipment-policy/.

Box Splint

Indications

- To immobilise a limb, typically due to a suspected fracture or dislocation.

Contraindications

- None – though consider whether other forms of immobilisation may be more appropriate, for example, a traction splint for isolated mid-shaft femur fracture.

Advantages

- Unlike vacuum splints, box splints are not easily damaged and will continue to work if minor damage is caused to the coverings.

Disadvantages

- Does not conform to the patient's limb, so may provide less effective immobilisation.
- Can only be used on straight limbs without significant deformity.

Procedure – Box Splint

Take the following steps to apply a box splint:

Action		Rationale
1.	If the patient is conscious, explain the procedure and obtain consent if appropriate to do so.	You must make sure that you have valid consent from service users or other appropriate authority before you provide care, treatment or other services (1,2).
2.	Don appropriate personal protective equipment (PPE), and undertake appropriate hand hygiene.	This reduces the risk of cross-infection (3).
3.	Ensure that all clothing is removed from the injured limb and a full neurovascular assessment has been completed. Any wounds should be dressed.	Injured limbs should be exposed so they can be fully assessed. No clothing should be included inside a box splint as this may contribute to a pressure injury. A neurovascular assessment will help to determine the injury and appropriate management. This should be completed before deciding to apply a splint.
4.	Choose an appropriately sized splint.	If possible, you should choose a splint that immobilises the joint above and below the anticipated injury. For example, if a tibial fracture is suspected, then the splint should be long enough to immobilise the tibia, knee and ankle.

Action		Rationale
5.	Ensure the patient has received adequate analgesia. 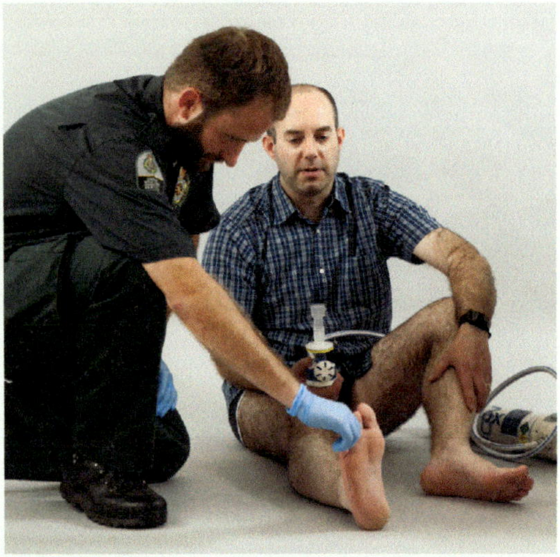	Splinting and moving the limb to apply a splint can be painful, so ensure appropriate analgesia has been administered.
6.	Open the splint and place it next to, or in line with, the injured limb with the Velcro pointing out towards you. Prepare additional padding in the form of a sheet, blanket or incontinence sheets, which may be required.	Prepare in advance so that once the limb is moved you are ready to insert the splint quickly and smoothly.
7.	In a coordinated move with other team members, lift the limb just enough to move the splint into position. Warn the patient in advance. 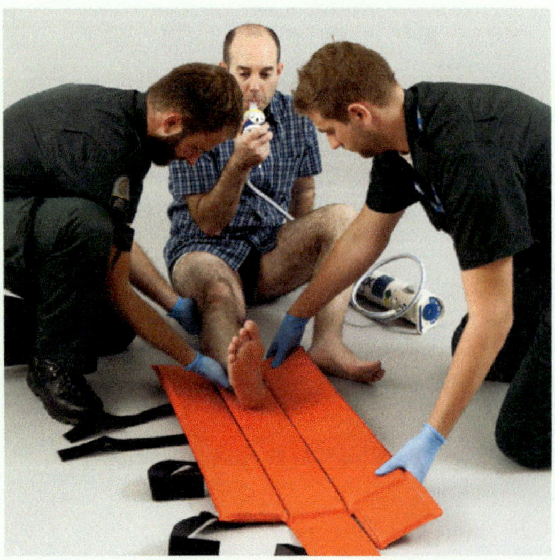	Minimal movement is important to avoid causing additional pain or worsening the injury.

Action		Rationale
8.	Once the splint is in position, lower the limb back on to the splint.	
9.	Lift the two side pieces to create an open box shape around the limb. If the splint is being applied to a lower limb, there may be a foot plate. This should be lifted so that it sits against the sole of the foot. All of these pieces should be firm but not tight against the skin of the limb. 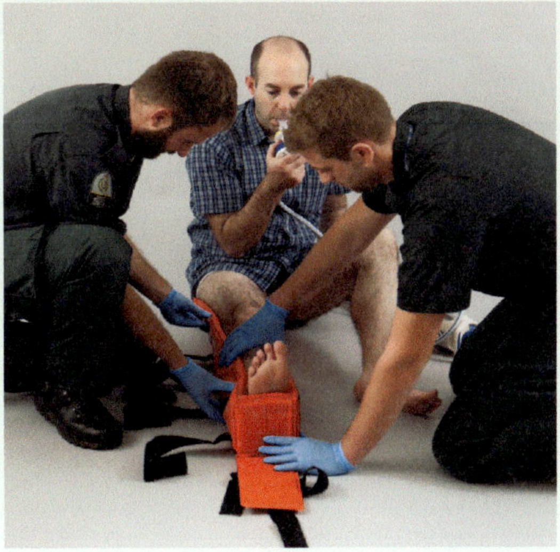	These sections provide the stability of the splint so should be firmly in place, though not so tight as to potentially cause a pressure injury.

Action		Rationale
10.	Gently fasten the Velcro straps to the opposite side of the splint, taking care to avoid placing straps directly over the site of the injury. Straps from the foot plate should cross over the top of the foot to provide additional lateral strength to the splint. 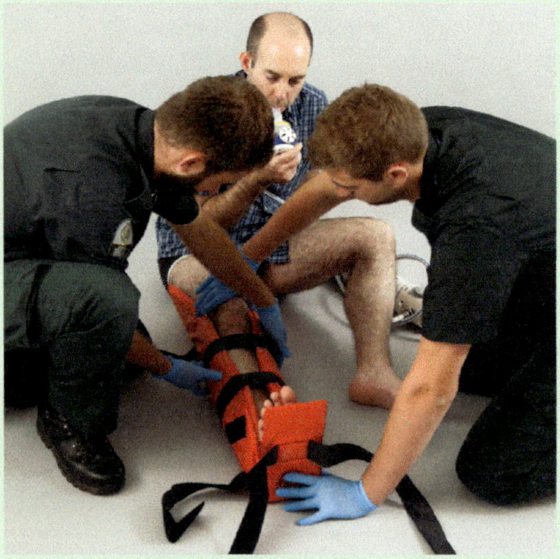	These straps will provide the ongoing stability of the splint so should be firmly stuck down. Avoid placing straps directly over the injury as this may apply pressure, causing more pain and potentially worsening the injury.
11.	If there are large gaps around the limb inside the splint, consider padding the voids with soft items such as incontinence sheets for transport.	Movement of fractured limbs caused by extrication and transport can be very painful and potentially cause further injury. Padding may help to reduce this, though this must be balanced against the potential risk of causing a pressure injury. If padding is used, it should be removed upon arrival at hospital.

Action		Rationale
12.	Recheck distal pulse and sensation for any change in neurovascular status now the limb has been immobilised. You may need to reposition the limb if neurovascular status has been compromised during immobilisation. 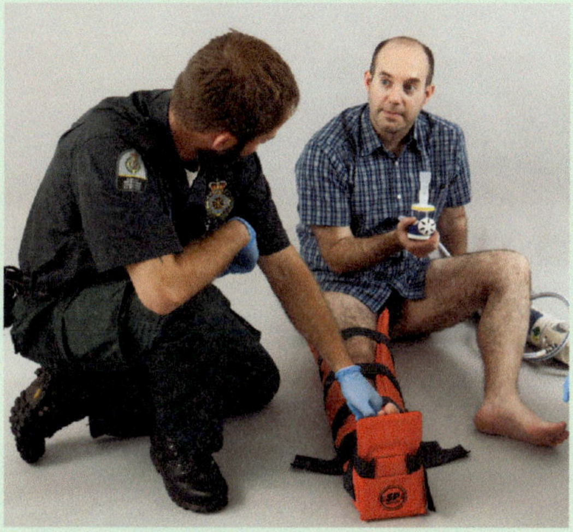	Neurovascular compromise can result in long-term injury to the limb or in the worst cases death of the limb tissue, rendering the limb unsalvageable.
13.	Document the procedure.	You must keep full, clear and accurate records for everyone you care for, treat, or provide other services to (2).

References

1. British Medical Association. Ethics – General information [Internet]. 2018 [cited 2019 Dec 29]. Available from: www.bma.org.uk/advice/employment/ethics/consent/consent-tool-kit/2-general-information.
2. Health and Care Professions Council. Standards of conduct, performance and ethics [Internet]. 2016 [cited 2022 Jul 16]. Available from: www.hcpc-uk.org/standards/standards-of-conduct-performance-and-ethics/.
3. NHS England. Standard infection control precautions: National hand hygiene and personal protective equipment policy [Internet]. 2019 [cited 2022 Feb 13]. Available from: www.england.nhs.uk/publication/standard-infection-control-precautions-national-hand-hygiene-and-personal-protective-equipment-policy/.

Vacuum Splint

Indications

- To immobilise a limb, typically due to a suspected fracture or dislocation.

Contraindications

- None – though consider whether other forms of immobilisation may be more appropriate, for example, a traction splint for isolated mid-shaft femur fracture.

Advantages

- Conforms to the patient's anatomy, resulting in a comfortable and rigid splint.

Disadvantages

- Requires a proprietary hand pump or suction unit to remove air from the splint.
- The splints are easily damaged; when damaged, they do not retain the vacuum and inflate, which results in a loss of immobilisation.

Procedure – Vacuum Splint

Take the following steps to apply a vacuum splint (1,2):

Action		Rationale
1.	If the patient is conscious, explain the procedure and obtain consent if appropriate to do so.	You must make sure that you have valid consent from service users or other appropriate authority before you provide care, treatment or other services (3,4).
2.	Don appropriate personal protective equipment (PPE), and undertake appropriate hand hygiene.	This reduces the risk of cross-infection (5).
3.	Ensure that all clothing is removed from the injured limb and a full neurovascular assessment has been completed. Any wound should be dressed.	Injured limbs should be exposed so they can be fully assessed. No clothing should be included inside a vacuum splint as this may contribute to a pressure injury. A neurovascular assessment will help to determine the injury and appropriate management. This should be completed before deciding to apply a splint.
4.	Choose an appropriately sized splint (generally, the joint above and below the injury should be immobilised too) and check it is working in advance.	Splints are easily damaged and it is not uncommon to find broken ones in kits. Test in advance that the splint holds its vacuum; finding out there is a leak after applying it means you will have to move the injured limb for a second time to replace it with a splint that is working.

Action		Rationale
5.	Ensure the patient has adequate analgesia.	Splinting and particularly moving the limb to apply a splint can be painful, so ensure appropriate analgesia has been administered.
6.	Open the splint and place it next to the injured limb with the valve pointing towards you. Open the valve to allow air to enter and use your hand to evenly distribute the polystyrene ball bearings inside so that the splint is flat. Securely close the valve.	Preparing the splint in advance will ensure it is ready to be applied to the patient. Distributing the polystyrene will ensure a flat and even splint that will provide even support all the way around the limb. Different manufactures use different valve designs, so study your specific vacuum splint to become familiar with the device you will be using.
7.	In a coordinated move with other team members, lift the limb just enough to slip the splint into position. Warn the patient in advance. 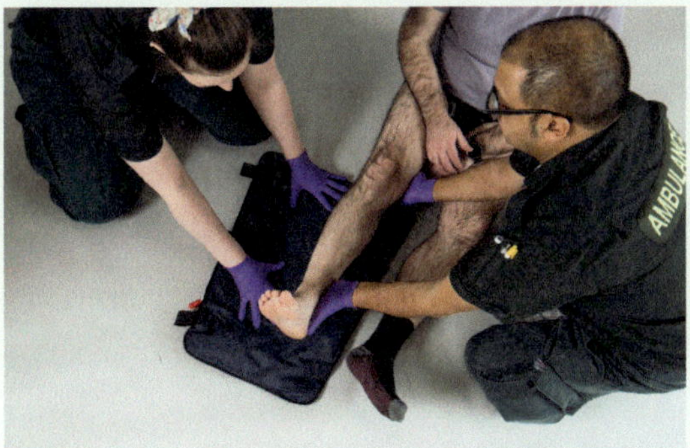	Minimal movement is important to avoid causing additional pain or potentially worsening the injury.

Action		Rationale
8.	Once the splint is in position, lower the limb back on to the splint. 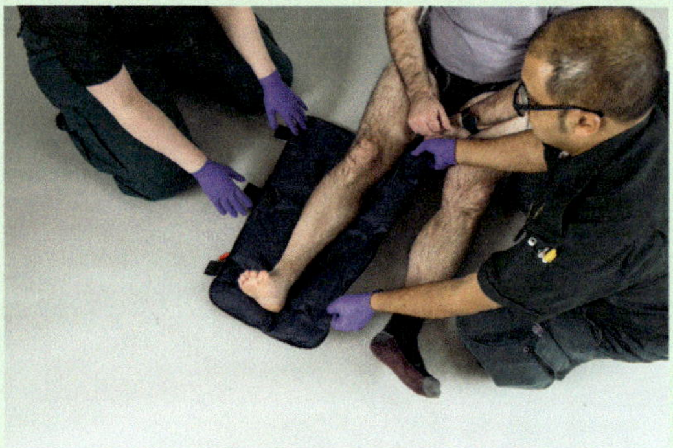	
9.	Form the splint around the injured limb. Try to leave the end of the splint open and a small gap of approximately 2.5 cm (1 in) along the top of the splint so the limb can still be visualised. If required, the straps can be loosely placed at this point to help keep the splint in shape. 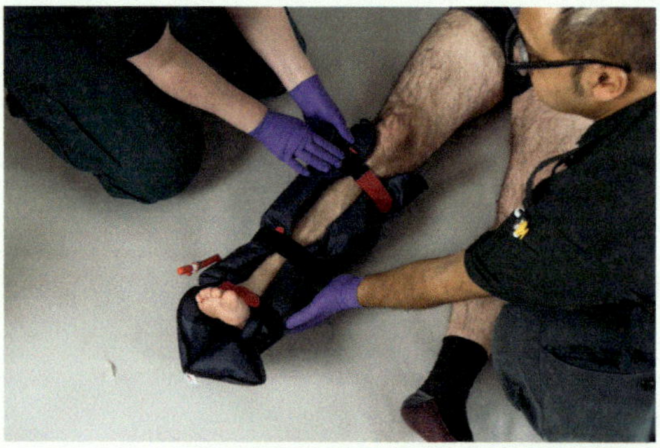	Forming the splint around the limb ensures it will be tight to the skin before the air is removed. Leaving a gap allows for easy reassessment once the splint has been tightened.

Action		Rationale
10.	Attach the pump to the valve and, while the splint is being held in position, another team member should operate the pump until the splint becomes firm. 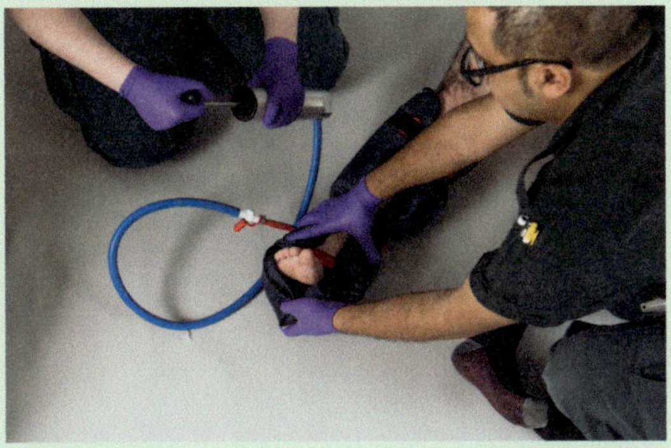	This will ensure that the vacuum splint remains closely conformed to the limb and maximise immobilisation once the air has been removed.
11.	Once the splint is firm, remove the pump. 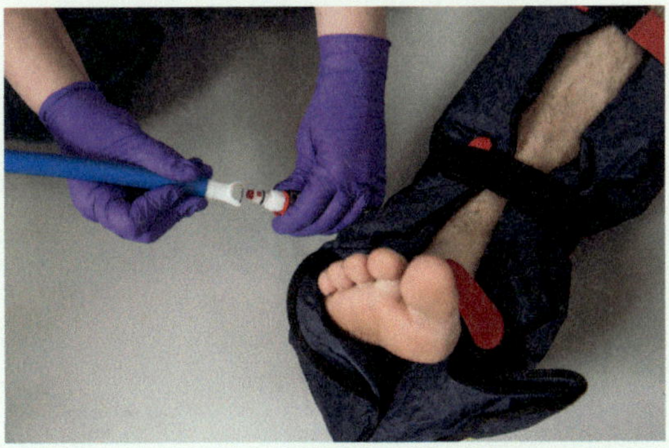	
12.	Wrap the Velcro straps around the now rigid splint. 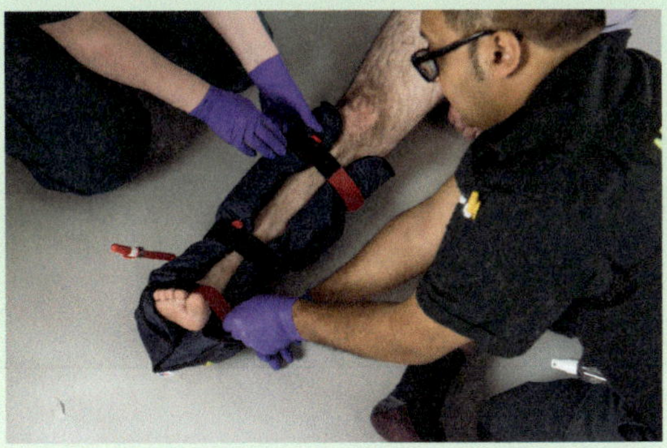	These provide additional support to the splint during extrication and transport.

Action		Rationale
13.	Recheck the limb distally for any change in neurovascular status now it has been immobilised. You may need to reposition the limb if neurovascular status has been compromised during immobilisation.	Neurovascular compromise can result in long-term injury to the limb or in the worst cases death of the limb tissue, rendering the limb unsalvageable.
14.	Regularly check the splint during transport. If it is becoming loose, then use the pump and remove air until it becomes firm again.	Vacuum splints can develop small leaks, resulting in a loss of splint integrity over time.
15.	Document the procedure.	You must keep full, clear and accurate records for everyone you care for, treat, or provide other services to (4).

References

1. Hartwell Medical. Evac-u-splint application guidelines [Internet]. 2021 [cited 2022 Jul 18]. Available from: www.hartwellmedical.com/wp-content/uploads/2021/08/EVAC-U-SPLINT_AppGuide_ENGLISH_AGEV_7-21.pdf.
2. Queensland Ambulance Service. Trauma/Orthopaedic splinting – vacuum. 2020 [cited 2022 Jul 18]; Available from: www.ambulance.qld.gov.au/docs/clinical/cpp/CPP_Orthopaedic%20splinting_vacuum.pdf.
3. British Medical Association. Ethics – General information [Internet]. 2018 [cited 2019 Dec 29]. Available from: www.bma.org.uk/advice/employment/ethics/consent/consent-tool-kit/2-general-information.
4. Health and Care Professions Council. Standards of conduct, performance and ethics [Internet]. 2016 [cited 2022 Jul 16]. Available from: www.hcpc-uk.org/standards/standards-of-conduct-performance-and-ethics/.
5. NHS England. Standard infection control precautions: National hand hygiene and personal protective equipment policy [Internet]. 2019 [cited 2022 Feb 13]. Available from: www.england.nhs.uk/publication/standard-infection-control-precautions-national-hand-hygiene-and-personal-protective-equipment-policy/.

Kendrick Traction Device

Indications
- Mid-shaft femur fractures.

Contraindications
- Fractures of the lower limb other than mid-shaft femur.

Advantages
- Can be used where there is suspicion of a co-existing pelvic fracture (apply pelvic binder first).
- Compact, lightweight device.
- Applying traction may help to (1):
  - Reduce discomfort by anatomically realigning the fractured sections.
  - Reduce ongoing bleeding.
  - Reduce the risk of fat embolus.

Disadvantages
- Requires training and familiarisation to apply appropriately.
- Once applied, it extends beyond the foot of the patient, which can make moving or conveying in an aircraft challenging.

Procedure – Kendrick Traction Device

Take the following steps to apply a Kendrick Traction Device (2):

Action		Rationale
1.	If the patient is conscious, explain the procedure and obtain consent if appropriate to do so.	You must make sure that you have valid consent from service users or other appropriate authority before you provide care, treatment or other services (3,4).
2.	Don appropriate personal protective equipment (PPE), and undertake appropriate hand hygiene.	This reduces the risk of cross-infection (5).

	Action	Rationale
3.	Ensure all the patient's clothing has been removed from the leg.	Devices should be applied at skin level. If there is no suspicion of a pelvic injury, it may be appropriate to leave underwear in situ to protect modesty.
4.	Ensure that all parts are present. 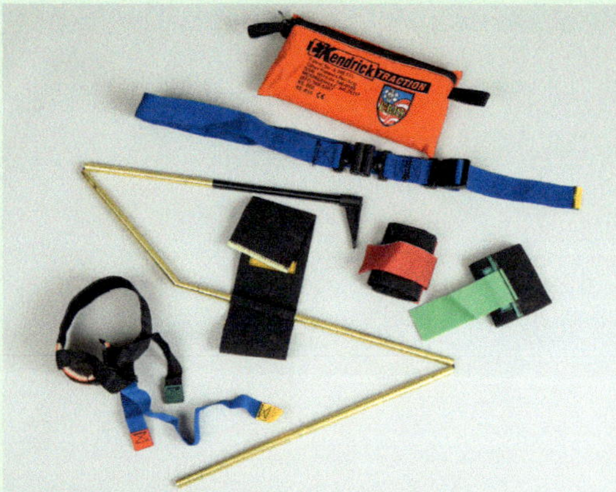 	Making certain that all required components are present at this early stage will ensure application is faster and easier. The kit also includes a boot holster which has been removed here, as is not required unless applying the traction splint with a boot remaining on the patient. This would only be appropriate if exposing the limb were to cause further complications, such as on a ski slope where the cold may cause further injury.
5.	Apply the ankle strap by passing the padded part of the strap around the back of the ankle. Secure the strap firmly with the Velcro. 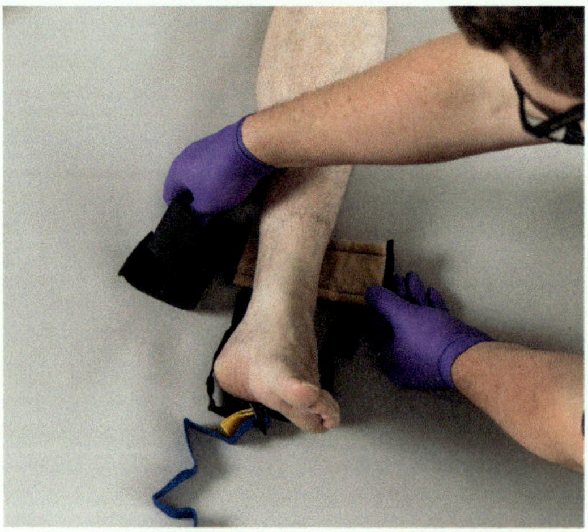	If applied the wrong way around, the device is likely to still work but be less comfortable. The ankle strap must be securely fixed to prevent it slipping off when traction is applied.

Action		Rationale
6.	Place the thigh strap under the back of the knee. 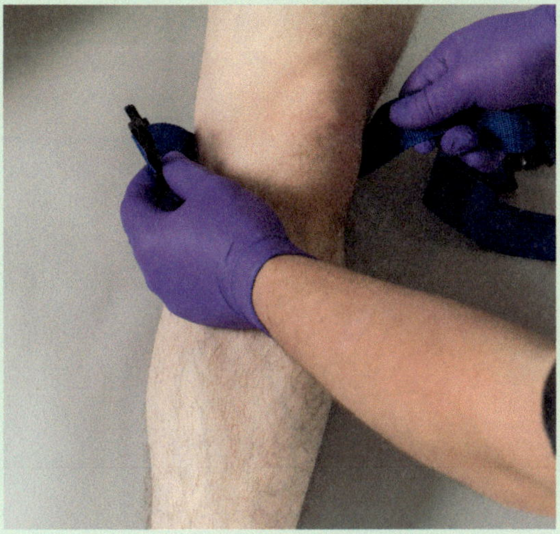	Placing the strap under the knee and sliding it up will result in less movement to the injured limb than trying to pass it immediately under the thigh area.
7.	Slide the thigh strap so that it is high in the groin.	The strap needs to be well seated in the groin to ensure that it is effective when traction is applied.
	Ensure that genitals are not trapped under the strap.	When traction is applied, significant pressure can be exerted by the strap. Crushing genitals underneath the strap will be painful and may cause further injury.
	Clip the buckle so it is on the superior aspect of the limb.	The buckle should be secured on the superior aspect so it can be easily accessed and adjusted, if required.
	Adjust the strap so that the pole receptacle is at the level of the iliac crest. Note: While underwear has been left on in these images, it would be more common to perform this at skin level. 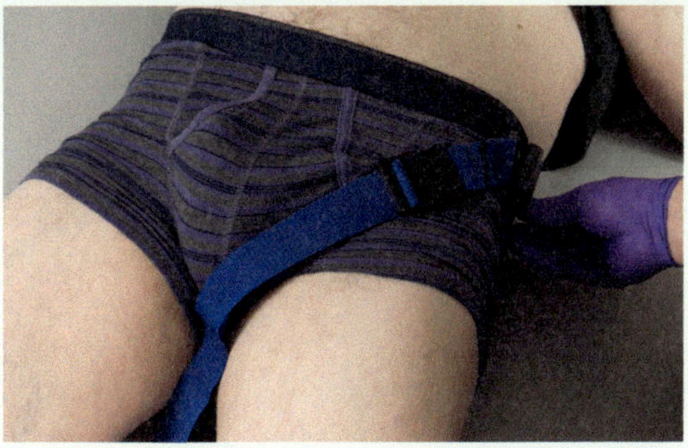	This is the recommendation of the manufacturer (5).

	Action	Rationale
8.	Take the pole and straighten it out. Then place it next to the patient and ensure that at least one full section of pole extends beyond the foot. 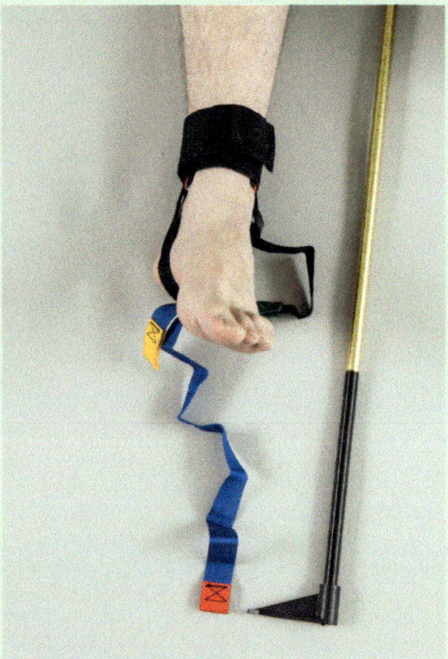	There needs to be a sufficient amount of pole extending beyond the foot to allow for tension to be applied later. In the image, the black section of the pole is fully beyond the foot.
9.	Once the pole is in the correct position the length can be adjusted. Once set to the correct length, it is inserted into the receptacle. 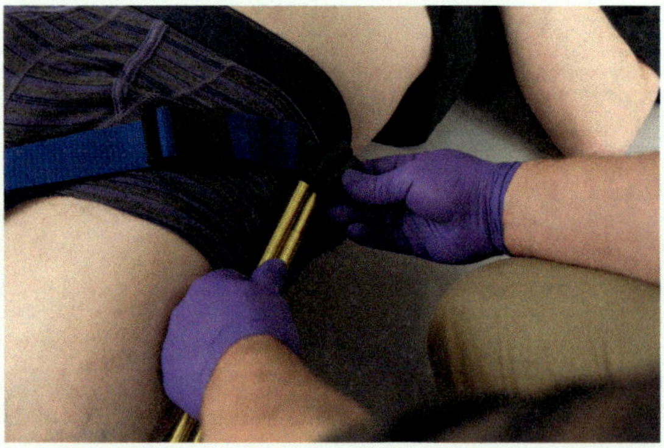	

	Action	Rationale
10.	Place the yellow strap around the knee and secure – this is the strap that comes pre-attached to the pole. 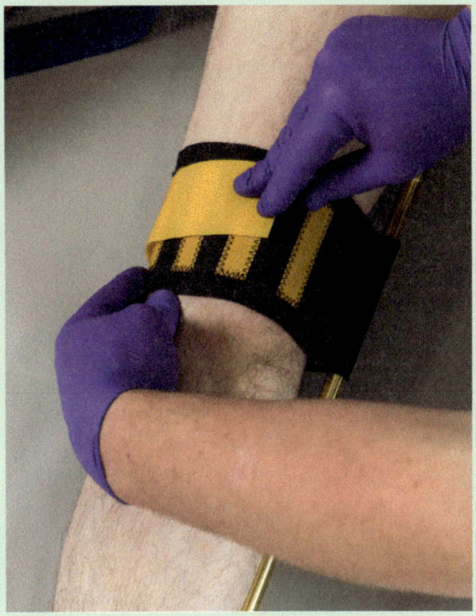	The strap helps to keep the pole in the correct alignment when tension is applied.
11.	Place the dart at the end of the black pole through the yellow loop on the section of strap that hangs down from the foot. 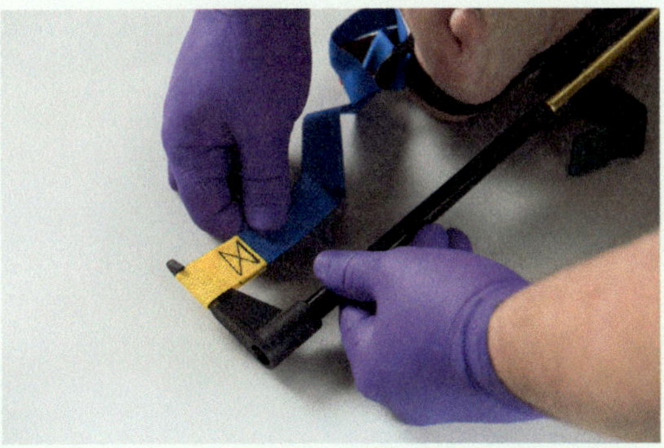	The loop needs to be secure to ensure it does not slip off the pole once traction is applied.
12.	Apply traction by simultaneously pulling down on the red tab on the foot strap and feeding the other side of the strap with the yellow tab through the buckle. Apply traction until normal anatomical alignment or significant reduction in pain is achieved.	The manufacturer recommends tension should be applied to approximately 10% of body weight to a maximum of approximately 7 kg (4). In reality this is very hard to determine when applying manual traction, so normal anatomical alignment and a significant reduction in pain are more measurable in the prehospital setting.

Action		Rationale
	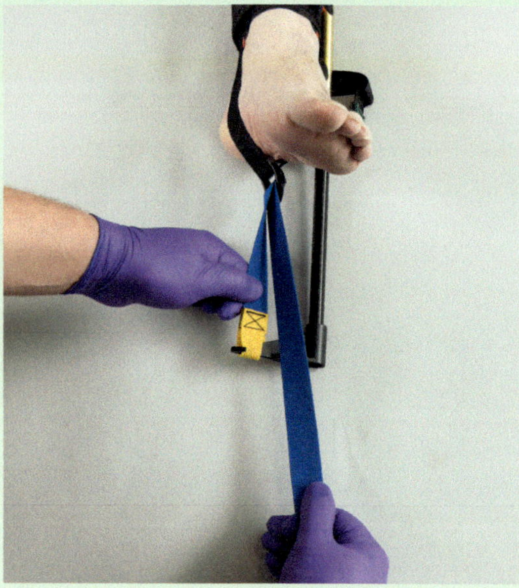	
13.	Apply straps over the thigh and ankle following the traffic light colour system: red at the top and green at the bottom. 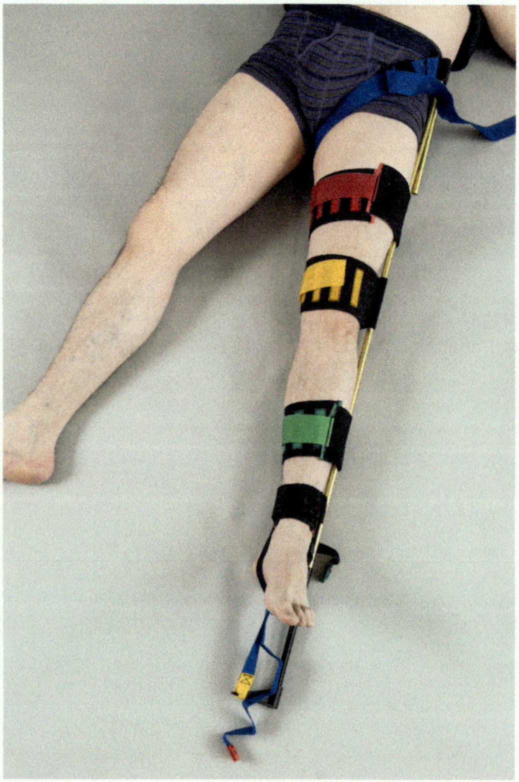	Straps keep the pole aligned and in place during transfer. The straps are different sizes to fit at the different positions on the leg. Avoiding place straps directly over the site of injury or any wounds.

Action		Rationale
14.	Assess the pulse, movement and sensation distally on the limb.	Assess for new or worsening neurovascular deficit after traction has been applied.
15.	Document the procedure and be sure to hand over at the hospital the suspected fracture and application of a traction splint.	You must keep full, clear and accurate records for everyone you care for, treat, or provide other services to (4).

References

1. Greaves I, Porter K, Wright C. *Trauma Care Pre-hospital Manual*. London: CRC Press; 2019.
2. Kendrick EMS. Kendrick Traction Device application instructions [Internet]. [cited 2021 Jan 31]. Available from: http://www.kentronmedical.com/files/KENDRICK_APPLICATION.pdf.
3. British Medical Association. Ethics – General information [Internet]. 2018 [cited 2019 Dec 29]. Available from: https://www.bma.org.uk/advice/employment/ethics/consent/consent-tool-kit/2-general-information.
4. Health and Care Professions Council. Standards of conduct, performance and ethics [Internet]. 2018 [cited 2019 Dec 29]. Available from: https://www.hcpc-uk.org/standards/standards-of-conduct-performance-and-ethics/.
5. NHS England. Standard infection control precautions: national hand hygiene and personal protective equipment policy [Internet]. 2019 [cited 2022 Feb 13]. Available from: https://www.england.nhs.uk/publication/standardinfection-control-precautions-national-hand-hygiene-andpersonal-protective-equipment-policy/.

Pelvic Binders

A fractured pelvis is a major injury, often caused by a high-energy mechanism and associated with other significant injuries, and has a high mortality, typically as a result of internal haemorrhage (1). The use of external compression devices has been shown to reduce severe fractures without causing further displacement (2). It is theorised that their use decreases internal haemorrhage (3). As a result, the application of pelvic binders (also known as pelvic slings) is recommended early in cases where pelvic bleeding is suspected following blunt high-energy trauma (3,4). Despite this, there remains no high-quality literature to demonstrate that pelvic binders alone improve patient outcomes (5).

While there is minimal evidence of benefit, there is some evidence that they can be harmful, causing soft-tissue injury due to pressure the device exerts on the skin once tightened (2,6). Pelvic binders should **therefore** not be applied as a purely precautionary measure (4) without indications for injury being present. When a binder is indicated, consider it to be a treatment intervention and not just a packaging device, and apply it early (during the primary survey where possible) (3).

Numerous commercial binders exist and it is important that clinicians are familiar with the device available to them. Recent observational studies have shown that binders placed by UK paramedics are located too high in as many as 40% of applications (7), which could potentially worsen bleeding. Hands-on training and familiarity are key to ensuring successful application.

References

1. Holstein JH, Culemann U, Pohlemann T. What are predictors of mortality in patients with pelvic fractures? *Clinical Orthopaedics and Related Research*. 2012; 470(8):2090–2097.
2. Knops SP, Schep NWL, Spoor CW, et al. Comparison of three different pelvic circumferential compression devices: A biomechanical cadaver study. *Journal of Bone and Joint Surgery – Series A*. 2011;93(3):230–240.
3. Scott I, Porter K, Laird C, et al. The prehospital management of pelvic fractures: Initial consensus statement. *Trauma*. 2015;17(2):151–154.
4. National Institute for Health and Care Excellence. Fractures (complex): Assessment and management NG37 [Internet]. 2017 [cited 2020 Mar 1]. Available from: https://www.nice.org.uk/guidance/ng37/chapter/recommendations.
5. Bakhshayesh P, Boutefnouchet T, Tötterman A. Effectiveness of non invasive external pelvic compression: A systematic review of the literature. *Scandinavian Journal of Trauma, Resuscitation and Emergency Medicine*. 2016;24:73.
6. Prasarn ML, Horodyski MB, Schneider PS, et al. Comparison of skin pressure measurements with the use of pelvic circumferential compression devices on pelvic ring injuries. *Injury*. 2016. E1398–1402.
7. Naseem H, Nesbitt P, Sprott D, et al. An assessment of pelvic binder placement at a UK major trauma centre. *Annals of the Royal College of Surgeons of England*. 2018;100(2):101–105.

SAM Pelvic Sling

Indications

- Suspected ongoing bleeding due to pelvic fracture.
- Local guidelines indicate application of a pelvic binder. An example of local guidelines for application would be:
  - Mechanism of injury that suggests a pelvic fracture **and** is accompanied by **any** of the following:
    - haemodynamic instability or signs of shock
    - deformity on examination
    - suspected open pelvic fracture, including bleeding from the urethra (PU), vagina (PV) or rectum (PR), or scrotal haematoma.

Contraindications

- Isolated neck of femur fracture.
- Patient who has an impaled object which would be covered by the binder.

Advantages

- Reduces fractures of the pelvis.
- May help to reduce bleeding associated with pelvic fractures.
- Simple to apply in the prehospital setting.

Disadvantages

- Pelvic binders utilise pressure to reduce the fracture. This pressure can be sufficient to cause soft-tissue injury (1).
- Can cause pelvis to not align appropriately if applied incorrectly.
- Accurate placement is challenging and binders often end up in the wrong place (typically too high) (2).
- Three sizes exist, which means having to carry multiple devices to accommodate all patients.

Procedure – SAM Pelvic Sling

Take the following steps to apply a SAM pelvic sling (3):

Action		Rationale
1.	If the patient is conscious, explain the procedure and obtain consent if appropriate to do so.	You must make sure that you have valid consent from service users or other appropriate authority before you provide care, treatment or other services (4,5).
2.	Don appropriate personal protective equipment (PPE), and undertake appropriate hand hygiene.	This reduces the risk of cross-infection (6).
3.	Check all the patient's clothing (including underwear) has been removed.	Binders should be applied at skin level as this helps to confirm location and means the binder will not need to be removed on arrival at hospital to remove underwear (8).

<table>
<tr><th colspan="2">Action</th><th>Rationale</th></tr>
<tr><td>4.</td><td>Choose the correctly sized binder, as there are three sizes available based on patient waist size:
• Small: 27–45 in (69–114 cm)
• Medium: 32–50 in (81–127 cm)
• Large: 36–54 in (91–137 cm).</td><td>Choosing an incorrect size means the binder may not fit properly.</td></tr>
<tr><td>5.</td><td>Locate the level of the greater trochanter by identifying the iliac crest and then moving down on the lateral side of the leg to the next obvious underlying bone structure. This is the greater trochanter.
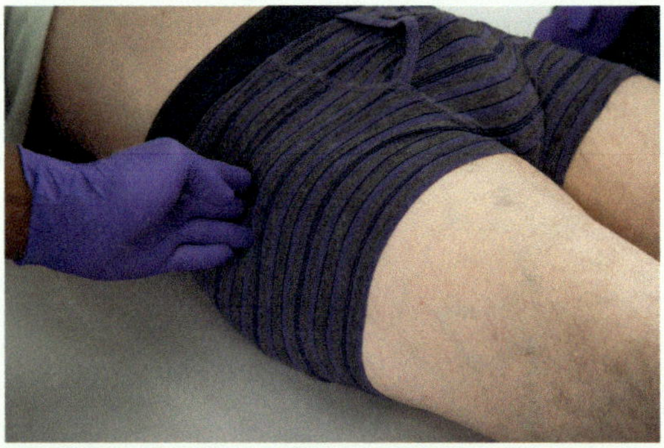</td><td>The binder must be applied at trochanter level to help ensure the pelvis is appropriately reduced; if applied too high, it can distort the shape of the pelvis when pressure is applied (2).</td></tr>
<tr><td>6.</td><td>As long as there are no other injuries that may be made worse, strap the feet together using a triangle bandage (or similar) in a figure of eight.
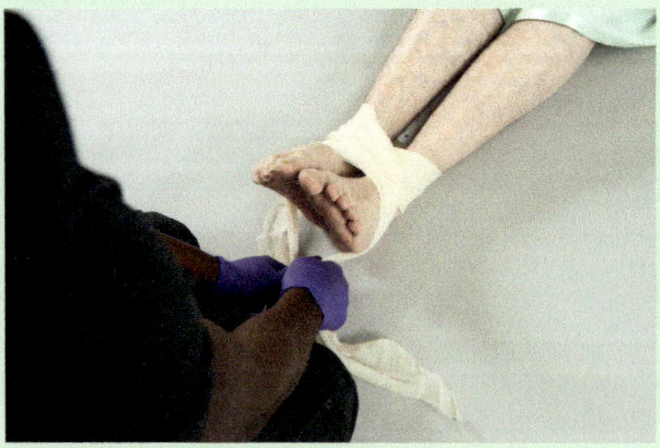</td><td>This brings the legs into normal alignment prior to applying the binder.</td></tr>
</table>

	Action	Rationale
7.	Insert the binder under the legs. 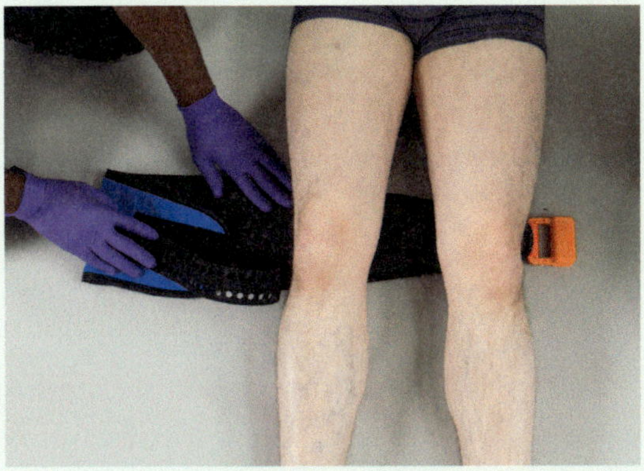	Binders are typically placed too high (8), so inserting them under the legs and moving up into position may help to prevent this.
8.	Slide the binder up into position and confirm the centre of the binder is in line with the greater trochanters. You may need to just 'lift' the hips a very small amount to help the binder get to the correct position. 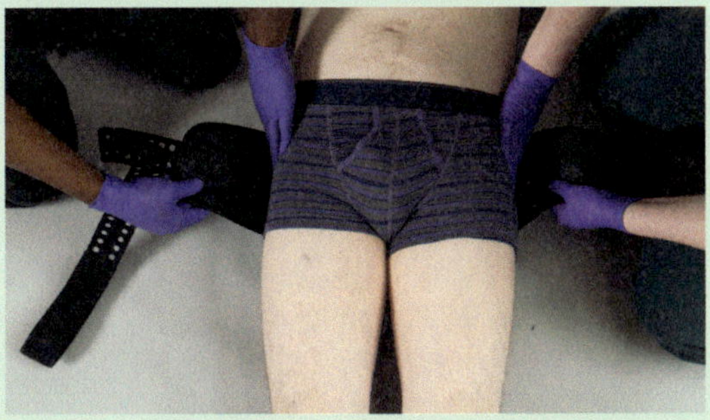	Be careful to minimise pelvis movement to prevent any potential further disruption and associated bleeding.
9.	Pull the strap through the orange buckle, and ensure that there is an equal amount of binder on each side of the patient. 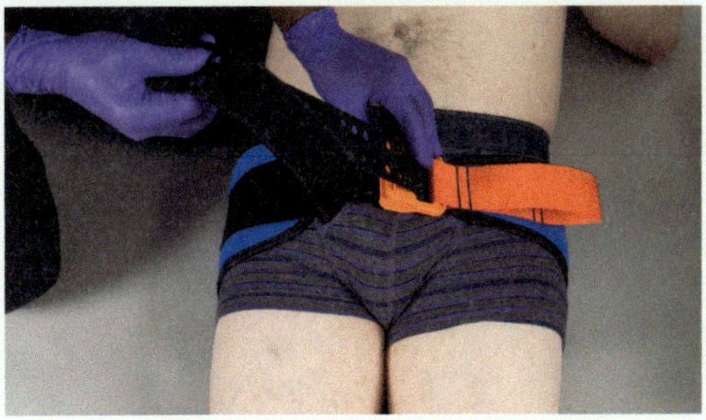	Ensuring the binder is located appropriately should help with applying an even force when the device is tightened (3).

Action		Rationale
10.	With one person on each side, pull the black strap and orange handle in opposite directions until the buckle clicks. Maintain tension and secure the Velcro of the black strap to the splint. Do not be concerned if the buckle clicks again during this manoeuvre. 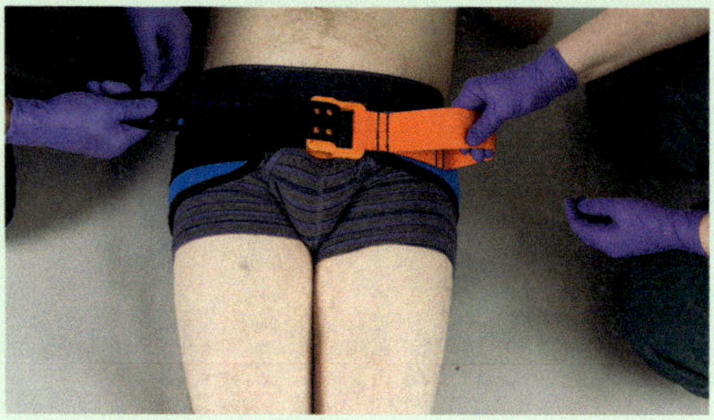	The buckle click indicates a 150 N tensional force, which is more than sufficient to realign the pelvis (9). This is the expected behaviour of the device (3).
11.	Document the time of application and ensure this is communicated at handover.	You must keep full, clear and accurate records for everyone you care for, treat, or provide other services to (5).

References

1. Prasarn ML, Horodyski MB, Schneider PS, et al. Comparison of skin pressure measurements with the use of pelvic circumferential compression devices on pelvic ring injuries. *Injury*. 2016 Mar;47(3):717–720.
2. Bonner TJ, Eardley WGP, Newell N, et al. Accurate placement of a pelvic binder improves reduction of unstable fractures of the pelvic ring. *Journal of Bone and Joint Surgery – Series B*. 2011;93(11):1524–1528.
3. SAM Medical. SAM PELVIC SLING II [Internet]. SAM Medical Store. 2021 [cited 2021 Aug 24]. Available from: https://www.sammedical.com/blogs/training/sam-pelvic-sling-ii.
4. British Medical Association. Ethics – General information [Internet]. 2018 [cited 2019 Dec 29]. Available from: https://www.bma.org.uk/advice/employment/ethics/consent/consent-tool-kit/2-general-information.
5. Health and Care Professions Council. Standards of conduct, performance and ethics [Internet]. 2018 [cited 2019 Dec 29]. Available from: https://www.hcpc-uk.org/standards/standards-of-conduct-performance-and-ethics/.
6. NHS England. Standard infection control precautions: national hand hygiene and personal protective equipment policy [Internet]. 2019 [cited 2022 Feb 13]. Available from: https://www.england.nhs.uk/publication/standard infection-control-precautions-national-handhygiene-andpersonal-protective-equipment-policy/.
7. Scott I, Porter K, Laird C, et al. The prehospital management of pelvic fractures: Initial consensus statement. *Trauma*. 2015;17(2):151–154.
8. Naseem H, Nesbitt PD, Sprott DC, et al. An assessment of pelvic binder placement at a UK major trauma centre. *Annals of the Royal College of Surgeons of England*. 2018;100(2):101–105.
9. Knops SP, van Riel MPJM, Goossens RHM, et al. Measurements of the exerted pressure by pelvic circumferential compression devices. *Open Orthopaedics Journal*. 2010;4:101–106.

T-POD® Stabilisation Device

Indications

- Suspected ongoing bleeding due to pelvic fracture.
- Local guidelines indicate application of a pelvic binder. An example of local guidelines for application would be:
    - Mechanism of injury that suggests a pelvic fracture **and** is accompanied by **any** of the following:
        - Haemodynamic instability or signs of shock
        - Deformity on examination
        - Suspected open pelvic fracture, including bleeding from the urethra (PU), vagina (PV) or rectum (PR), or scrotal haematoma.

Contraindications

- Isolated neck of femur fracture.
- Patient who has an impaled object which would be covered by the binder.

Advantages

- Reduces fractures of the pelvis.
- May help to reduce bleeding associated with pelvic fractures.
- Simple to apply in the prehospital setting.

Disadvantages

- Pelvic binders utilise pressure to reduce the fracture. This pressure can be sufficient to cause soft-tissue injury (1).
- Can cause pelvis to not align appropriately if applied incorrectly.
- Accurate placement is challenging and binders often end up in the wrong place (typically too high) (2).

Procedure – Apply a T-POD® Stabilisation Device

Take the following steps to apply a T-POD® stabilisation device (3):

Action		Rationale
1.	If the patient is conscious, explain the procedure and obtain consent if appropriate to do so.	You must make sure that you have valid consent from service users or other appropriate authority before you provide care, treatment or other services (4,5).
2.	Don appropriate personal protective equipment (PPE), and undertake appropriate hand hygiene.	This reduces the risk of cross-infection (6).
3.	Check all the patient's clothing (including underwear) has been removed.	Binders should be applied at skin level as this helps to confirm location and means the binder will not need to be removed on arrival at hospital to remove underwear (7).

Action		Rationale
4.	Ensure all parts are present and that the pulley system has been fully opened up and is not twisted. 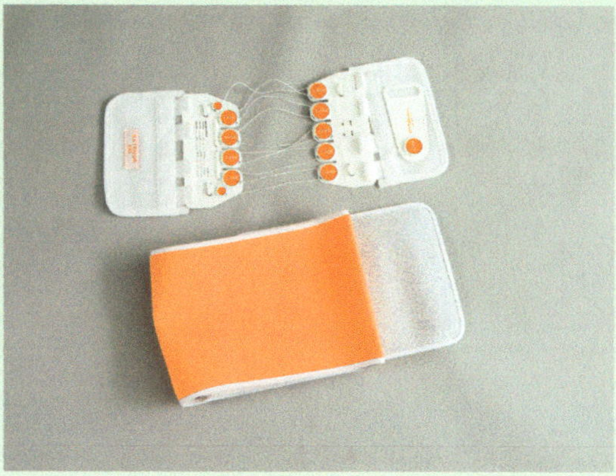	This will make the final application faster and simpler.
5.	As long as there are no other injuries that may be made worse, strap the feet together using a triangle bandage (or similar) in a figure of eight. 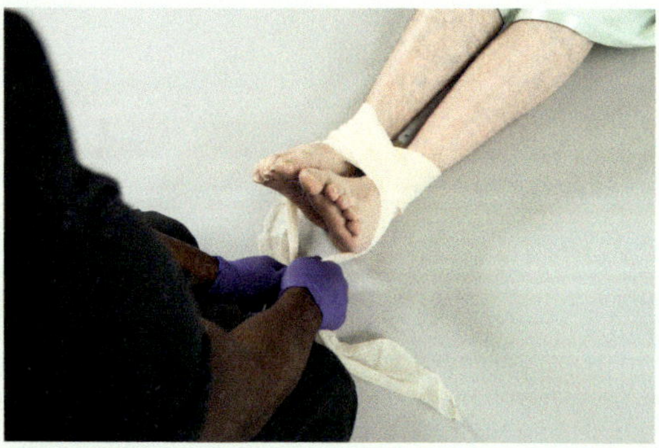	This brings the legs into normal alignment prior to applying the binder.

	Action	Rationale
6.	Locate the level of the greater trochanter by identifying the iliac crest and then moving down on the lateral side of the leg to the next obvious underlying bone structure. This is the greater trochanter. 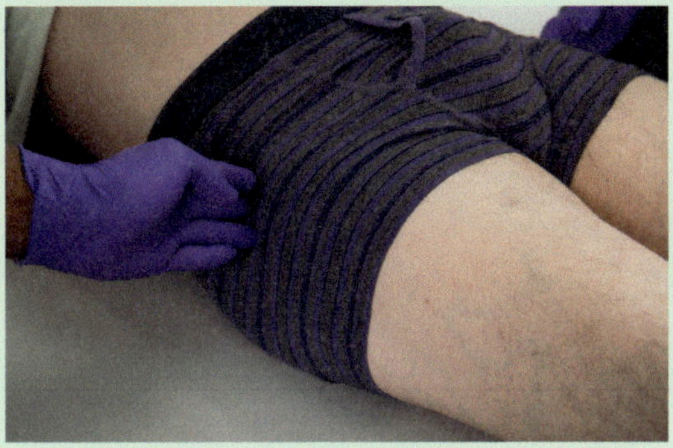	The binder must be applied at trochanter level to help ensure the pelvis is appropriately reduced; if applied too high, it can distort the shape of the pelvis when pressure is applied (2).
7.	Insert the belt under the legs, with the white side facing the patient. 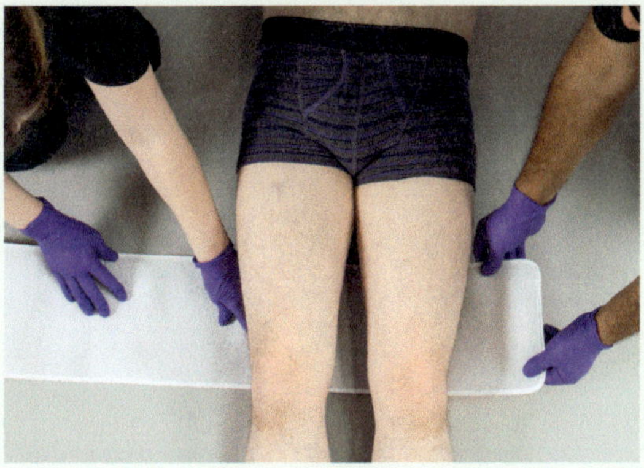	Binders are typically placed too high (8). Inserting them under the legs and moving up into position can help to prevent this.

Action		Rationale
8.	Slide the binder up into position and confirm the centre of the binder is in line with the greater trochanters. You may need to just 'lift' the hips a very small amount to help the binder get to the correct position. 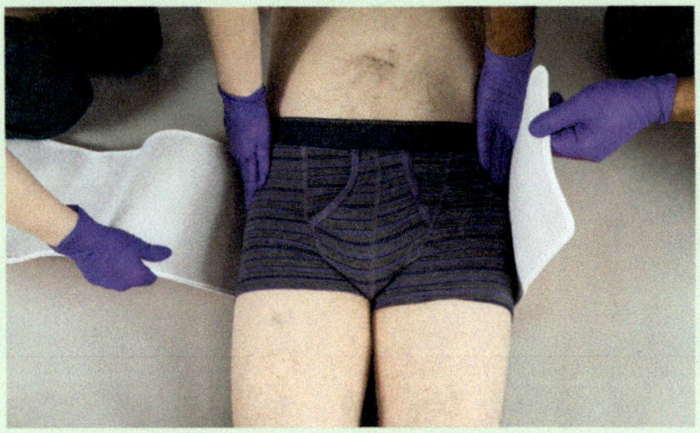	This helps to confirm the correct location. Be careful to minimise pelvis movement to prevent any potential further disruption and associated bleeding.
9.	Cut the excess belt, so there is a 15–20 cm (6–8 in) gap over the centre of the pelvis. Do not fold the material back on itself. 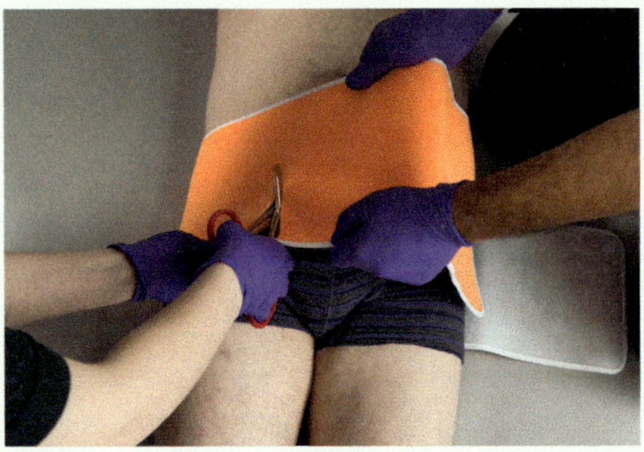	Leave a sufficient gap for when the belt is tightened using the pulley system. Folded material will increase the risk of soft-tissue pressure injury.

Action		Rationale
10.	Place the pulley system on the belt, ensuring that the Velcro is stuck down well. 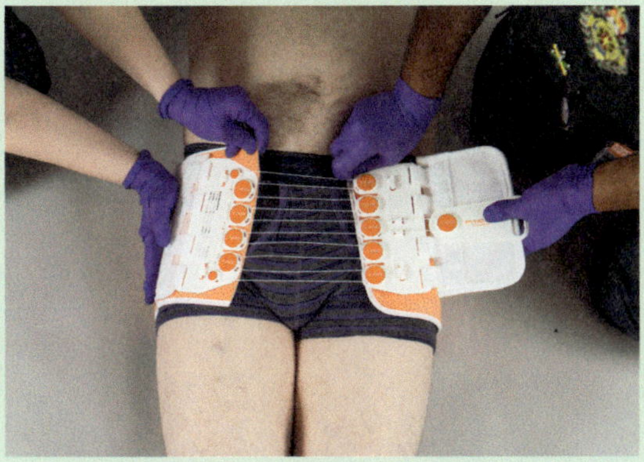	This will be used to apply tension and needs to be firmly in place so it is not dislodged when tension is applied.
11.	Gently apply tension to the pull cord by pulling on the attached tab, which will apply circumferential pressure to the pelvis. 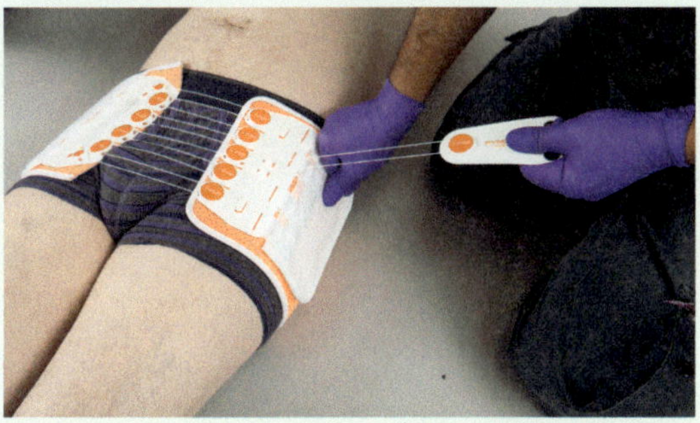	There is no clear guidance on how much tension should be applied. A good rule of thumb is to apply sufficient tension to achieve normal anatomical alignment.
12.	Once appropriate tension has been applied, wrap the excess pull cord around the vertical posts located next to the pulleys until the excess cord has been wrapped up sufficiently for the plastic tab to be conveniently stuck to the Velcro. 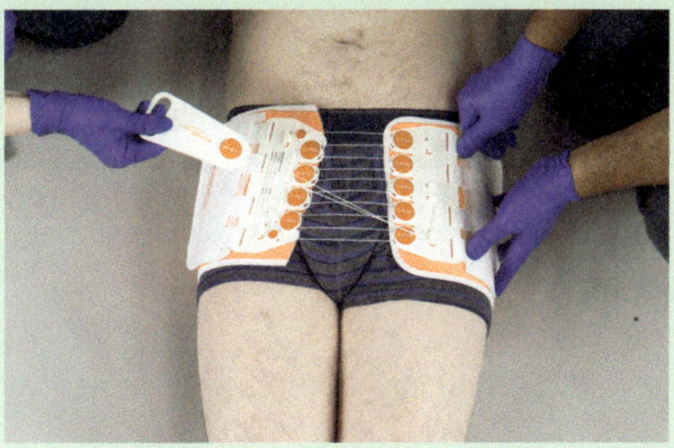	This will prevent the binder from loosening.

<table>
<tr><th colspan="2">Action</th><th>Rationale</th></tr>
<tr><td>13.</td><td>Stick the plastic tab down so it is secure. It needs to be in an easily accessible location.
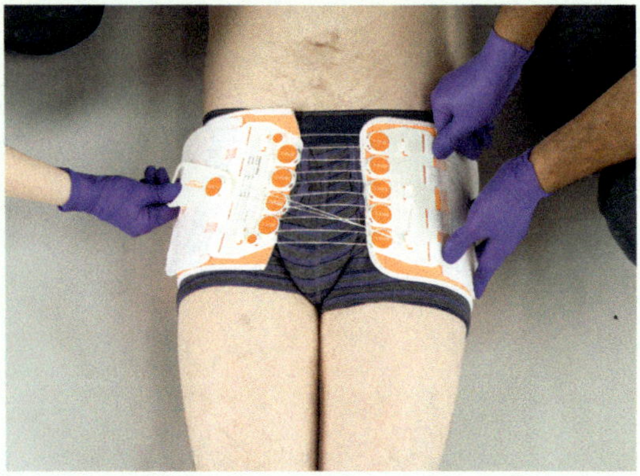</td><td>The tab needs to be secure to prevent tension being released.
It may be necessary to adjust the tension. If the tab is easily accessible, this can be achieved without difficulty.</td></tr>
<tr><td>14.</td><td>Document the time of application and ensure this is communicated at handover.</td><td>You must keep full, clear and accurate records for everyone you care for, treat, or provide other services to (5).</td></tr>
</table>

References

1. Prasarn ML, et al. Comparison of skin pressure measurements with the use of pelvic circumferential compression devices on pelvic ring injuries. *Injury*. 2016;47(3):717–20.
2. Bonner TJ, et al. Accurate placement of a pelvic binder improves reduction of unstable fractures of the pelvic ring. *Journal of Bone and Joint Surgery – Series B*. 2011;93(11):1524–8.
3. PYNG Medical. T-POD pelvic stabilization device [Internet]. 2011 [cited 2022 Jul 31]. Available from: https://sovmed.com/wp-content/uploads/2019/10/T-POD-Training-PowerPoint-Presentation.pdf.
4. British Medical Association. Ethics – General information [Internet]. 2018 [cited 2019 Dec 29]. Available from: https://www.bma.org.uk/advice/employment/ethics/consent/consent-tool-kit/2-general-information/.
5. Health and Care Professions Council. Standards of conduct, performance and ethics [Internet]. 2016 [cited 2022 Jul 16]. Available from: https://www.hcpc-uk.org/standards/standards-of-conduct-performance-and-ethics/.
6. NHS England. Standard infection control precautions: National hand hygiene and personal protective equipment policy [Internet]. 2019 [cited 2022 Feb 13]. Available from: https://www.england.nhs.uk/publication/standard-infection-control-precautions-national-hand-hygiene-and-personal-protective-equipment-policy/.
7. Scott I, et al. The prehospital management of pelvic fractures: initial consensus statement. *Trauma*. 2015;30(12):1070– 1072.
8. Naseem H, et al. An assessment of pelvic binder placement at a UK major trauma centre. *RCS Annals*. 2018;100(2):101– 105.

Manual In-Line Stabilisation

Indications

- Spinal immobilisation is indicated according to local procedure.
- While awaiting definitive cervical spine immobilisation.

Contraindications

- Distressed and agitated patients where performing manual in-line stabilisation (MILS) may cause further distress and movement.

Advantages

- Rapid technique to immobilise the cervical spine.
- Requires no equipment.

Disadvantages

- Requires a member of the clinical team to be dedicated to the task of providing MILS.
- Can make airway management more challenging.

Procedure – Manual In-Line Stabilisation

Take the following steps to apply MILS immobilisation (1):

Action		Rationale
1.	If the patient is conscious, explain the procedure and obtain consent if appropriate to do so.	You must make sure that you have valid consent from service users or other appropriate authority before you provide care, treatment or other services (2,3).
2.	Don appropriate personal protective equipment (PPE), and undertake appropriate hand hygiene.	This reduces the risk of cross-infection (4).
3.	Advise the patient not to move their head and explain you are going to hold their head to help keep it still.	Explaining the procedure to the patient should avoid inadvertent head movement when they are surprised by a clinician clasping their head!
4.	Place yourself in a comfortable position behind the patient; this should be either kneeling behind the patient or lying behind the patient. Rest your arms on the floor, on your knees or other objects that will help to stabilise them.	MILS will likely need to be applied for a prolonged period. You want to remain stable to prevent your arms from moving due to fatigue.

Action		Rationale
5.	Place your hands either side of the head and over the mastoid process. This should result in your hands being positioned under the ears, and not covering them. If necessary, move one finger to above the ear, as shown here. 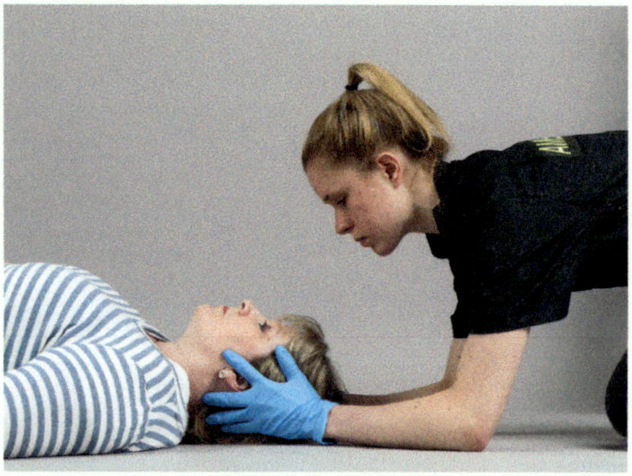	The spine connects to the skull at the same height from the floor as the mastoid process. Covering the patient's ears will reduce what they can hear, which can be frightening and can complicate history-taking.
6.	If the patient's head is not facing forwards and the patient is conscious, ask them to slowly move their head into a neutral, in-line position (eyes looking straight ahead and nose in line with umbilicus). If the patient is unconscious, gently move the head into a neutral position. Movement to the neutral position should cease if there is: • Resistance to movement • Neck muscle spasm • Increased pain • An increase in neurological deficit (numbness, tingling, etc.). In any of these cases the neck should be immobilised in the position that it presents in.	Where possible, patients should always be managed in neutral alignment as this is the anatomically normal position of the spine. It is thought that it is less likely that further injury will occur if the spine can be managed in this position. Returning to the neutral position should be ceased if problems develop, as there is a small risk further damage may be caused by moving the neck.
7.	MILS should be maintained until: • The patient is fully immobilised • It is decided that immobilisation is no longer required.	
8.	Document the procedure, including the time it was undertaken and any complications.	You must keep full, clear and accurate records for everyone you care for, treat, or provide other services to (2).

References

1. National Association of Emergency Medical Technicians. *PHTLS Prehospital Trauma Life Support*. 9th edition. NAEMT, editor. Burlington, MA: Jones & Bartlett Learning; 2019.
2. Health and Care Professions Council. Standards of conduct, performance and ethics [Internet]. 2016 [cited 2022 Jul 16]. Available from: www.hcpc-uk.org/standards/standards-of-conduct-performance-and-ethics/.
3. British Medical Association. Ethics – General information [Internet]. 2018 [cited 2019 Dec 29]. Available from: www.bma.org.uk/advice/employment/ethics/consent/consent-tool-kit/2-general-information.
4. NHS England. Standard infection control precautions: National hand hygiene and personal protective equipment policy [Internet]. 2019 [cited 2022 Feb 13]. Available from: www.england.nhs.uk/publication/standard-infection-control-precautions-national-hand-hygiene-and-personal-protective-equipment-policy/.

Helmet Removal

Indications

- To assess and manage a patient wearing a motorcycle helmet following a traumatic incident.

Contraindications

- Single rescuers should not attempt this procedure unless immediate interventions which could not be completed with the helmet in situ are required, for example clearing or maintaining an airway.

Advantages

- Removes helmet with minimal movement of the spine.
- Allows for full assessment of the patient's face and airway.

Disadvantages

- Requires two rescuers to complete.

Note: Manufactures of motorcycle helmets have evolved designs significantly over the years. Many dedicated safety technologies now exist, including helmet airbags and Emergency Helmet Removal Systems (EHRS) which you should be familiar with.

Another commonly found feature is the emergency quick release system (EQRS), which is typically two red straps built into the padding around the base of the chin. If these are present, pulling on them will easily remove some of the padding around the lower face making helmet removal simpler. Inspect for these prior to following the procedure below; if they are present, incorporate their removal into step 5.

Procedure – Helmet Removal

Take the following steps to remove a motorcycle helmet (1,2):

Action		Rationale
1.	If the patient is conscious, explain the procedure and obtain consent if appropriate to do so.	You must make sure that you have valid consent from service users or other appropriate authority before you provide care, treatment or other services (3,4).
2.	Don appropriate personal protective equipment (PPE), and undertake appropriate hand hygiene.	This reduces the risk of cross-infection (5).
3.	The clinician leading the procedure should verbalise their plan and ensure that others involved are clear on the process and their roles.	To avoid confusion and ensure the procedure is a smooth process, brief the team in advance on their roles.
4.	One rescuer should position themselves at the head end and take a grip of the helmet by placing their hands on either side of the head and curling their fingers under the edges of the helmet.	This will give a strong grip of the helmet and good control of the head and neck.

Action		Rationale
5.	From the side, a second rescuer should remove the face shield if present and release the chin strap or padding where possible. Remove EQRS padding, if present. 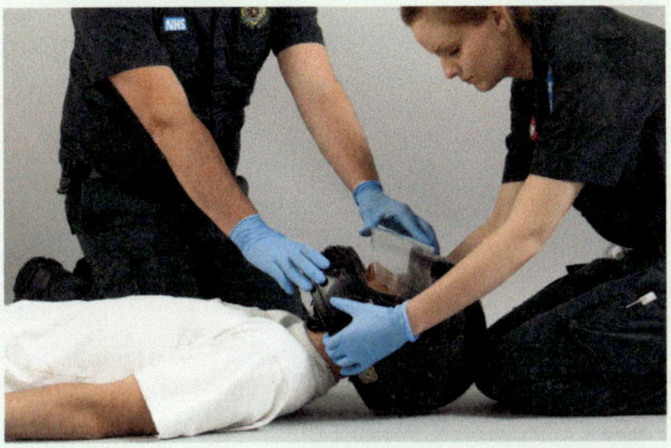	Loosening the helmet and removing any accessible padding will make it easier to remove the helmet.
6.	The second rescuer should take control of the head by placing their upper hand around the patient's mandible, in a 'c grip', and the lower hand under the back of the head, reaching up towards the occiput. Once in position with a firm grip, this rescuer should say 'I'm on' to indicate they have a firm grip and are controlling movement of the neck. The other rescuer can now release their grip. 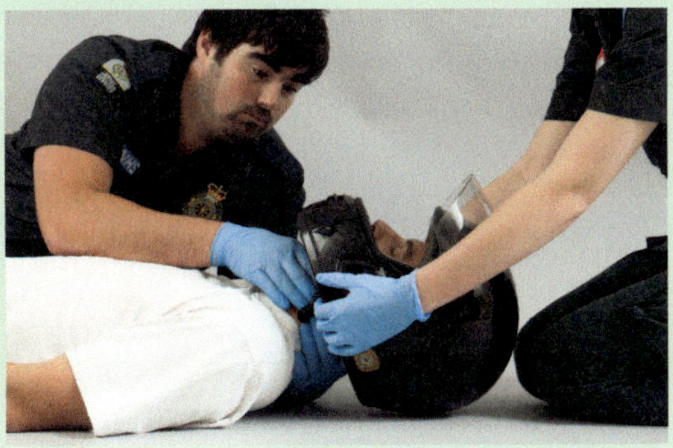	This will give a firm support of the neck to prevent rotational movement whilst the helmet is removed. Note how the forearm of the upper hand is in contact with the patient's chest; this improves stability of the grip.

	Action	Rationale
7.	Rescuer one can now gently rock the helmet back and forth whilst pulling the sides of the helmet slightly apart and applying traction. Be careful when going past the nose that the helmet does not jam against it. 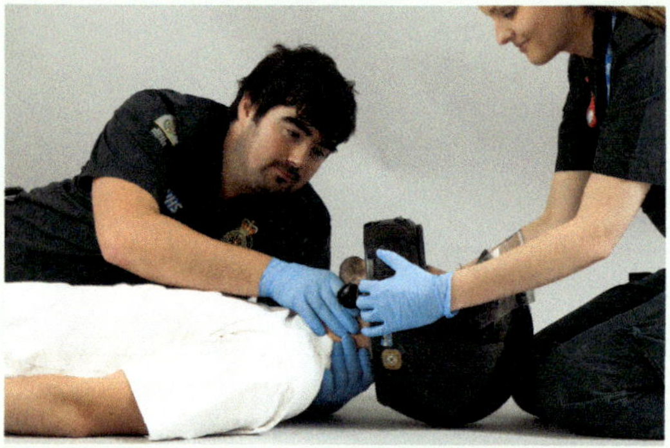	A gentle rocking action should result in minimal movement of the head. Observe the head and neck whilst undertaking this process. If significant patient head movement occurs, stop and consider how to proceed without causing such movement.
8.	Once the helmet is approximately halfway off, rescuer one should stop moving the helmet and adjust their hands, so they can take over control of the head and neck through the helmet. Once they have control, they should say 'I'm on'.	This will enable rescuer two to reposition their hands in anticipation of the helmet being fully removed.
9.	Rescuer two should adjust their hands to ensure they have a good grip. The hand against the back of the head should be moved up to take control of the occiput. It may be helpful to brace the elbow of the lower hand against the floor at this point. Once in position, with a firm grip controlling the head and neck, rescuer two should declare 'I'm on'. 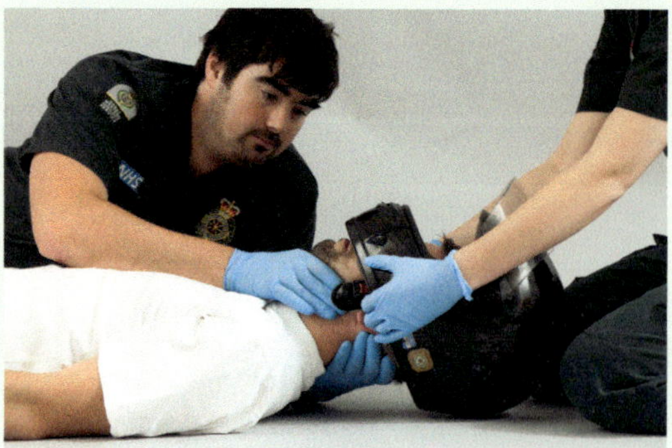	In the next move, the head will be released from the helmet and the weight of the head (it is heavy!) will need to be supported by rescuer two. Bracing elbows on the floor will help to manage the weight when it transfers to the rescuer's hands.

Action		Rationale
10.	Rescuer one should continue to rock the helmet whilst applying traction until the head is released. Once this happens, set the helmet to one side ready to convey to hospital with the patient. 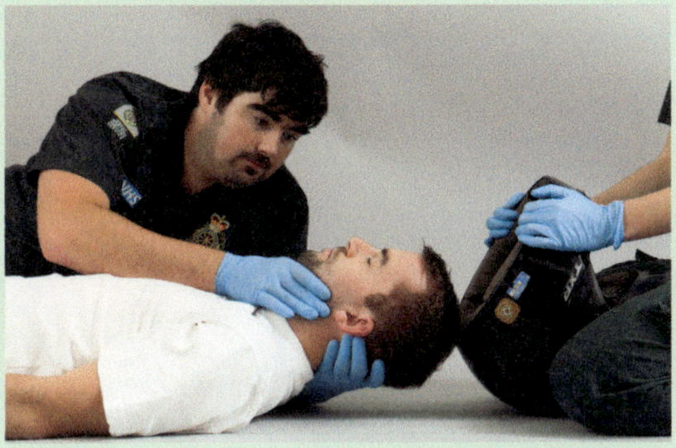	Damage to helmets may help to predict patterns of injury and should always be conveyed along with the patient.
11.	Rescuer one should now apply manual in-line stabilisation (MILS) and in a co-ordinated move (on 'Move' of 'Ready, Set, Move') lower the head to neutral alignment along with rescuer two. This may require a small amount of padding to be placed under the occiput. If any resistance is felt whilst lowering to neutral alignment, cease immediately and pad in the current position. 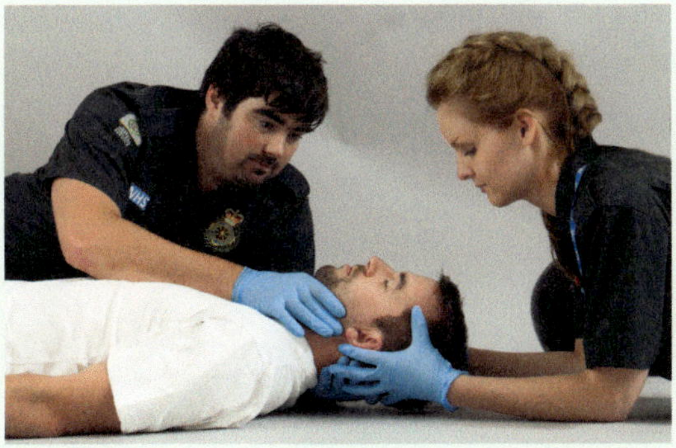	Unless it is not possible to achieve for some reasons, patients should normally be immobilised in neutral alignment.
12.	Document the procedure.	You must keep full, clear and accurate records for everyone you care for, treat, or provide other services to (4).

References

1. National Association of Emergency Medical Technicians (NAEMT). *PHTLS Prehospital Trauma Life Support*. 9th Edition. NAEMT, editor. Burlington: Jones & Bartlett Learning; 2019.
2. Queensland Ambulance Service. Trauma: Helmet Removal [Internet]. 2019 [cited 2022 Aug 1]. Available from: https://www.ambulance.qld.gov.au/docs/clinical/cpp/CPP_Helmet%20removal.pdf.
3. British Medical Association. Ethics - General information [Internet]. 2018 [cited 2019 Dec 29]. Available from: https://www.bma.org.uk/advice/employment/ethics/consent/consent-tool-kit/2-general-information.
4. Health and Care Professions Council. Standards of conduct, performance and ethics [Internet]. 2016 [cited 2022 Jul 16]. Available from: https://www.hcpc-uk.org/standards/standards-of-conduct-performance-and-ethics/.
5. NHS England. Standard infection control precautions: national hand hygiene and personal protective equipment policy [Internet]. 2019 [cited 2022 Feb 13]. Available from: https://www.england.nhs.uk/publication/standard-infection-control-precautions-national-hand-hygiene-and-personal-protective-equipment-policy/.

Cervical Collar – Adults

The use of semi-rigid cervical collars to minimise the movement of the cervical spine when a traumatic injury of that area is suspected, has been a mainstay of trauma management for many decades and remains a treatment intervention in modern trauma management guidelines (1,2). Despite this, no high-quality studies have demonstrated an outcome benefit for patients when collars are utilised as part of prehospital immobilisation; moreover, in recent years an increasing number of concerns have been raised over the safety and consequences of their use (3).

National guidelines are beginning to acknowledge the limitations of cervical collars (4). However, in the absence of high-quality evidence, their use by some ambulance services in the UK is likely to remain a part of prehospital spinal care treatment guidelines for some time, so knowing how to utilise them correctly to minimise potentially harmful situations caused by mis-sizing or poor application is important.

Their use in paediatric patients is no longer recommended due to a lack of evidence for benefit and concerns that, among other issues, their application may lead to distress, causing a child to move their cervical spine more, rather than less (5).

Indications
- To minimise movement of the cervical spine of an adult as part of spinal immobilisation.

Contraindications
- Do not attempt to apply a collar when the patient has abnormal spinal anatomy (such as severe kyphosis).
- Where applying a collar is likely to cause distress that could result in increased cervical movement.

Advantages
- Helps to reduce rotational movement of the cervical spine.
- Provides a clear visual indictor that there is a concern for a potential cervical spine injury.

Disadvantages
- Raises intracranial pressure in head-injured patients (6).
- Can complicate airway management (7).
- Can cause pressure sores (8).
- Does not fully immobilise the cervical spine.

Procedure – Apply a Cervical Collar

Take the following steps to apply an Ambu® Perfit ACE cervical collar (**Figure 6.1**) (9):

Note that other types of collars may have different fitting instructions.

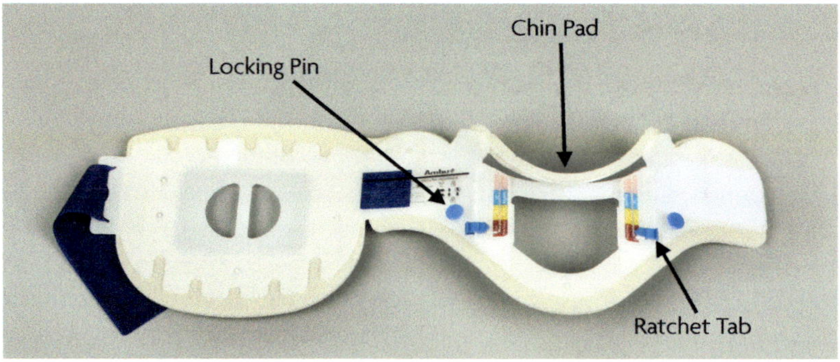

Figure 6.1 C-spine collar.

Action		Rationale
1.	Explain the procedure to the patient and obtain consent unless the patient is unable to do so, for example due to being unconscious.	You must make sure that you have valid consent from service users or other appropriate authority before you provide care, treatment or other services (10,11).
2.	Don appropriate personal protective equipment (PPE), and undertake appropriate hand hygiene.	This reduces the risk of cross-infection (12).
3.	Ensure you have the correct equipment and, where possible, three people available to apply the collar.	To minimise movement, the procedure requires three people: one to maintain manual in-line stabilisation (MILS) and two who will apply the collar.
4.	Ensure the head is in a neutral position. This can only be accurately assessed by looking from the side of, and at the level of, the patient. Assign a rescuer to maintain MILS while the collar is applied.	If the head is not in neutral alignment prior to collar application, the neck may be immobilised in an incorrect position, increasing the risk of hyperflexion or extension.
5.	Size the collar by measuring the distance with your fingers between an imaginary line drawn horizontally and immediately below the patient's chin, and another immediately on top of the patient's shoulder. To help illustrate this, the patient here is shown sitting. 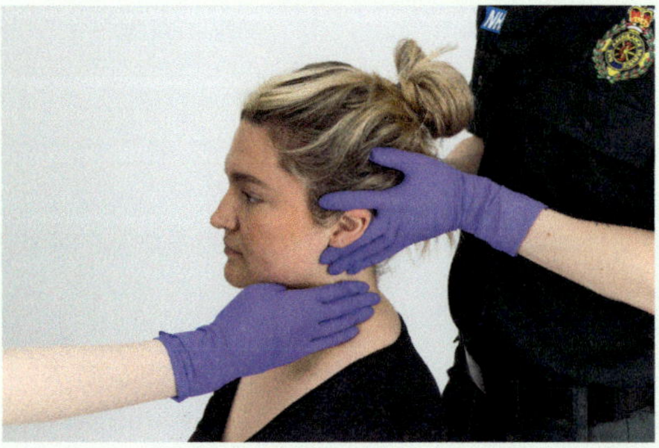	These are the locations given by the manufacturer of the device to gain a measurement of the patient that will correlate to the sizing guide on the collar.

Action		Rationale
6.	Compare the distance measured in step 5 with the space on the collar between the sizing line and the lower aspect of the plastic part of the collar body (not the foam). 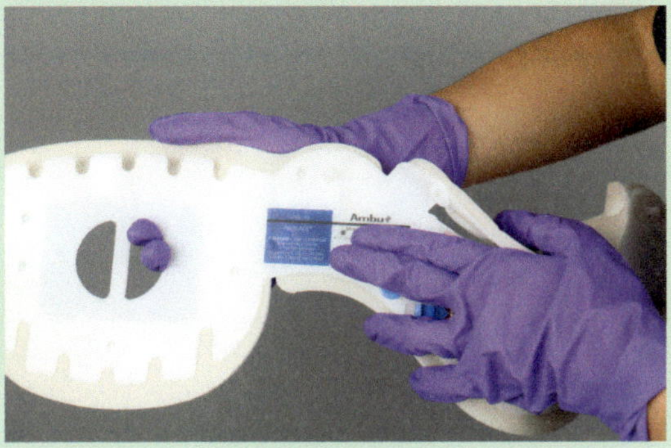	
7.	To initially increase the size of the collar: Disengage the locking pins by pulling them up. Adjust the collar to the appropriate size by pulling it apart until the distance between the sizing line and the collar body equals your finger measurements. Engage the locking pins by pushing them down. 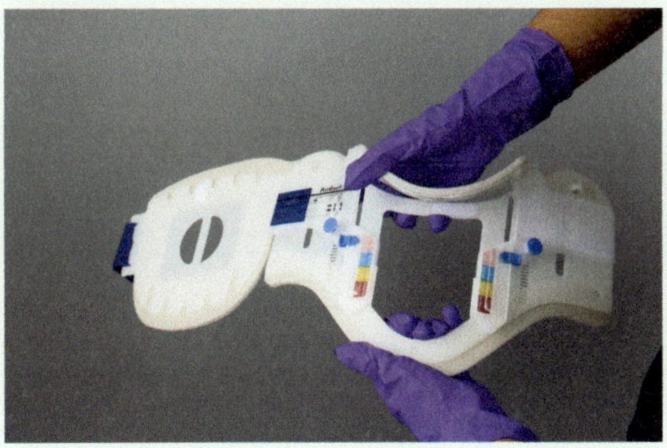	The collar comes in the smallest configuration and normally only needs to be adjusted up. To do this, the ratchet tabs can be left in place; they only need to be disengaged if the size of the collar needs to be reduced again.

Action		Rationale
8.	Ensure the chin piece has been flipped over from its storage position and is pointing towards the front of the device. 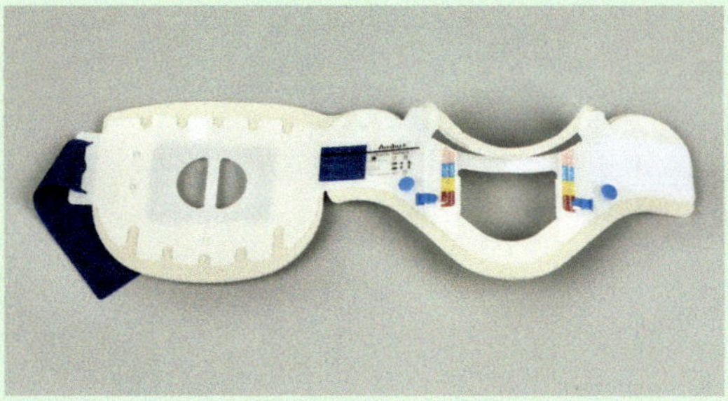	The collar can accidentally be applied without the chin piece having been flipped over, which will allow much more movement than should be possible.
9.	Offer the front of the collar up to the patient's chin and chest in order to see if the size is correct.	Checking the size prior to applying the collar will help to reduce the risk of causing accidental flexion or extension when applying the device.
10.	If you need to adjust from the original size: Disengage the locking tabs by pulling them up. Pull the ratchet tabs out. Adjust the collar to the correct size by sliding the ratchet tabs up or down.	There are a total of 16 positions the collar can be secured in. Making appropriate adjustments will help to ensure it is optimally sized for the patient.
11.	Once the size is correct, ensure all ratchet tabs and the locking tabs are secured. 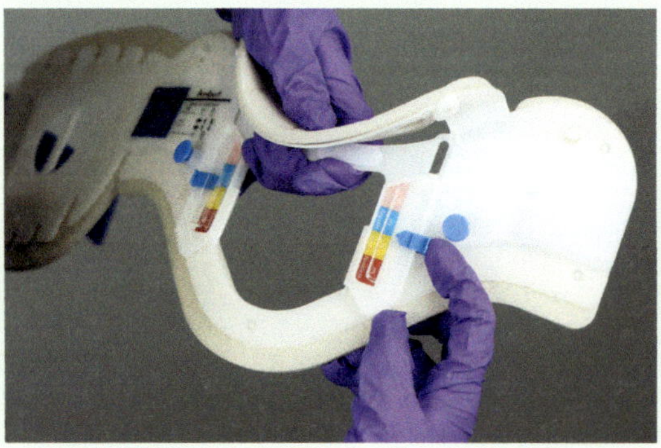	Ensure all locking tabs are in place to prevent movement once applied to the patient.

<table>
<tr><th colspan="2">Action</th><th>Rationale</th></tr>
<tr><td>12.</td><td>Roll the collar up to pre-form it prior to application.
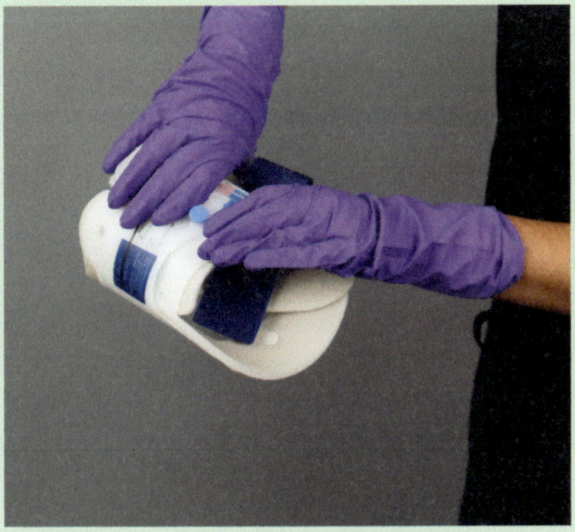</td><td>Collars come packed flat and rolling them prior to application can help them to conform to the natural shape of the patient's neck once applied.</td></tr>
<tr><td>13.</td><td>Slide the back part of the collar under the patient's neck until the Velcro can be seen appearing on the other side.
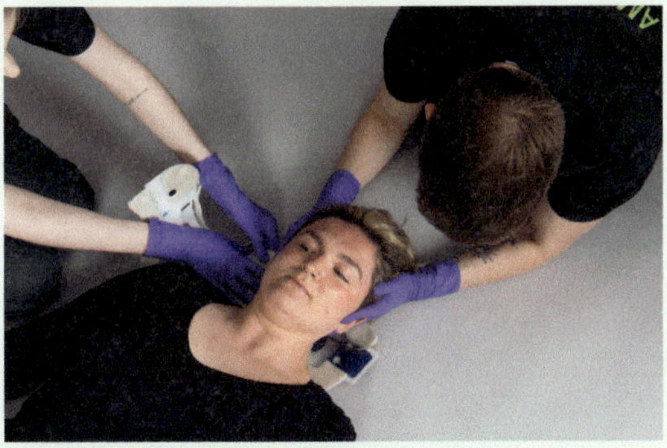</td><td>If you place the chin piece on first, it will cause movement of the neck while you slide the back piece around the neck.</td></tr>
<tr><td>14.</td><td>Position the chin piece under the chin.
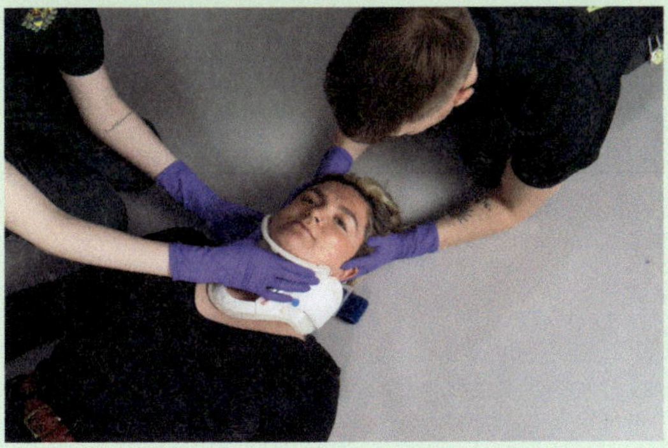</td><td></td></tr>
</table>

Action		Rationale
15.	While keeping the front of the collar in the correct position with one hand, attach the Velcro with your other hand to achieve a secure fit.	This secures the collar in place.
	Maintain MILS until the patient's neck is fully immobilised in a vacuum mattress or similar appropriate device. 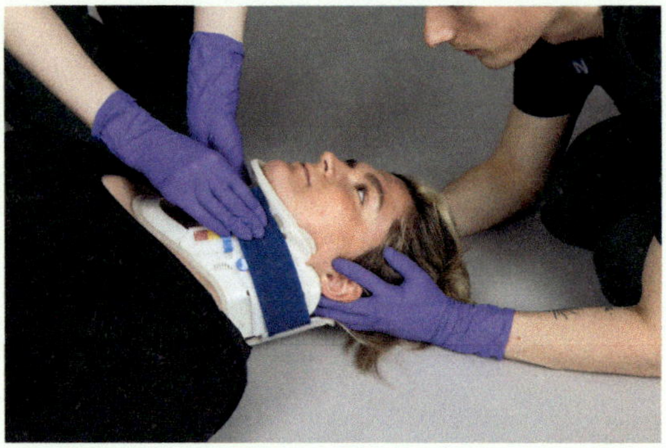	A collar does not fully immobilise the cervical spine, so MILS must be maintained until full spinal immobilisation is in place.
16.	Document the procedure and the time it was completed.	You must keep full, clear and accurate records for everyone you care for, treat, or provide other services to (13).

References

1. Henry S. *Advanced Trauma Life Support*. 10th edition. ACS American College of Surgeons; 2018.
2. JRCALC. *JRCALC Clinical Guidelines 2019*. Bridgwater: Class Publishing; 2019.
3. Sundstrøm T, Asbjørnsen H, Habiba S, et al. Prehospital use of cervical collars in trauma patients: A critical review. *Journal of Neurotrauma*. 2014;31(6):531–540.
4. Conner D, Greaves I, Porter K, et al. Pre-hospital spinal immobilisation: An initial consensus statement. *Journal of Paramedic Practice*. 2014;6(5):242–246.
5. Royal College of Emergency Medicine. Position statement paediatric trauma – Stabilisation of the cervical spine [Internet]. 2019 [cited 2021 Dec 4]. Available from: https://rcem.ac.uk/wp-content/uploads/2021/10/Paediatric_Trauma_Stabilisation_of_the_Cervical_Spine_Jan20.pdf.
6. Núñez-Patiño RA, Rubiano AM, Godoy DA. Impact of cervical collars on intracranial pressure values in traumatic brain injury: A systematic review and meta-analysis of prospective studies. *Neurocritical Care*. 2019;32(2):469-477.
7. Austin N, Krishnamoorthy V, Dagal A. Airway management in cervical spine injury. *International Journal of Critical Illness and Injury Science*. 2014 Jan;4(1):50–56.
8. Ham W, Schoonhoven L, Schuurmans MJ, et al. Pressure ulcers from spinal immobilization in trauma patients: A systematic review. *Journal of Trauma and Acute Care Surgery*. 2014;76(4):1131–1141.
9. Ambu. Instructions for use Ambu Perfit ACE [Internet]. 2020 [cited 2021 Dec 4]. Available from: file:///Users/krislethbridge/Downloads/492280000-IFU-Ambu-Perfit-Ace-V08-052020-10791_-Multi.pdf.
10. British Medical Association. Ethics – General information [Internet]. 2018 [cited 2019 Dec 29]. Available from: https://www.bma.org.uk/advice/employment/ethics/consent/consent-tool-kit/2-general-information.
11. Health and Care Professions Council. Standards of conduct, performance and ethics [Internet]. 2018 [cited 2019 Dec 29]. Available from: https://www.hcpc-uk.org/standards/standards-of-conduct-performance-and-ethics/.
12. NHS England. Standard infection control precautions: national hand hygiene and personal protective equipment policy [Internet]. 2019 [cited 2022 Feb 13]. Available from: https://www.england.nhs.uk/publication/standardinfection-control-precautions-national-handhygiene-andpersonal-protective-equipment-policy/.
13. Health and Care Professions Council. Standards of conduct, performance and ethics. Health & Care Professions Council. 2016.

Scoop Stretcher

Indications

- To provide immobilisation and transport of a patient.

Contraindications

- Patient too heavy for device (weighs more than 227 kg (36 st)) (1).
- Any missing or defective components.
- Device regular inspection interval expired (check local policy).

Advantages

- Lightweight.
- Adjustable to suit most patients.
- Requires minimal casualty manoeuvring to position them on the stretcher (2).

Disadvantages

- Morbidly obese patients may not fit.
- Less comfortable and more likely to cause pressure injury than a vacuum mattress.

Procedure – Scoop Stretcher

Take the following steps to place a patient on a scoop stretcher (1):

Note: This device is also sometimes referred to as an orthopaedic stretcher.

Action		Rationale
1.	If the patient is conscious, explain the procedure and obtain consent if appropriate to do so.	You must make sure that you have valid consent from service users or other appropriate authority before you provide care, treatment or other services (3,4).
2.	Don appropriate personal protective equipment (PPE), and undertake appropriate hand hygiene.	This reduces the risk of cross-infection (5).
3.	If indicated, ensure manual in-line stabilisation (MILS) is being applied and a cervical collar has been fitted. 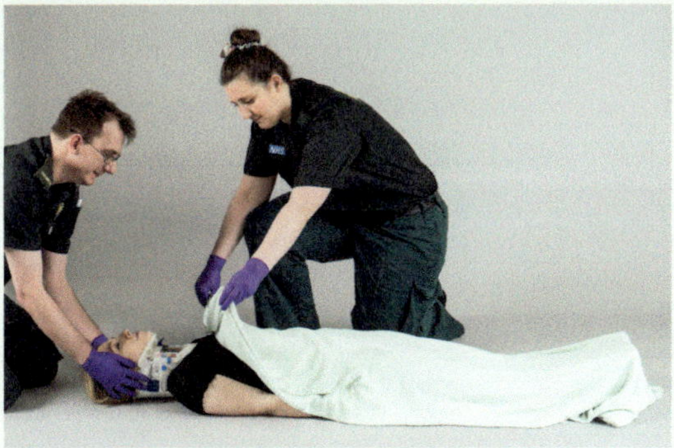	Where cervical spinal immobilisation is indicated, it should be continued throughout the process of transferring a patient onto a scoop stretcher.

Action		Rationale
4.	Ensure that the patient is exposed appropriately (being mindful of maintaining dignity) and any other equipment required has been gathered.	To place a patient on to a scoop stretcher, small positional movements (rolls) will be required. Any other outstanding procedures that require a roll (such as examination of the back) should be completed at the same time to minimise movement.
5.	Place the scoop on the ground next to the patient so that the head is in line with the area that is designed to accommodate the head on the scoop stretcher. 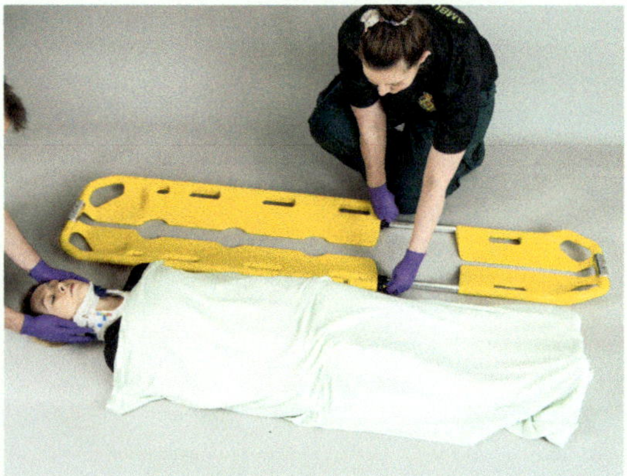	This will allow you to accurately adjust the size of the scoop stretcher to match the patient in advance.
6.	Move the locking pins on either side of the stretcher to the upright position. Adjust the length of the stretcher by pulling on the foot section until the scoop stretcher is the desired length. 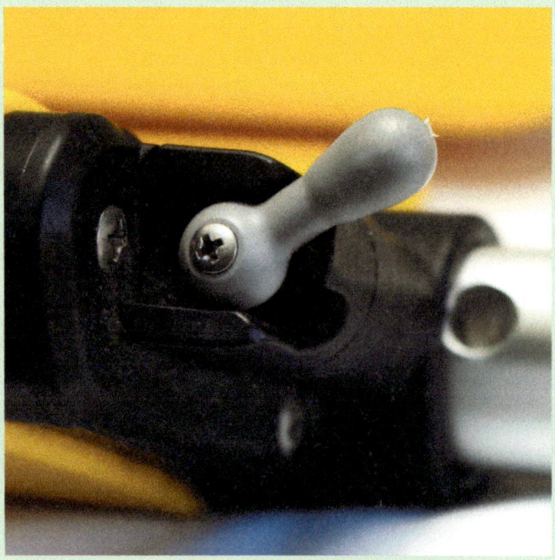	

Action		Rationale
7.	Move the locking pins to the downward position. Gently move the foot section up and down until it locks into place. 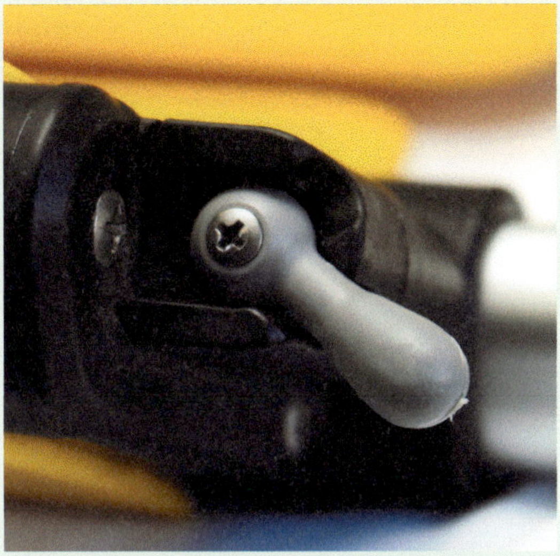	
8.	Separate the scoop stretcher by pressing the tabs on the Twin Safety Lock system at both the head and foot ends. Pull the two halves away from each other. 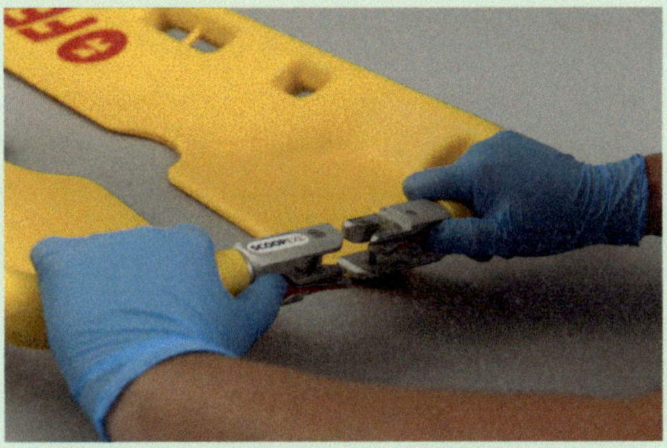	
9.	Ensure you have enough people to undertake the procedure. You will require people for each of the following: • MILS (if indicated). • Two people to undertake the roll. • One person to insert the scoop stretcher. The team leader should brief everyone as to their role and the steps involved.	Placing a patient onto a scoop stretcher should be performed in a controlled fashion to avoid unnecessary movement. Not everyone involved needs to be a clinician. Someone from the fire or police service could insert the scoop stretcher under the patient on the instructions of the team leader, for example.

	Action	Rationale
10.	Position the rescuers: • One clinician should be positioned at the head of the patient to maintain MILS. • Two clinicians should kneel on the side the patient is being rolled towards, level with the patient's chest and hips and legs. • Another person with the scoop stretcher should position themselves on the other side of the patient, ready to insert the first half of the board. All rescuers should consider the principles of safe moving and roll in a straight line with their back as straight as possible.	It has traditionally been taught that the clinicians undertaking the roll should cross arms as this can help to ensure spinal alignment. There is no strong evidence to support this and most organisations are moving away from this and no longer teach crossing arms. The angle of the roll should be as small as possible. The patient only needs to be rolled to create a gap of 5 cm (2 in) to enable the scoop stretcher to be inserted underneath. In practice it is common to see patients rolled much more than they need to be.
11.	When all rescuers are ready, the clinician at the head end of the patient should issue the command: 'Ready, Set, Move.' On 'move', the clinicians should conduct a coordinated roll. Once completed, the scoop stretcher should be inserted under the patient. 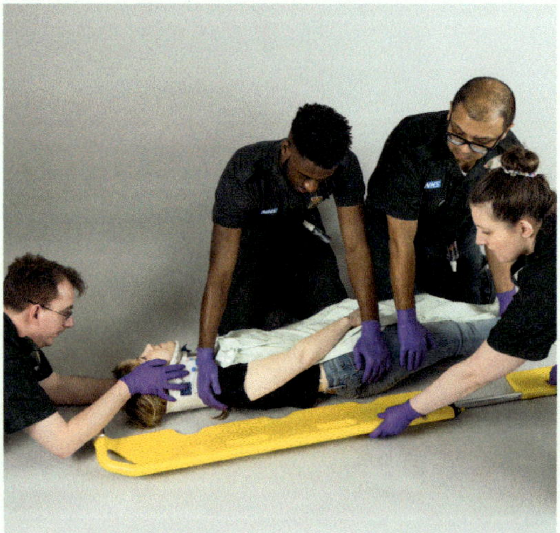	A coordinated move should ensure the patient's spine remains in line.

Action		Rationale
12.	Once the scoop stretcher has been inserted, the patient should be lowered using the same 'Ready, Set, Move' command issued by the clinician at the head end of the patient. 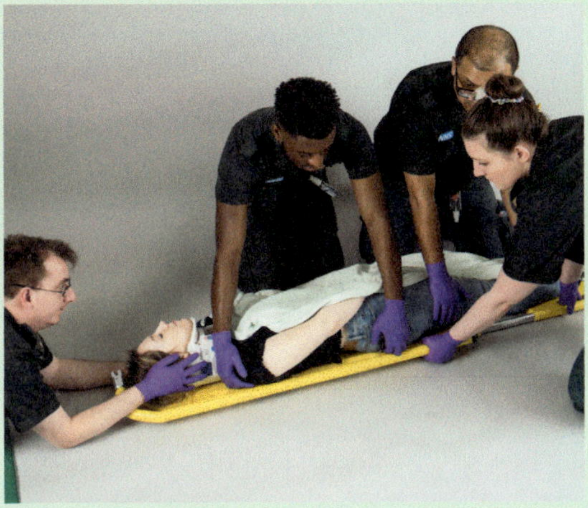	Lowering movements should also be coordinated to reduce rotation of the spine.
13.	Repeat the procedure on the other side. Once both sections are in place, push the brackets of the Twin Safety Lock together until clicked into position. Start with the bracket at the head end.	Bringing the brackets together can cause some movement to occur. By fixing the head first, any movement from the second and normally more difficult bracket will occur at the foot end instead of the neck.
14.	Secure the patient to the stretcher by attaching the chest straps first. If possible, ask the patient to take a deep breath and to hold it before tightening the chest straps. 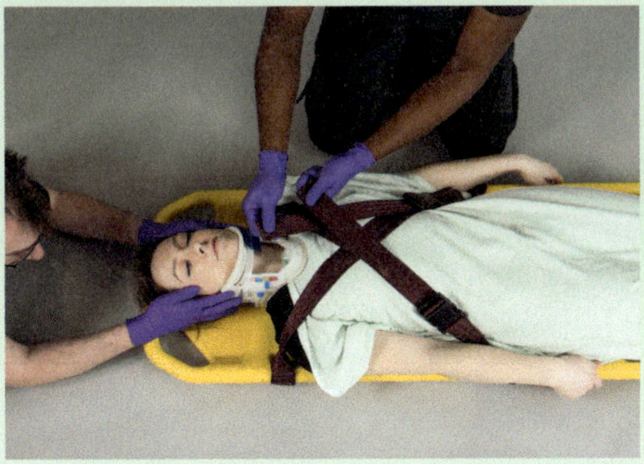	The buckles should go at the lower end by the flanks rather than over the shoulders as they are less likely to cause a pressure injury here. Asking the patient to breathe in before tightening the chest straps should ensure they are not so tight as to interfere with chest expansion during breathing.

Action		Rationale
15.	Apply the hip strap and secure. 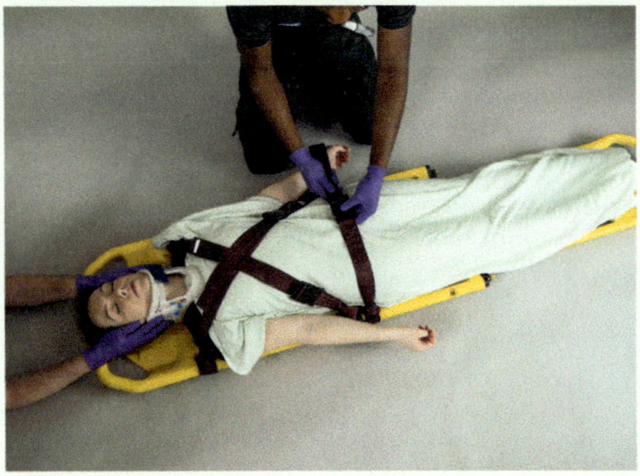	
16.	Apply the foot strap in a figure-of-eight configuration. 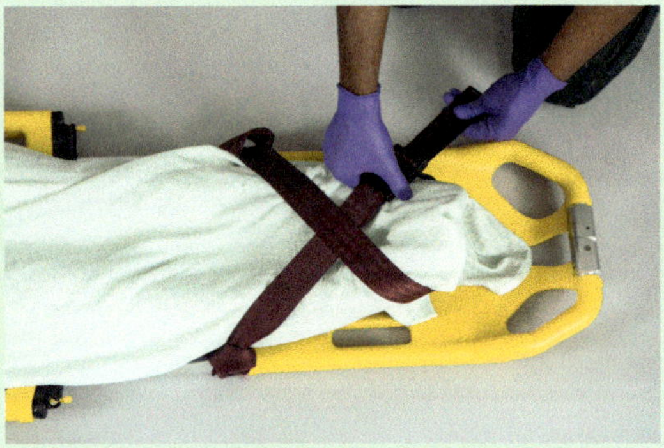	A figure of eight will keep the patient more secure and may also help to reduce vertical movement if the stretcher has to be tilted at all during extrication.
17.	Secure the head using a system designed for use with a scoop stretcher. Here a disposable system is used. 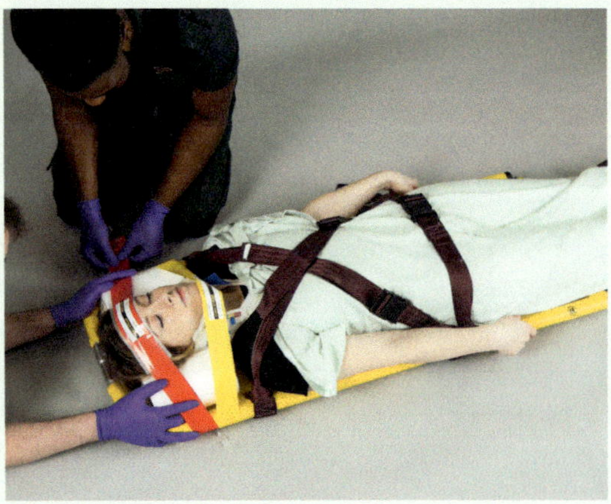	Ad hoc securing such as using tape and upside-down blocks should be avoided as this is not an approved technique for keeping the neck immobilised, and this method frequently fails.

Action		Rationale
18.	Document the procedure.	You must keep full, clear and accurate records for everyone you care for, treat, or provide other services to (4).

References

1. Ferno. User and Maintenance Manual SCOOP EXL Atraumatic Stretcher [Internet]. 2019 [cited 2022 Jul 25]. Available from: https://www.ferno.it/upload/prodotti/99/mu-en_scoopex-PDF-20210525141714.pdf.
2. Krell JM, McCoy MS, Sparto PJ, et al. Comparison of the Ferno Scoop Stretcher with the long backboard for spinal immobilization. *Prehospital Emergency Care*. 2006;10(1):46–51.
3. British Medical Association. Ethics – General information [Internet]. 2018 [cited 2019 Dec 29]. Available from: www.bma.org.uk/advice/employment/ethics/consent/consent-tool-kit/2-general-information.
4. Health and Care Professions Council. Standards of conduct, performance and ethics [Internet]. 2016 [cited 2022 Jul 16]. Available from: www.hcpc-uk.org/standards/standards-of-conduct-performance-and-ethics/.
5. NHS England. Standard infection control precautions: National hand hygiene and personal protective equipment policy [Internet]. 2019 [cited 2022 Feb 13]. Available from: www.england.nhs.uk/publication/standard-infection-control-precautions-national-hand-hygiene-and-personal-protective-equipment-policy/.

Vacuum Mattress

Indications

- To provide immobilisation and transport of a patient.

Contraindications

- Patients should not be placed on a vacuum mattress for transport if they are time-critical and doing so would result in any delay. In this case they should be conveyed on the first device they are placed on (scoop stretcher).
- Cannot be used for extrication.

Advantages

- Reduced movement of the spine in comparison to other devices (1), though the clinical relevance of this is not clear.
- More comfortable for longer periods and lower chance of pressure injury than other immobilisation devices (2).
- May provide some degree of immobilisation to other injuries (for example, pelvic fracture).
- Can be shaped to fit the patient, so if a patient needs to be immobilised sitting up (due to a respiratory complaint, for example), a vacuum mattress can be used to achieve this.
- Patient can safely be tilted laterally (for example, if pregnant or if required due to vomiting).

Disadvantages

- Requires a proprietary hand pump or suction unit to remove air.
- Has less horizontal strength than other immobilisation devices, which can lead to flexing when carrying. It is not suitable for carrying a patient over long distances without some other device being used to provide support.
- The splints are easily damaged; when damaged, they do not retain the vacuum and inflate, resulting in a loss of immobilisation.

Procedure – Vacuum Mattress

Take the following steps to apply a vacuum mattress (3,4):

Action		Rationale
1.	If the patient is conscious, explain the procedure and obtain consent if appropriate to do so.	You must make sure that you have valid consent from service users or other appropriate authority before you provide care, treatment or other services (5,6).
2.	Don appropriate personal protective equipment (PPE), and undertake appropriate hand hygiene.	This reduces the risk of cross-infection (7).
3.	Lay the vacuum mattress out on the floor. Check which end is the head end and extend all the buckles on the straps so they are fully open prior to placing the patient in the device.	Having the straps laid out and fully extended will make application simpler once the patient has been placed in the device.

Action		Rationale
4.	Check the mattress has no leaks by quickly removing the air and ensuring it does not rapidly lose its vacuum effect.	These devices can be damaged easily, and it is not uncommon to find damaged ones on ambulances. Checking it is working prior to application will avoid the delay and extra movement that will result if you place a patient on a damaged mattress.
5.	Prepare the patient by removing clothing as necessary and use a scoop stretcher to transfer them into the mattress.	Patients should be transferred with minimal movement, best achieved with the use of a scoop stretcher (see Scoop Stretcher procedure). Note: A bed sheet can be used for comfort, but this increases the potential for extra movement, and is often used inappropriately to slide a patient out of the vacuum mattress on arrival at hospital. If a sheet is not required (as in this sequence where the patient remains clothed) then it should be avoided.
6.	With one person providing manual in-line stabilisation (MILS) of the cervical spine, one or two more clinicians should start to buckle up the straps, working from the chest down. The two chest straps cross over and are colour coded. 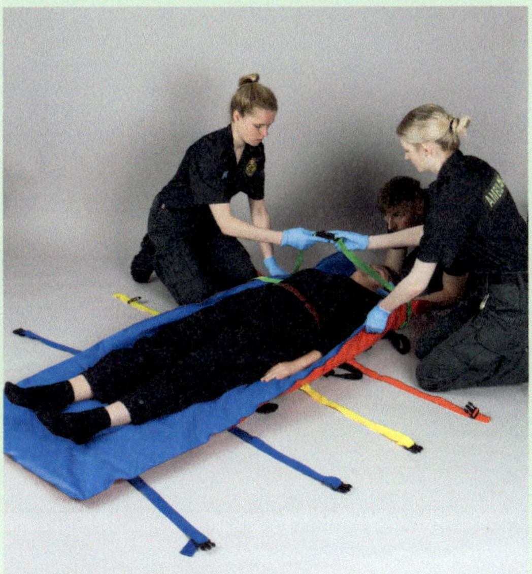	Like the scoop stretcher, straps are applied in the order of chest down to feet, returning to the head last.

Action		Rationale
7.	To tighten, two clinicians should apply equal opposing force to the buckle. While tightening the chest straps, ask the patient to take a deep breath in and hold it. 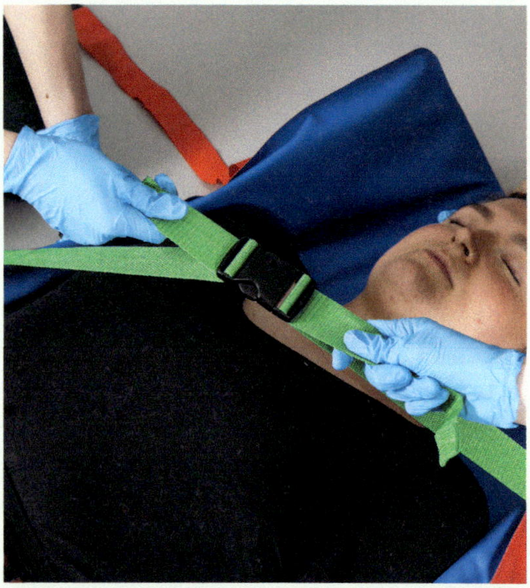	Working in opposition should result in smooth tightening and equal force. Asking the patient to breathe in before tightening the chest straps should ensure they are not so tight as to interfere with chest expansion during breathing.
8.	Secure the thigh strap (colour coded) and the two foot straps. 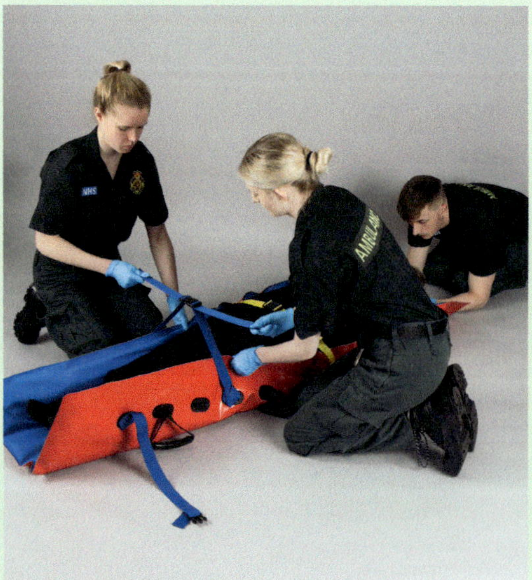	This secures the lower body.

Action		Rationale
9.	Another clinician should take control of the cervical spine by kneeling to the side of the patient and placing a hand each on the forehead and the chin, utilising a 'c grip' technique. 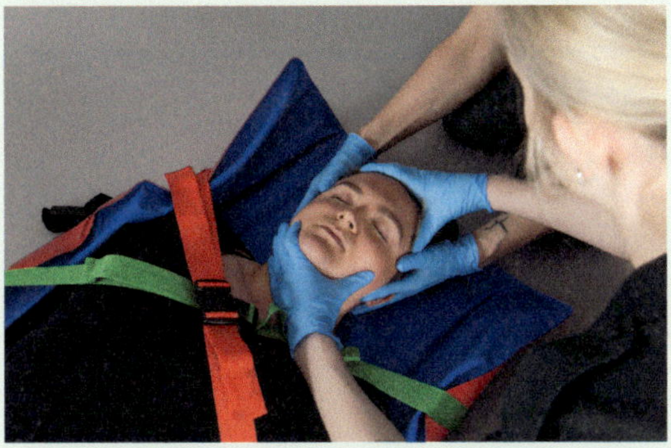	This will provide manual immobilisation of the spine while releasing the clinician currently controlling the head. The clinician providing MILS should not let go until the clinician taking over confirms 'I have control'.
10.	Once the hands on the sides of the head have been released, a device for immobilising the head can be inserted. 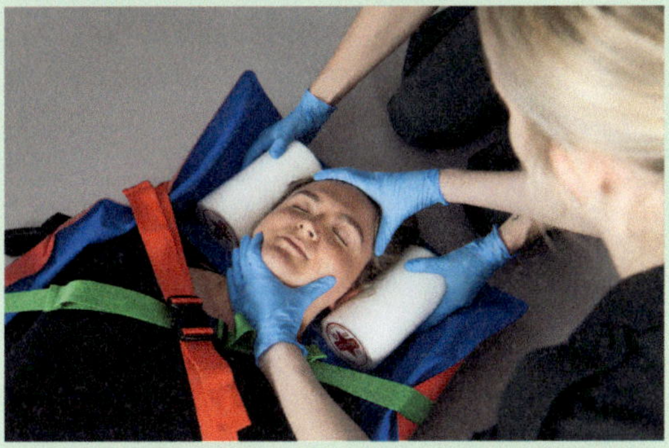	On some vacuum mattresses there are inbuilt 'head huggers'. That is not the case on the device shown here, so disposable blocks have been inserted to provide better immobilisation of the head inside the mattress.
11.	Form the vacuum mattress securely around the head blocks. Once the head is controlled from the sides through the mattress, the immobilisation of the forehead and chin can be released. 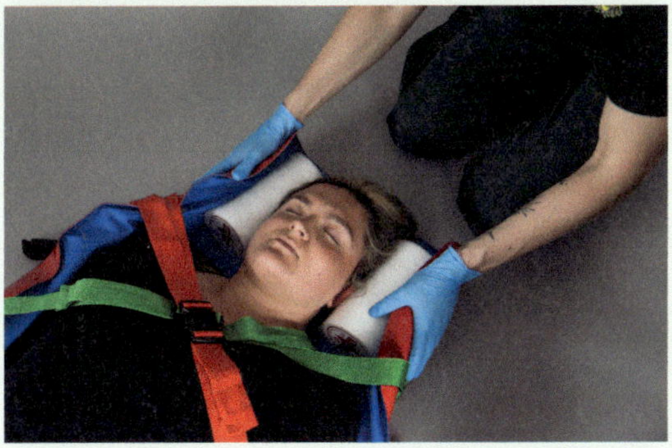	Forming the mattress around the head blocks will ensure adequate immobilisation is maintained after the air is removed.

	Action	Rationale
12.	Check that the valve is securely in the closed position and attach the pump which has been set up to extract air. 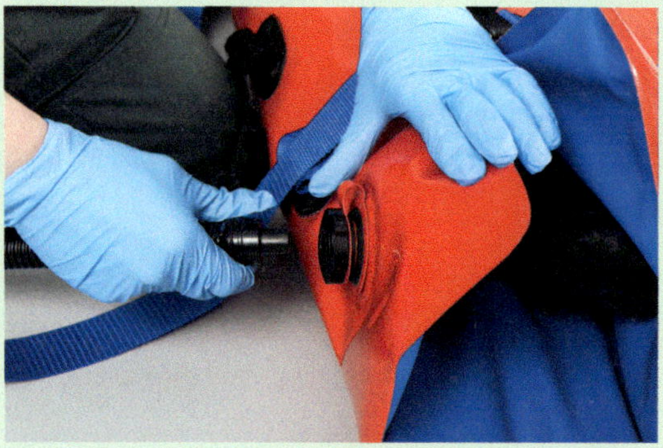	If the valve is not closed, it will leak, resulting in the mattress not becoming firm.
13.	With one person maintaining manual control of the head, another should pump the air out of the mattress. Any spare rescuers can help to gently form the body of the mattress to the patient. 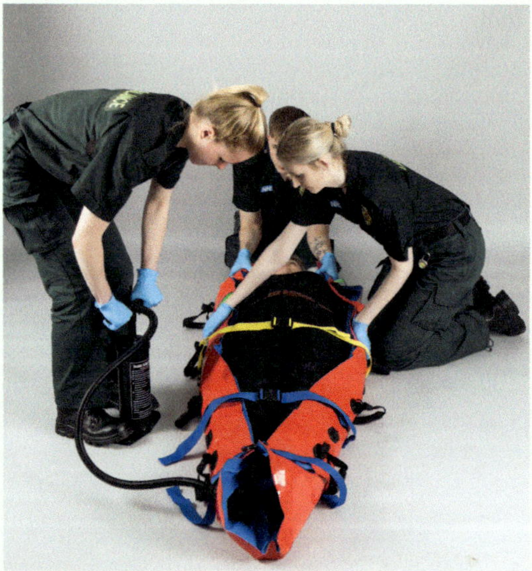	Forming the body of the mattress to the patient will help to ensure a firm fit as the air is removed. The provided pump can both inflate and deflate the mattress by adjusting the position the air hose is connected to the pump. If you are struggling to pump air out of the mattress, check the hose is connected to the correct port on the pump.
14.	Continue to remove air until the mattress becomes firm and can no longer be easily reshaped by hand.	Once firm, the mattress should provide adequate immobilisation.

Action		Rationale
15.	Check the straps; if any have become loose, retighten now. 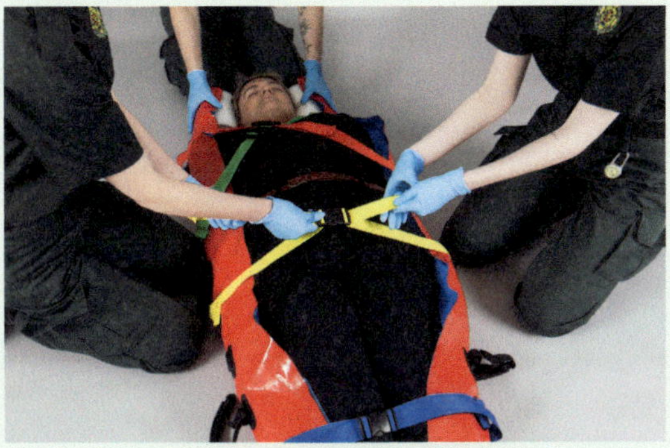	As air is removed, it is common for the straps to become slack. Retightening after air has been removed will help to ensure the mattress provides adequate immobilisation.
16.	Strap the head down using appropriate straps or tape. 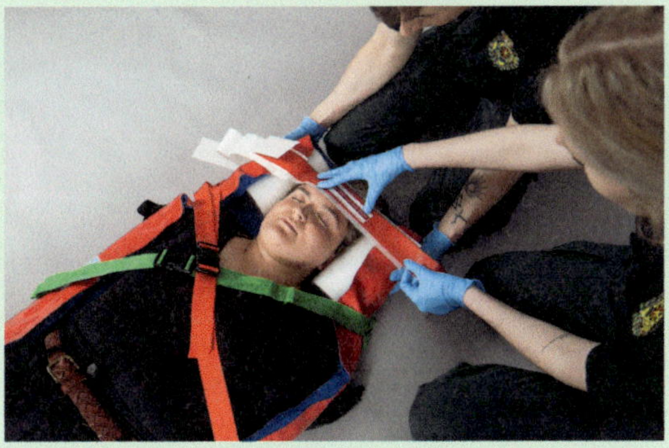	Here disposable straps are used. Once the straps have been applied, the manual control of the head can be released.
17.	If the patient subsequently requires removing from the mattress, a scoop stretcher should be used.	The patient should not be slid sideways using a bed sheet and patient slide. There is little point in taking care to keep patients immobilised by following the above procedure to then apply uncontrolled lateral movement of the spine by sliding the patient sideways during the transfer at hospital.
18.	Document the procedure.	You must keep full, clear and accurate records for everyone you care for, treat, or provide other services to (6).

References

1. Prasarn ML, Hyldmo PK, Zdziarski LA, et al. Comparison of the vacuum mattress versus the spine board alone for immobilization of the cervical spine injured patient. *Spine* (Philadelphia, PA 1976). 2017;42(24):E1398–1402.
2. Ahmad M. Spinal boards or vacuum mattresses for immobilisation. *Emergency Medicine Journal*. 2014;31(9).
3. Queensland Ambulance Service. Clinical practice procedures: Trauma/Orthopaedic splinting – EasyFIX

PLUS vacuum mattress [Internet]. 2021 [cited 2022 Jul 31]. Available from: www.ambulance.qld.gov.au/docs/clinical/cpp/CPP_Orthopaedic%20splinting_EasyFIX%20PLUS%20vaccuum%20matress.pdf.
4. Ferno. Directions for use: EasyFIX PLUS vacuum mattress [Internet]. 2019 [cited 2022 Jul 31]. Available from: www.fernonorden.dk/Files/Images/Ecom/PDF/GE23271511001_D_ALL_2019-04-02.pdf.
5. British Medical Association. Ethics – General information [Internet]. 2018 [cited 2019 Dec 29]. Available from: www.bma.org.uk/advice/employment/ethics/consent/consent-tool-kit/2-general-information.
6. Health and Care Professions Council. Standards of conduct, performance and ethics [Internet]. 2016 [cited 2022 Jul 16]. Available from: www.hcpc-uk.org/standards/standards-of-conduct-performance-and-ethics/.
7. NHS England. Standard infection control precautions: National hand hygiene and personal protective equipment policy [Internet]. 2019 [cited 2022 Feb 13]. Available from: www.england.nhs.uk/publication/standard-infection-control-precautions-national-hand-hygiene-and-personal-protective-equipment-policy/.

Chapter

7 Cardiac Arrest

Cardiac arrest is the ultimate medical emergency, but you will have the ability to undertake the two most effective treatments for this: cardiopulmonary resuscitation (more commonly called basic life support or BLS in healthcare circles) and defibrillation. However, the role of the ambulance service is just one link in a chain that maximises the patient's chances not only of a return of spontaneous circulation (ROSC), but also of surviving to hospital discharge neurologically intact (with normal or near-normal brain function) (1). That chain is known as the chain of survival (2).

The chain of survival encompasses four key principles that are required if a resuscitation is to be successful in adults (**Figure 7.1**) (1):

- Early recognition and call for help
- Early bystander cardiopulmonary resuscitation (CPR)
- Early defibrillation
- Early advanced life support (ALS) and standardised post-resuscitation care.

In this chapter, we have assumed that you'll be working within an ambulance service and have at least one colleague to support your resuscitation effort. Because of this, we have not separated BLS from defibrillation, since both should be available to you and their seamless integration is important for patient survival. As always, follow local guidelines and take advantage of any specialist clinicians who may be available in your service to support you and your patient.

References

1. Semeraro F, Greif R, Böttiger BW, et al. European Resuscitation Council Guidelines 2021: systems saving lives. *Resuscitation*. 2021 Apr 1;161:80–97.
2. Nolan J, Soar J, Eikeland H. The chain of survival. *Resuscitation*. 2006 Dec;71(3):270–271.

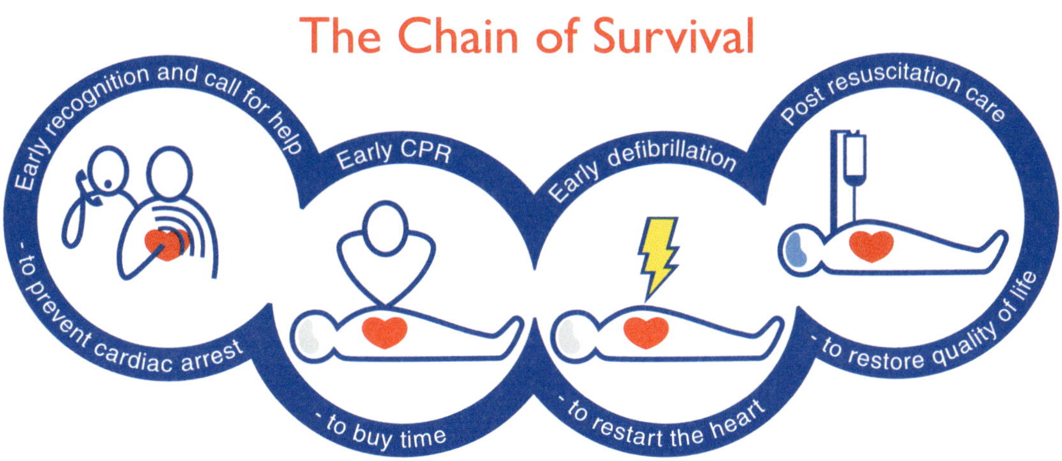

Figure 7.1 The chain of survival.

Reproduced with the kind permission of Laerdal Medical.

Newborn Life Support

Indications
- Newborn baby undergoing physiological transition from foetus to infant.

Contraindications
- None.

Advantage
- Likely to result in a successful resuscitation, often with little intervention from clinicians (1).

Disadvantage
- Different from the resuscitation of infants and children which clinicians are likely to be more familiar with.

Procedure – Newborn Life Support

Take the following steps to perform newborn life support (**Figure 7.2**) (1,2):

Action		Rationale
1.	Ensure the scene is safe for you, your colleague, the patient and other bystanders. Ensure that the immediate environment is warm (ideally 23–25°C).	Your safety and that of your colleagues is your primary concern. Newborns are prone to hypothermia, particularly if the environment is cool and draughty, as this will exacerbate heat loss (3).
2.	Don appropriate personal protective equipment (PPE), and undertake appropriate hand hygiene.	Childbirth can be messy, with copious amounts of bodily fluids. Wearing PPE will reduce the risk of cross-infection (4).
3.	Note the time and dry the newborn with a towel. Discard that towel and wrap them with a fresh, dry towel and put on a newborn hat, if available. 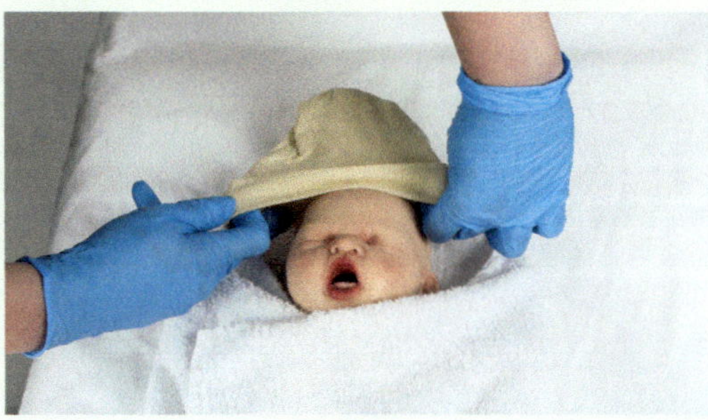	Newborns become hypothermic easily if they are not dried and wrapped early, which can be forgotten during a resuscitation attempt.

	Action	Rationale
4.	Do not rush to clamp or tie the cord unless it is broken, the position of the mother makes ongoing management impossible, or the newborn requires resuscitation. Leave the cord intact until it stops pulsating where possible.	Delayed cord clamping can result in an additional 30 ml/kg of blood transferred from the placenta to the newborn, improving levels of iron and red blood cell counts and reducing the need for subsequent blood transfusions (1). This can take up to 10–20 minutes, but anything over 60 seconds is beneficial. Auto-transfusion will still occur even when the newborn is chest to chest or abdomen with the mother (5).
5.	Assess tone, colour, adequacy of breathing and the heart rate. This can be undertaken with step 2 since drying the newborn provides tactile stimulation. Remember to re-assess every 30 seconds.	This will help you decide whether there is a need for medical intervention. Signs of a healthy newborn will include good tone, and while they may initially be cyanosed, they will become pink within 1–2 minutes. They will also spontaneously breathe within a minute of the birth and their heart rate will be greater than 100 beats per minute within 2 minutes (6). An ill newborn will be pale and floppy, with no respiratory effort and a heart rate of less than 60 beats per minute (6).
6.	If breathing is inadequate (or absent), place the newborn on their back with the head in a neutral position. A jaw thrust may be required if the newborn has poor tone (is floppy). A 2 cm-thick pad can be placed under the shoulders to facilitate correct head position. 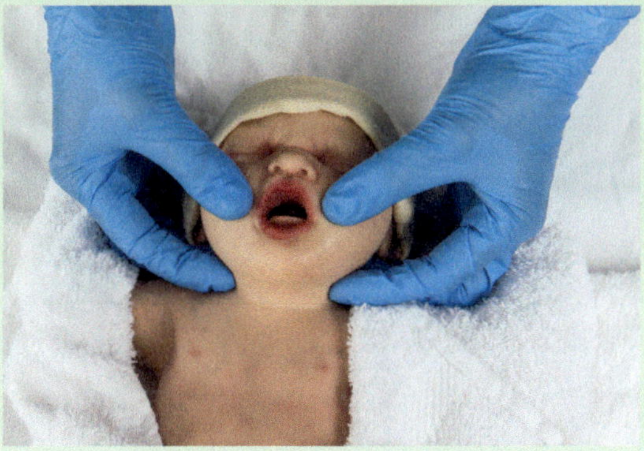	A newborn will be unable to maintain their own airway if they have poor tone and ventilations will be less effective if the airway is not fully open.

Action		Rationale
7.	If opening the airway has not resulted in adequate breathing, provide five inflation breaths. These are higher pressure (30 cm H_2O) ventilations given over 2–3 seconds each time. The chest may not rise until several ventilations have been administered. Do not administer supplemental oxygen with these ventilations. 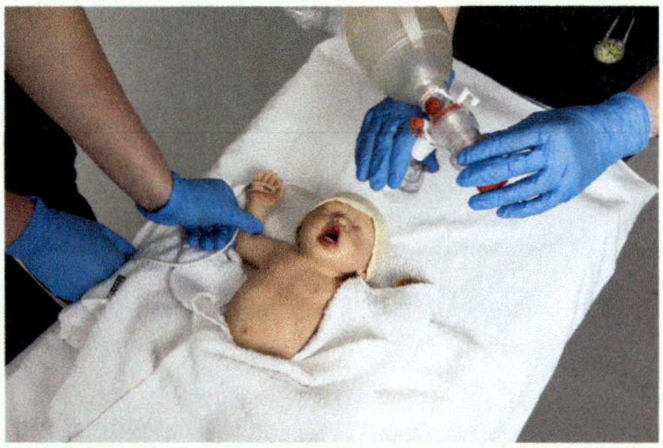	The newborn lungs are typically filled with fluid, which is rapidly cleared by aeration of the lungs caused by spontaneous breathing and crying. In the event that the newborn is not breathing effectively, inflation ventilations will do this instead. However, fluid-filled lungs have a higher resistance than air-filled lungs, which require higher and more sustained ventilatory pressures to be effective. Resuscitation of the newborn with air rather than oxygen appears to lead to a significant reduction in short-term mortality (7,8). In addition, while the cord is pulsating, oxygenated blood is still being transferred from mother to newborn.
8.	Reassess colour, tone, breathing and heart rate. 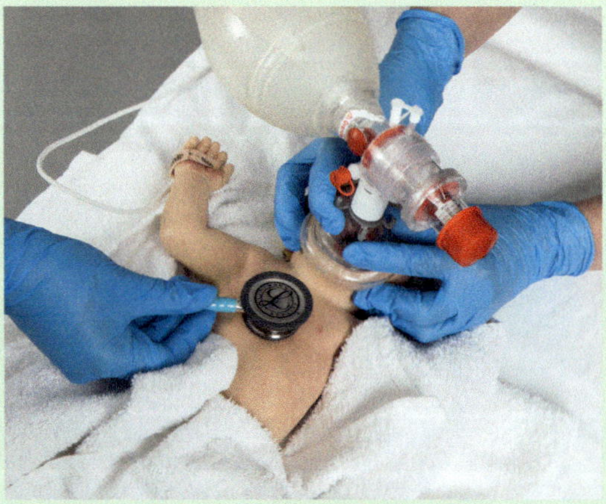	
9a.	If the chest is not moving recheck the airway and repeat the inflation breaths. After 30 seconds return to step 8.	The most likely reason that the chest is not moving is because the lungs have not been sufficiently aerated. Without adequate lung aeration, chest compressions will not be effective (2).

Action		Rationale
9b.	If the chest is moving but the heart rate is not increasing, continue to ventilate at a rate of 30 per minute and reassess after 30 seconds (1). 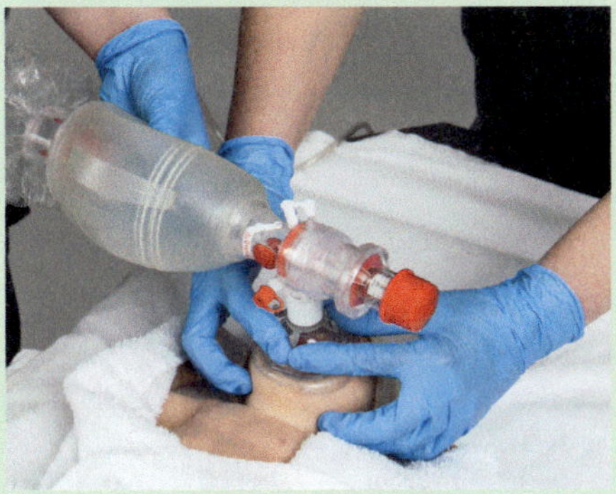	This should improve oxygenation which in turn should encourage spontaneous breathing and an increase in heart rate.
9c.	If the chest is moving, but heart sounds are absent or the heart rate is less than 60 beats per minute following 30 seconds of effective ventilation, provide chest compressions with ventilations at a ratio of three chest compressions to every ventilation and provide supplemental oxygen at 100%. 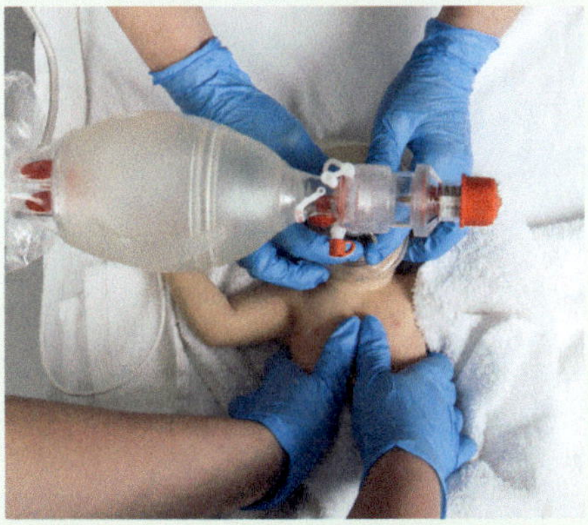	The ratio of 3:1 is advocated in newborn life support in order to provide more breaths per minute (9).
10.	Provide a time-critical transfer to the nearest emergency department with an obstetric unit (6). If there is sufficient capacity in the team, consider vascular access and drug administration as long as this does not distract from CPR and ventilation.	
11.	Document the procedure.	You must keep full, clear, and accurate records for everyone you care for, treat, or provide other services to (10).

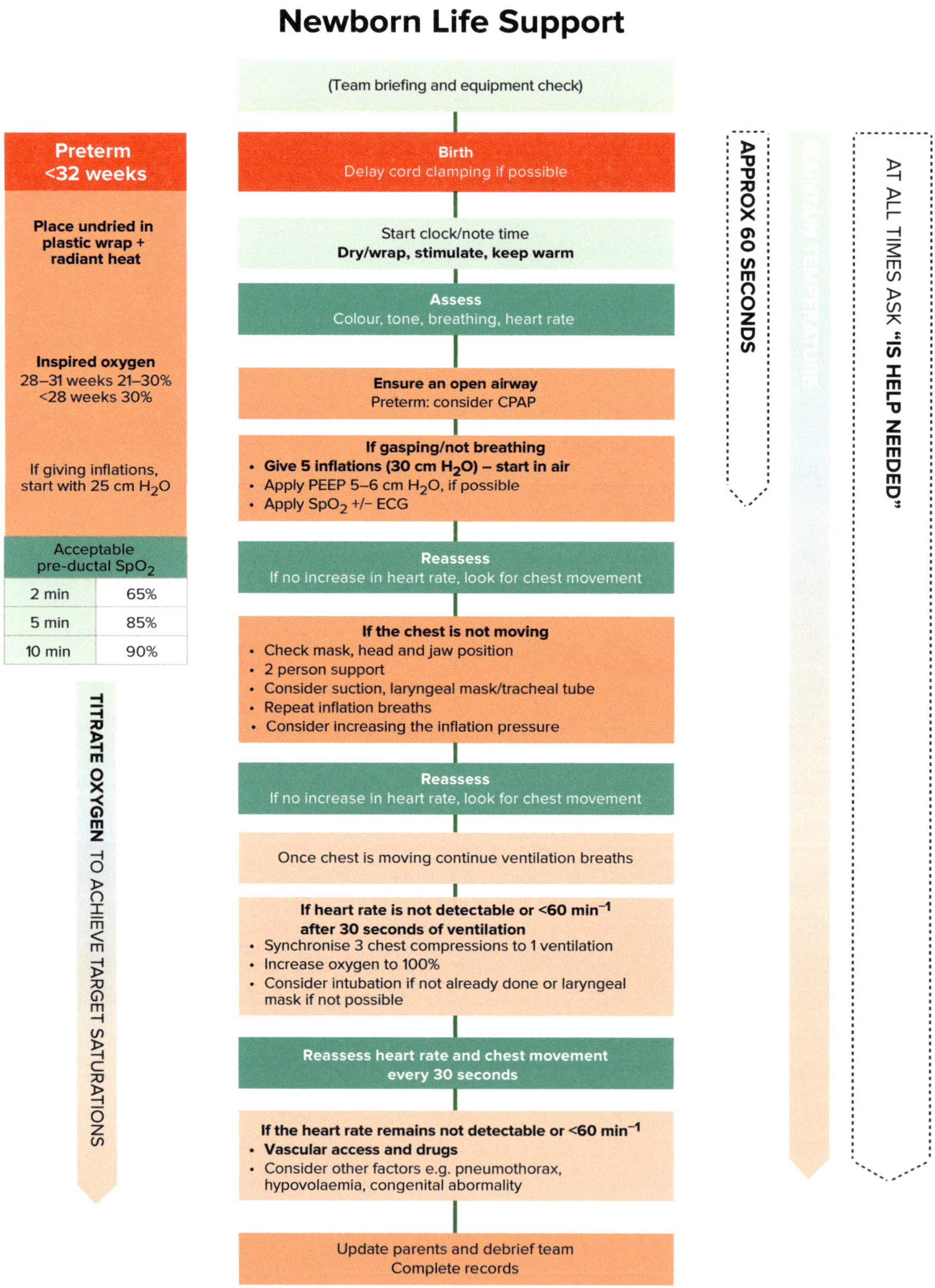

Figure 7.2 Newborn Life Support, Resuscitation Council UK (2021).
Reproduced with the kind permission of Resuscitation Council UK.

References

1. Madar J, Roehr CC, Ainsworth S, et al. European Resuscitation Council Guidelines 2021: newborn resuscitation and support of transition of infants at birth. *Resuscitation*. 2021 Apr 1;161:291–326.
2. Fawke J, Wylie J, Madar J, et al. Newborn resuscitation and support of transition of infants at birth guidelines [Internet]. Resuscitation Council UK. 2021 [cited 2022 May 15]. Available from: https://www.resus.org.uk/library/2021-resuscitation-guidelines/newborn-resuscitation-and-support-transition-infants-birth.
3. Trevisanuto D, Testoni D, de Almeida MFB. Maintaining normothermia: why and how? *Seminars in Fetal Neonatal Medicine*. 2018 Oct 1;23(5):333–339.
4. NHS England, NHS Improvement. Standard infection control precautions: national hand hygiene and personal protective equipment policy [Internet]. 2019 [cited 2021 Nov 11]. Available from: https://www.england.nhs.uk/publication/standard-infection-control-precautions-national-hand-hygiene-and-personal-protective-equipment-policy/.
5. Vain NE, Satragno DS, Gorenstein AN, et al. Effect of gravity on volume of placental transfusion: a multicentre, randomised, non-inferiority trial. *The Lancet*. 2014 Jul;384(9939):235–240.
6. Joint Royal Colleges Ambulance Liaison Committee, Association of Ambulance Chief Executives. JRCALC clinical guidelines. Cited from JRCALC Plus (Version 1.2.13) [Mobile application software]. Bridgwater: Class Publishing Ltd; 2021.
7. Welsford M, Nishiyama C, Shortt C, et al. Room air for initiating term newborn resuscitation: a systematic review with meta-analysis. *Pediatrics*. 2019 Jan 1;143(1):e20181825.
8. Davis PG, Tan A, O'Donnell CP, Schulze A. Resuscitation of newborn infants with 100% oxygen or air: a systematic review and meta-analysis. *The Lancet*. 2004 Oct 9;364(9442):1329–1333.
9. Resuscitation Council UK. *European Paediatric Advanced Life Support*. 5th edition. London: Resuscitation Council UK; 2021.
10. Health and Care Professions Council. Standards of conduct, performance and ethics [Internet]. 2018 [cited 2019 Dec 29]. Available from: https://www.hcpc-uk.org/standards/standards-of-conduct-performance-and-ethics/.

Infant Basic Life Support with Automated External Defibrillation

Indications
- Infant (0–12 months) patient with no apparent signs of life.

Contraindicationss
- Newborn who requires resuscitation (follow Newborn Life Support guideline).
- Patient whose condition is unequivocally associated with death.
- Patient has a Recommended Summary Plan for Emergency Care and Treatment (ReSPECT), relevant to their current clinical presentation, indicating that cardiopulmonary resuscitation (CPR) attempts are not recommended (1).
- Patient has a valid 'do not attempt cardiopulmonary resuscitation' (DNACPR) form (2).

Advantages
- Provides blow flow to the brain and other vital organs (3).
- Good chance of a return of spontaneous circulation (ROSC) if the primary cause is cardiac (although less common in infants).

Disadvantages
- Unlikely to lead to ROSC without other interventions, particularly effective ventilation and oxygenation, and treatment for reversible causes.

Procedure – Infant Basic Life Support with Automated External Defibrillation

Take the following steps to perform basic life support (BLS) on an infant with an automated external defibrillator (AED) (3):

Action		Rationale
1.	Ensure the scene is safe for you, your colleague, the patient and other bystanders.	Your safety and that of your colleagues is your primary concern. Some causes of cardiac arrest can present a risk to the rescuer, for example drowning and electrocution.
2.	Don appropriate personal protective equipment (PPE), and undertake appropriate hand hygiene.	This reduces the risk of cross-infection (4).

	Action	Rationale
3.	Check for responsiveness by placing a hand on the infant's forehead to stabilise it and tug their hair while calling their name. If they have no hair, apply another method of tactile stimulation. 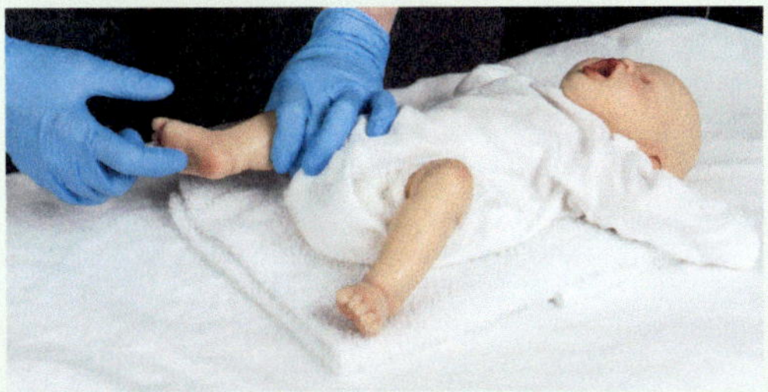	Not every patient who appears to be unresponsive is in cardiac arrest.
4.	If the patient responds, assess the infant's ABCDE, call for assistance and reassess regularly. If they do not respond, summon additional assistance and remove outer clothing.	All cases where infants have experienced a period of unresponsiveness or collapse should be taken seriously. The management of peri-arrest infants is a team effort (1).
5.	Open the infant's airway by placing one hand on their forehead and gently tilt it back until it is in a neutral position (3). Perform a chin lift by placing the fingertips of your other hand on the bony part of the lower jaw and lift upwards. Do not compress the soft tissues under the jaw as this will occlude the airway. Placing a towel under the infant's shoulders and upper body can help keep their head in a neutral position (5). 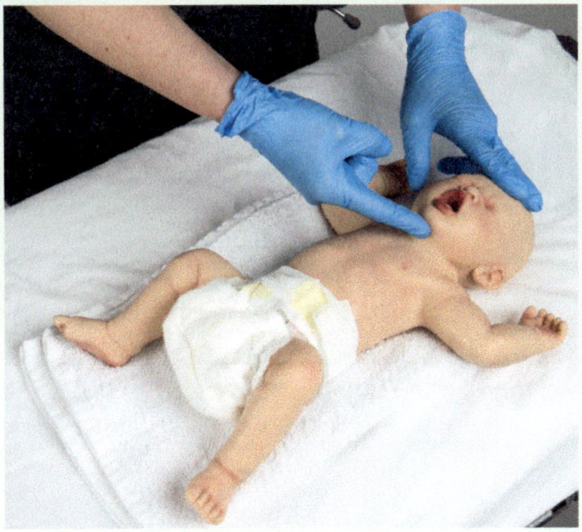	The infant's head is disproportionately large compared to their body. Since they have a prominent occiput, when you place an infant on their back, the neck will flex, potentially obstructing their airway. Obstruction can also occur if the head is over-extended, hence the current guidance advocating a neutral position (1).

Action		Rationale
6.	If a head tilt–chin lift does not effectively open the airway or you suspect a cervical spinal injury, you can use a jaw thrust to open the airway: • Position yourself behind the infant. • Place one or two fingers under both angles of the jaw. • Rest your thumbs on the infant's cheeks. • Lift the jaw upwards. 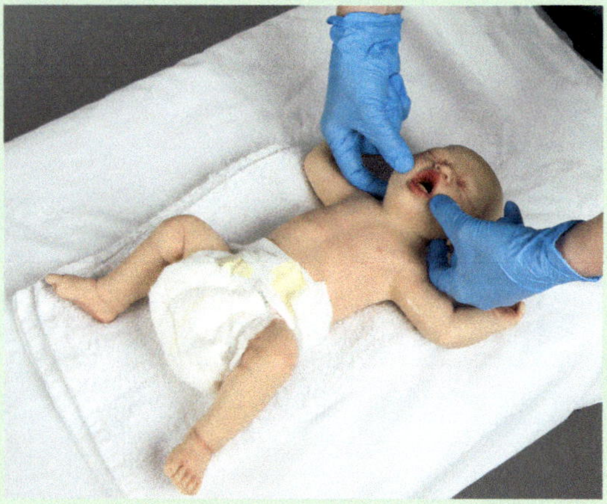	A jaw thrust results in less (but not zero) movement of the neck (1).
7.	Look, listen and feel for normal breathing and check for signs of life (swallowing, vocalising, coughing or normal breathing) for no longer than 10 seconds, by placing your face close to the infant's face: • Look for chest and abdominal movements. • Listen for airflow at the mouth and nose. • Feel for airflow at the mouth and nose. 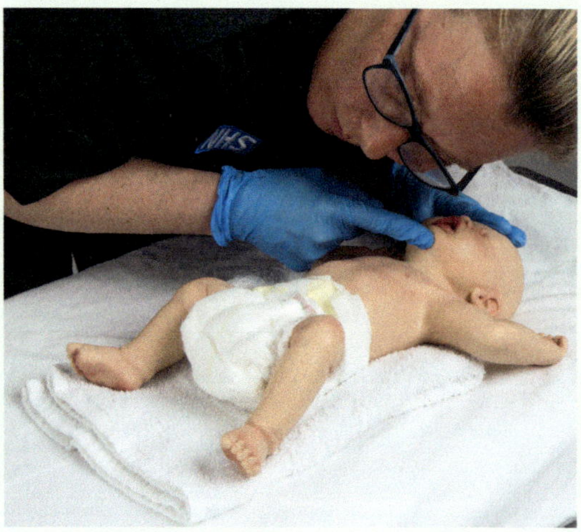	

	Action	Rationale
8.	If the infant is breathing normally, place them into the recovery position.	This should enable free drainage of any airway secretions or vomit (3).
9.	If the infant is not breathing or there are no signs of life (no swallowing, vocalising, coughing or normal breathing), check for and carefully remove any airway obstruction, and provide five rescue breaths:	There is equipoise about whether the sequence for BLS should be chest compressions first or ventilations first. Since ventilations first has been previously advocated for paediatric patients, the current guidance is that this should remain the case (6–10).
	• Where possible, use a two-handed bag-valve-mask (BVM) technique and ensure the bag is connected to high-flow oxygen.	The two-handed technique results in a better seal and may be less fatiguing than a one-handed technique (11–13).
	• Ventilate the chest steadily for one second, just enough to make the chest rise. • Maintain head tilt–chin lift and watch the chest fall. 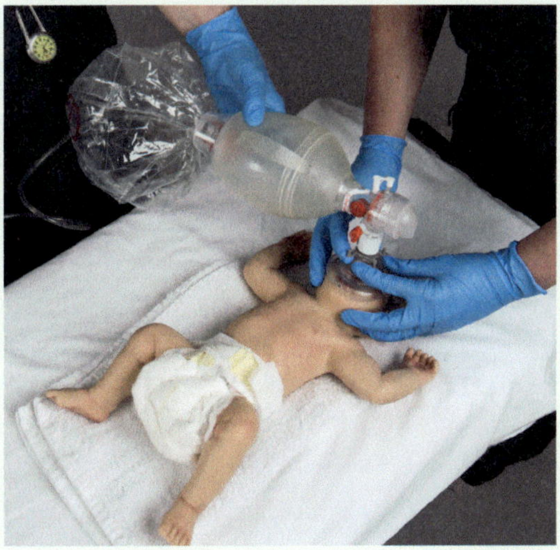	Excessive ventilation is commonly performed during CPR. Hyperventilation can lead to increased intrathoracic pressure and reduced coronary and cerebral perfusion, although the effect this has on survival is not clear (14–19).

Action		Rationale
10.	If the infant's chest is not rising and falling in a similar fashion to normal breathing, open the infant's mouth and check for any visible obstruction. Do not blindly sweep in the infant's mouth. Reposition the head, using a jaw thrust if the head tilt–chin lift manoeuvre is not effective. The use of an airway adjunct, such as an oropharyngeal airway may help too (2). Make no more than five attempts to achieve effective ventilation before moving on to chest compressions. 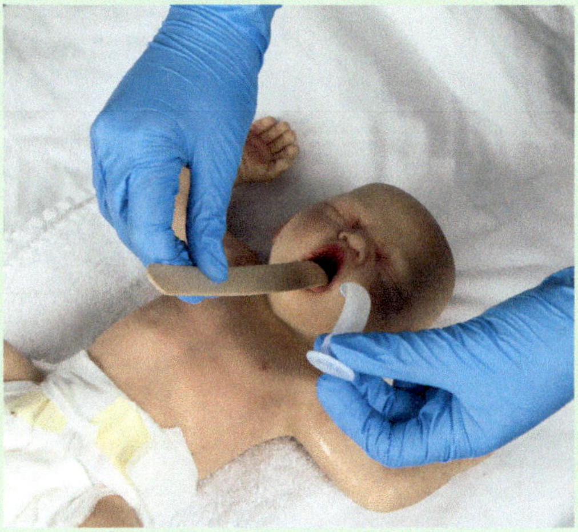	
11.	Check for signs of life (swallowing, vocalising, coughing or normal breathing) and if they are absent (or you are not sure), start chest compressions. If there are signs of life, continue ventilation until the infant starts breathing effectively on their own.	Signs of life are prioritised over pulse checks to recognise cardiac arrest. This is because palpation of pulses to confirm cardiac arrest is unreliable in paediatric patients, even among healthcare professionals (20,21).

	Action	Rationale
12.	If there are no signs of life (or you are unsure), start chest compressions: • If you are on your own, use the tips of two fingers; otherwise, adopt the encircling technique by placing both thumbs side by side on the lower sternum and spreading the remaining fingers around to the infant's back.	
	• Avoid compressing the abdomen by placing your fingers one finger's width above the xiphisternum.	Compressing the abdomen instead of the chest will result in ineffective chest compressions and may result in abdominal injury.
	• Compress the sternum at least one-third of the depth of the chest (or by 4 cm) and then fully release the pressure while maintaining contact with the sternum. If this is difficult, use the two-handed technique as you would for adults.	Allowing full chest re-expansion after a chest compression improves return of blood to the heart (22).
	• Repeat the compressions at a rate of 100–120 per minute for 15 compressions and then give 2 ventilations.	Data from observational studies suggest that a rate of 100–120 compressions per minute results in improved blood pressures (22).
	• Continue compressions and ventilations at a ratio of 15:2. 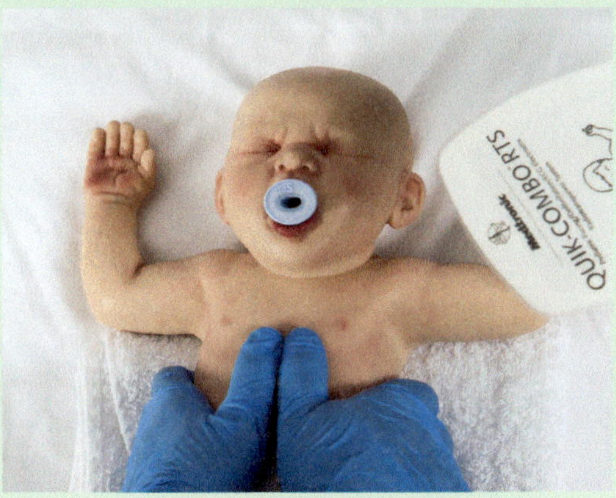	Low-quality evidence suggests that alternating between chest compressions and ventilation is better than chest compressions alone (9). There is no good evidence for a ratio of 15:2 versus 30:2 in infants (23), although a ratio of 15:2 results in a greater number of ventilations provided.

Action		Rationale
13.	Once BLS is established, your colleague should expose the infant's chest and ensure that the pad sites are free from jewellery, piercings, medication patches, pacemakers, wounds and tumours.	There is a small theoretical risk to defibrillators and the myocardium if shocks are delivered over a pacemaker or implantable cardioverted-defibrillator (ICD). This can be minimised by placing pads more than 8 cm from such devices, where possible (24). Patches with plastic backing are unlikely to cause explosions, even with glyceryl trinitrate (GTN), but may adversely affect the defibrillator pad's contact with the skin (24,25).
14.	Switch on the AED and attach the pads to the patient, ensuring they make a good contact. Use paediatric pads if available. In infants, it may be more practical to place the pads in the anterior-posterior position in order to provide enough gap between the pads. 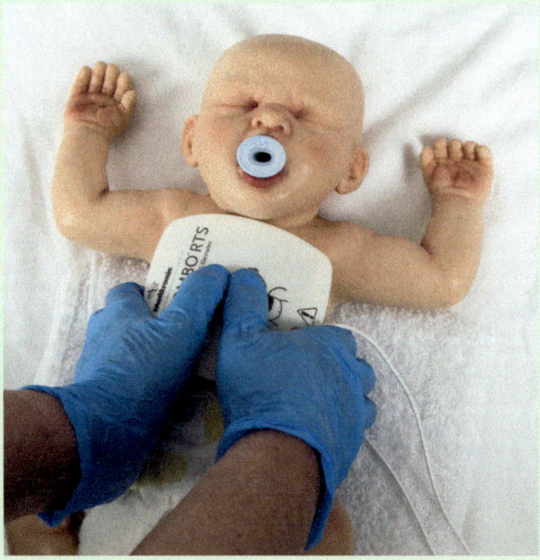	Effective defibrillation is dependent, in part, on good contact between the pads and the skin. There is some evidence that using paediatric attenuated pads in children less than 8 years old, results in higher survival rates. However, it is acceptable to use standard adult pads if that is all that is available (3).

Action		Rationale
15.	Follow visual and voice prompts, ensuring that no one touches the patient while the AED is analysing the rhythm. 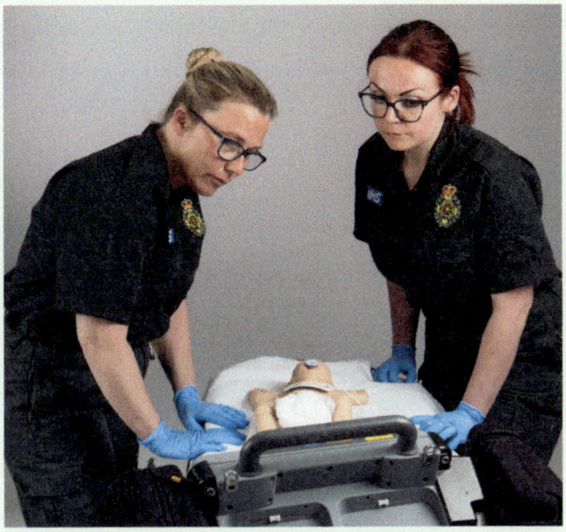	If the AED detects movement, it may result in a longer rhythm interpretation time and hence delay in defibrillation.
16.	If a shock is advised, make sure everyone is clear of the patient, oxygen is kept at least 1 metre away from the patient and push the shock button. If a shock is not advised, skip to step 17. 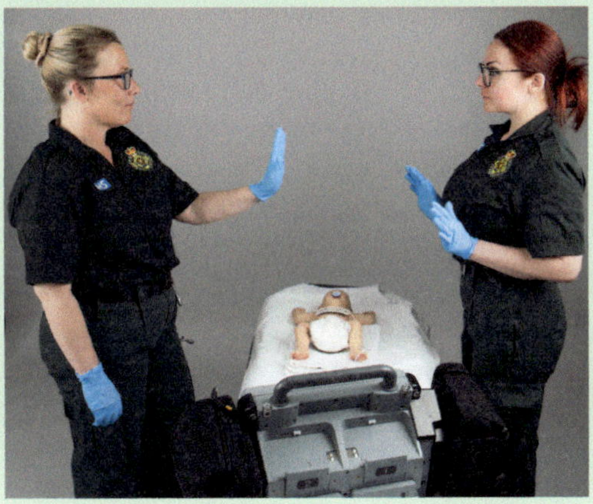	Removing the source of oxygen reduces the risk of combustion due to an oxygen-rich environment.

Action		Rationale
17.	Immediately restart CPR at a ratio of 15:2. You should alternate chest compressions with your colleague every 2 minutes, but keep the changeover time to a minimum. 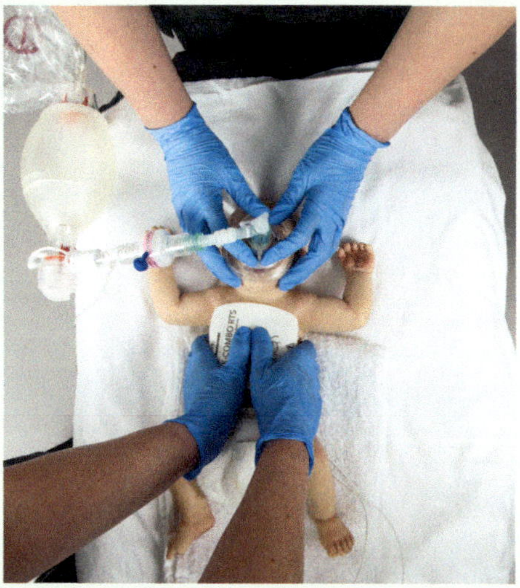	Manikin studies have demonstrated rescuer fatigue as evidenced by decreasing chest compression depth after 2 minutes (3 minutes with real-time feedback devices), so regular breaks are recommended (26).
18.	Continue to follow visual and voice prompts from the AED, ensuring that no one touches the patient while the AED is analysing the rhythm, and that oxygen is kept at least 1 metre away from the patient if defibrillation is required.	
19.	Document the procedure.	You must keep full, clear, and accurate records for everyone you care for, treat, or provide other services to (27).

References

1. Resuscitation Council UK. *European Paediatric Advanced Life Support*. 5th edition. London: Resuscitation Council UK; 2021.
2. Joint Royal Colleges Ambulance Liaison Committee, Association of Ambulance Chief Executives. JRCALC clinical guidelines. Cited from JRCALC Plus (Version 1.2.13) [Mobile application software]. Bridgwater: Class Publishing Ltd; 2021.
3. Voorde PV de, Turner NM, Djakow J, et al. European Resuscitation Council Guidelines 2021: paediatric life support. *Resuscitation*. 2021 Apr 1;161:327–387.
4. NHS England, NHS Improvement. Standard infection control precautions: national hand hygiene and personal protective equipment policy [Internet]. 2019 [cited 2021 Nov 11]. Available from: https://www.england.nhs.uk/publication/standard-infection-control-precautions-national-hand-hygiene-and-personal-protective-equipment-policy/.
5. Kovacs G, Law JA. *Airway Management in Emergencies*. 2nd edition. Shelton: McGraw-Hill Medical; 2011.
6. Sekiguchi H, Kondo Y, Kukita I. Verification of changes in the time taken to initiate chest compressions according to modified basic life support guidelines. *American Journal of Emergency Medicine*. 2013 Aug 1;31(8):1248–1250.
7. Marsch S, Tschan F, Semmer NK, et al. ABC versus CAB for cardiopulmonary resuscitation: a prospective, randomized simulator-based trial. *Swiss Medical Weekly*. 2013 Sep 6;143:w13856.
8. Lubrano R, Cecchetti C, Bellelli E, et al. Comparison of times of intervention during pediatric CPR maneuvers using ABC and CAB sequences: a randomized trial. *Resuscitation*. 2012 Dec;83(12):1473–1477.
9. de Caen AR, Maconochie IK, Aickin R, et al. Part 6: pediatric basic life support and pediatric

advanced life support. *Circulation*. 2015 Oct 20;132(16_suppl_1):S177–203.
10. Maconochie IK, Aickin R, Hazinski MF, et al. Pediatric life support: 2020 international consensus on cardiopulmonary resuscitation and emergency cardiovascular care science with treatment recommendations. *Circulation*. 2020 Oct 20;142(16_suppl_1):S140–184.
11. Otten D, Liao MM, Wolken R, et al. Comparison of bag-valve-mask hand-sealing techniques in a simulated model. *Annals of Emergency Medicine*. 2014 Jan 1;63(1): 6–12.e3.
12. Hart D, Reardon R, Ward C, Miner J. Face mask ventilation: a comparison of three techniques. *Journal of Emergency Medicine*. 2013 May;44(5):1028–1033.
13. Jin Y, Lee BN, Park JR, Kim YM. Comparison of two mask holding techniques for two person bag-valve-mask ventilation: a cross-over simulation study. *Resuscitation*. 2010 Dec 1;81(2):S59.
14. Del Castillo J, López-Herce J, Matamoros M, et al. Hyperoxia, hypocapnia and hypercapnia as outcome factors after cardiac arrest in children. *Resuscitation*. 2012 Dec;83(12):1456–1461.
15. Gazmuri RJ, Ayoub IM, Radhakrishnan J, et al. Clinically plausible hyperventilation does not exert adverse hemodynamic effects during CPR but markedly reduces end-tidal PCO_2. *Resuscitation*. 2012 Feb;83(2):259–264.
16. O'Neill JF, Deakin CD. Do we hyperventilate cardiac arrest patients? *Resuscitation*. 2007 Apr;73(1):82–85.
17. Wik L, Kramer-Johansen J, Myklebust H, et al. Quality of cardiopulmonary resuscitation during out-of-hospital cardiac arrest. *Journal of the American Medical Association*. 2005 Jan 19;293(3):299–304.
18. Aufderheide TP, Lurie KG. Death by hyperventilation: a common and life-threatening problem during cardiopulmonary resuscitation. *Critical Care Medicine*. 2004 Sep;32(9 Suppl):S345–351.
19. Aufderheide TP, Sigurdsson G, Pirrallo RG, et al. Hyperventilation-induced hypotension during cardiopulmonary resuscitation. *Circulation*. 2004 Apr 27;109(16):1960–1965.
20. Tibballs J, Russell P. Reliability of pulse palpation by healthcare personnel to diagnose paediatric cardiac arrest. *Resuscitation*. 2009 Jan;80(1):61–64.
21. Tibballs J, Weeranatna C. The influence of time on the accuracy of healthcare personnel to diagnose paediatric cardiac arrest by pulse palpation. *Resuscitation*. 2010 Jun;81(6):671–675.
22. Topjian AA, Raymond TT, Atkins D, et al. Part 4: pediatric basic and advanced life support: 2020 American Heart Association guidelines for cardiopulmonary resuscitation and emergency cardiovascular care. *Circulation*. 2020 Oct 20;142(16_suppl_2):S469–523.
23. Ashoor HM, Lillie E, Zarin W, et al. Effectiveness of different compression-to-ventilation methods for cardiopulmonary resuscitation: a systematic review. *Resuscitation*. 2017 Sep;118:112–125.
24. Resuscitation Council (UK). *Advanced Life Support*. London: Resuscitation Council (UK); 2021.
25. Liddle R, Richmond W. Investigation into voltage breakdown in glyceryl trinitrate patches. *Resuscitation*. 1998 Jun;37(3):145–148.
26. Perkins GD, Handley AJ, Koster RW, et al. European Resuscitation Council Guidelines for Resuscitation 2015. Section 2. Adult basic life support and automated external defibrillation. *Resuscitation*. 2015 Oct;95:81–99.
27. Health and Care Professions Council. Standards of conduct, performance and ethics [Internet]. 2018 [cited 2019 Dec 29]. Available from: https://www.hcpc-uk.org/standards/standards-of-conduct-performance-and-ethics/.

Infant Basic Life Support with Manual Defibrillation

Indications

- Infant (0–12 months) patient with no apparent signs of life.

Contraindications

- Newborn who requires resuscitation (follow Newborn Life Support guideline).
- Patient whose condition is unequivocally associated with death.
- Patient has a Recommended Summary Plan for Emergency Care and Treatment (ReSPECT), relevant to their current clinical presentation, indicating that cardiopulmonary resuscitation (CPR) attempts are not recommended (1).
- Patient has a valid 'do not attempt cardiopulmonary resuscitation' (DNACPR) form (2).

Advantages

- Provides blow flow to the brain and other vital organs (3).
- Good chance of a return of spontaneous circulation (ROSC) if the primary cause is cardiac (although less common in infants).
- Prompt and accurate rhythm interpretation by the clinician can result in a shorter pre-shock pause.

Disadvantages

- Unlikely to lead to ROSC without other interventions, particularly effective ventilation and oxygenation, and treatment for reversible causes.
- Relies on clinician to accurate interpret the rhythm.

Procedure – Infant Basic Life Support with Manual Defibrillation

Take the following steps to perform basic life support (BLS) on an infant with a manual defibrillator (3):

Action		Rationale
1.	Ensure the scene is safe for you, your colleague, the patient and other bystanders.	Your safety and that of your colleagues is your primary concern. Some causes of cardiac arrest can present a risk to the rescuer, for example drowning and electrocution.
2.	Don appropriate personal protective equipment (PPE), and undertake appropriate hand hygiene.	This reduces the risk of cross-infection (4).

Action		Rationale
3.	Check for responsiveness by placing a hand on the infant's forehead to stabilise it and tug their hair while calling their name. If they have no hair, apply another method of tactile stimulation. 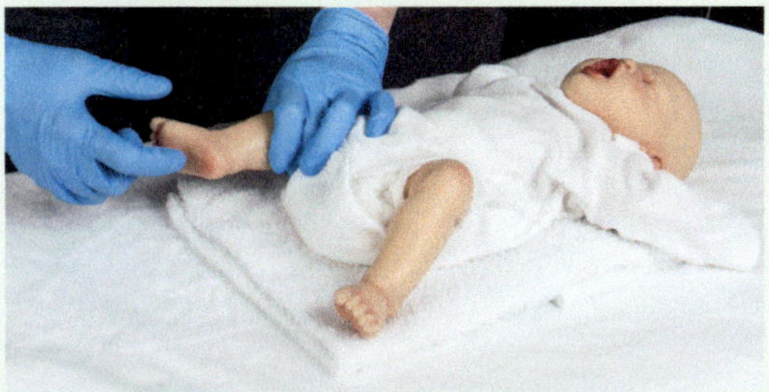	Not every patient who appears to be unresponsive is in cardiac arrest.
4.	If the patient responds, assess the infant's ABCDE, call for assistance and reassess regularly. If they do not respond, summon additional assistance.	All cases where infants have experienced a period of unresponsiveness or collapse should be taken seriously. The management of peri-arrest infants is a team effort (1).
5.	Open the infant's airway by placing one hand on their forehead and gently tilt it back until it is in a neutral position (3). Perform a chin lift by placing the fingertips of your other hand on the bony part of the lower jaw and lift upwards. Do not compress the soft tissues under the jaw as this will occlude the airway. Placing a towel under the infant's shoulders and upper body can help keep their head in a neutral position (5). 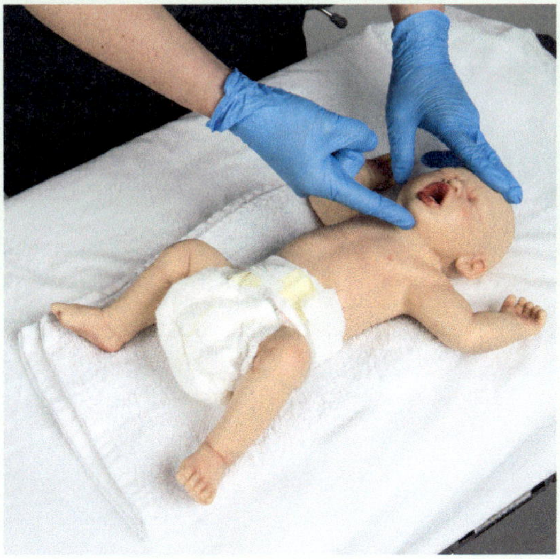	The infant's head is disproportionately large compared to their body. Since they have a prominent occiput, when you place an infant on their back, the neck will flex, potentially obstructing their airway. Obstruction can also occur if the head is over-extended, hence the current guidance advocating a neutral position (1).

Action		Rationale
6.	If a head tilt–chin lift does not effectively open the airway or you suspect a cervical spinal injury, you can use a jaw thrust to open the airway: • Position yourself behind the infant. • Place one or two fingers under both angles of the jaw. • Rest your thumbs on the infant's cheeks. • Lift the jaw upwards. 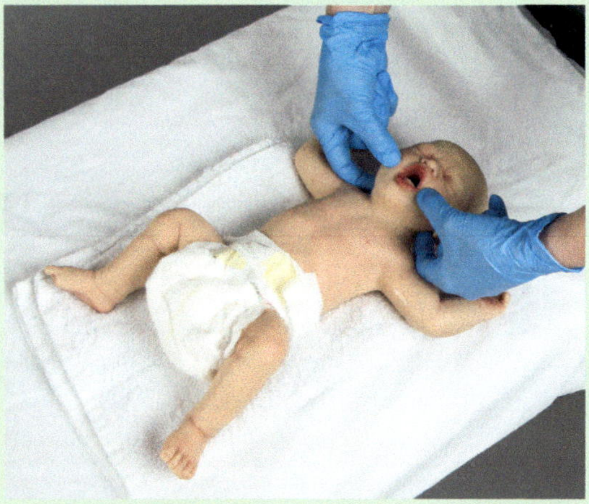	A jaw thrust results in less (but not zero) movement of the neck (1).
7.	Look, listen and feel for normal breathing and check for signs of life (swallowing, vocalising, coughing or normal breathing) for no longer than 10 seconds, by placing your face close to the infant's face: • Look for chest and abdominal movements. • Listen for airflow at the mouth and nose. • Feel for airflow at the mouth and nose. 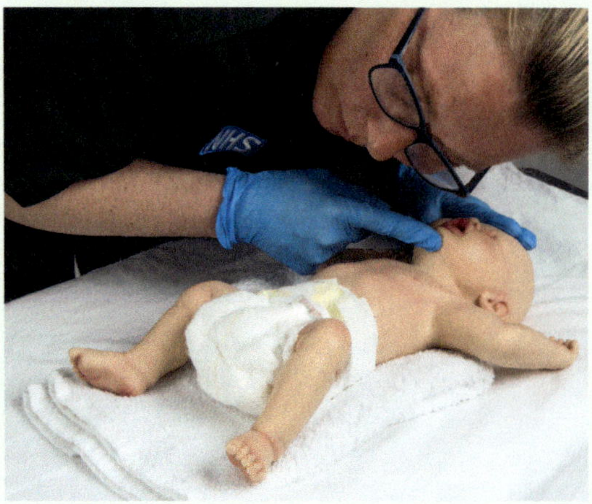	

Action		Rationale
8.	If the infant is breathing normally, place them into the recovery position.	This should enable free drainage of any airway secretions or vomit (3).
9.	If the infant is not breathing or there are no signs of life (no swallowing, vocalising, coughing or normal breathing), check for and carefully remove any airway obstruction, and provide five rescue breaths:	There is equipoise about whether the sequence for BLS should be chest compressions first or ventilations first. Since ventilations first has been previously advocated for paediatric patients, the current guidance is that this should remain the case (6–10).
	• Where possible, use a two-handed bag-valve-mask (BVM) technique and ensure the bag is connected to high-flow oxygen.	The two-handed technique results in a better seal and may be less fatiguing than a one-handed technique (11–13).
	• Ventilate the chest steadily for one second, just enough to make the chest rise. • Maintain head tilt–chin lift and watch the chest fall. 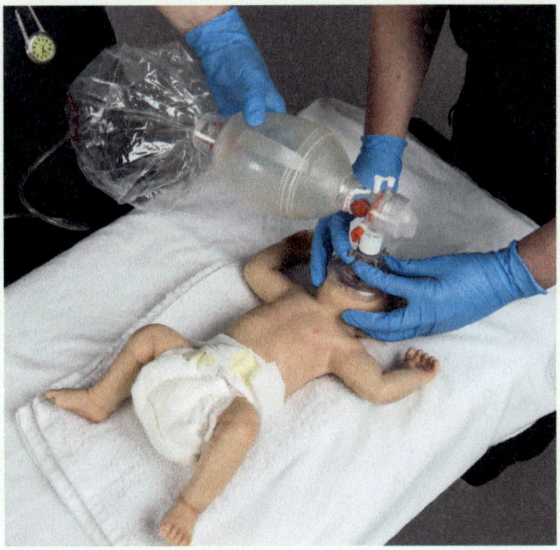	Excessive ventilation is commonly performed during CPR. Hyperventilation can lead to increased intrathoracic pressure and reduced coronary and cerebral perfusion, although the effect this has on survival is not clear (14–19).

	Action	Rationale
10.	If the infant's chest is not rising and falling in a similar fashion to normal breathing, open the infant's mouth and check for any visible obstruction. Do not blindly sweep in the infant's mouth. Reposition the head, using a jaw thrust if the head tilt–chin lift manoeuvre is not effective. The use of airway adjuncts such as an oropharyngeal airway may help too (2). Make no more than five attempts to achieve effective ventilation before moving on to chest compressions. 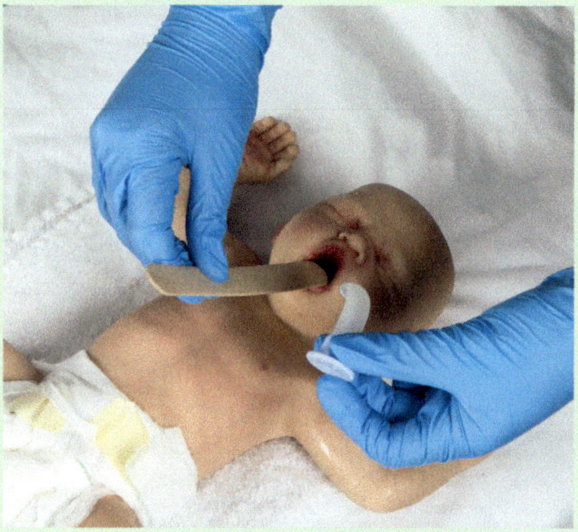	
11.	Check for signs of life (swallowing, vocalising, coughing or normal breathing) and if they are absent (or you are not sure), start chest compressions. If there are signs of life, continue ventilation until the infant starts breathing effectively on their own.	Signs of life are prioritised over pulse checks to recognise cardiac arrest. This is because palpation of pulses to confirm cardiac arrest is unreliable in paediatric patients, even amongst healthcare professionals (20,21).

<table>
<tr><th colspan="2">Action</th><th>Rationale</th></tr>
<tr><td>12.</td><td>If there are no signs of life (or you are unsure), start chest compressions:
• If you are on your own, use the tips of two fingers; otherwise, adopt the encircling technique by placing both thumbs side by side on the lower sternum and spreading the remaining fingers around to the infant's back.</td><td></td></tr>
<tr><td></td><td>• Avoid compressing the abdomen by placing your fingers one finger's width above the xiphisternum.</td><td>Compressing the abdomen instead of the chest will result in ineffective chest compressions and may result in abdominal injury.</td></tr>
<tr><td></td><td>• Compress the sternum at least one-third of the depth of the chest (or by 4 cm) and then fully release the pressure while maintaining contact with the sternum. If this is difficult, use the two-handed technique as you would for adults.</td><td>Allowing full chest re-expansion after a chest compression improves return of blood to the heart (22).</td></tr>
<tr><td></td><td>• Repeat the compressions at a rate of 100–120 per minute for 15 compressions and then give 2 ventilations.</td><td>Data from observational studies suggest that a rate of 100–120 compressions per minute results in improved blood pressures (22).</td></tr>
<tr><td></td><td>• Continue compressions and ventilations at a ratio of 15:2.

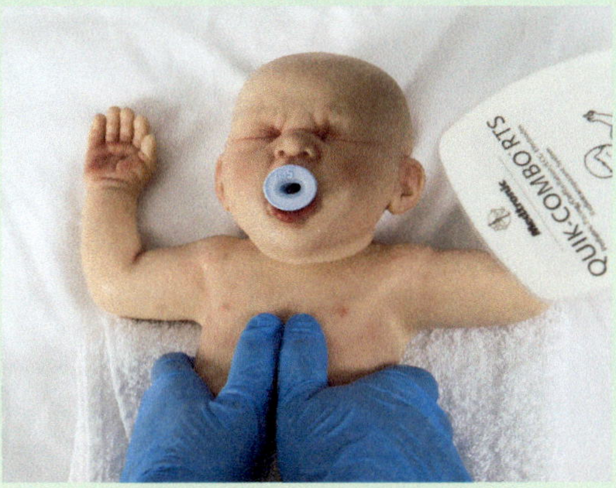

</td><td>Low-quality evidence suggests that alternating between chest compressions and ventilation is better than chest compressions alone (9). There is no good evidence for a ratio of 15:2 versus 30:2 in infants (23), although a ratio of 15:2 results in a greater number of ventilations provided.</td></tr>
</table>

	Action	Rationale
13.	Once BLS is established, your colleague should expose the infant's chest and ensure that the pad sites are free from jewellery, piercings, medication patches, pacemakers, wounds and tumours.	There is a small theoretical risk to the device and the myocardium if shocks are delivered over a pacemaker or implantable cardioverted-defibrillator (ICD). This can be minimised by placing pads more than 8 cm from such devices, where possible (24). Patches with plastic backing are unlikely to cause explosions, even with glyceryl trinitrate (GTN), but may adversely affect the defibrillator pad's contact with the skin (24,25).
14.	Switch on the defibrillator and attach the pads to the patient, ensuring they make a good contact. Use paediatric pads if available. In infants, it may be more practical to place the pads in the anterior-posterior position in order to provide enough gap between the pads. 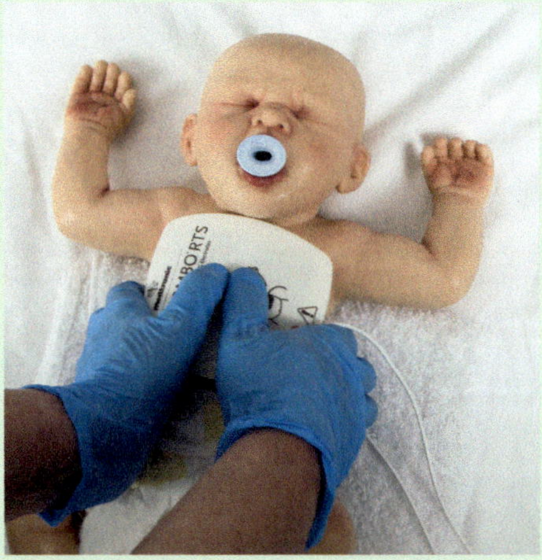	Effective defibrillation is dependent, in part, on good contact between the pads and the skin. There is some evidence that using paediatric attenuated pads in children less than 8 years old results in higher survival rates. However, it is acceptable to use standard adult pads if that is all that is available (3).
15.	Plan actions before pausing chest compressions for rhythm analysis and make sure all team members know their role and the sequence of actions.	Resuscitation guidelines suggest a target of less than 5 seconds to interpret the rhythm and decide a shock should be delivered.
16.	A clinician not performing chest compressions should palpate a brachial pulse to determine its location while chest compressions are being performed.	There is evidence that healthcare professionals cannot always reliably palpate pulses in cardiac arrest. This step is not in current resuscitation guidelines, but is a pragmatic step to aid in the detection of a pulse (if present), without incurring a delay, which can occur during a rhythm check and the rhythm is pulse electrical activity/ventricular tachycardia (PEA/VT).

Action		Rationale
17.	Stop chest compressions to analyse the rhythm. Confirm the presence or absence of a pulse and signs of life.	Most defibrillators do not filter chest compression interference from the electrocardiogram (ECG).
18.	If ventricular fibrillation (VF) or pulseless VT is present, follow instructions below. If the rhythm is asystole, PEA or the infant has a heart rate of less than 60 beats per minute, skip to step 19: • Immediately resume chest compressions. • The designated person should charge the defibrillator based on the infant's weight (4 J/kg). If the exact energy value cannot be selected, choose the closest, higher value (2). • While the defibrillator is charging, everyone except for the chest compressor should stand back and move oxygen 1 metre away. For safety, the clinician operating the defibrillator should keep their fingers away from the shock button. • Once the defibrillator is charged, the person defibrillating should tell the chest compressor to 'stand clear' and deliver the shock as soon as they have done so. 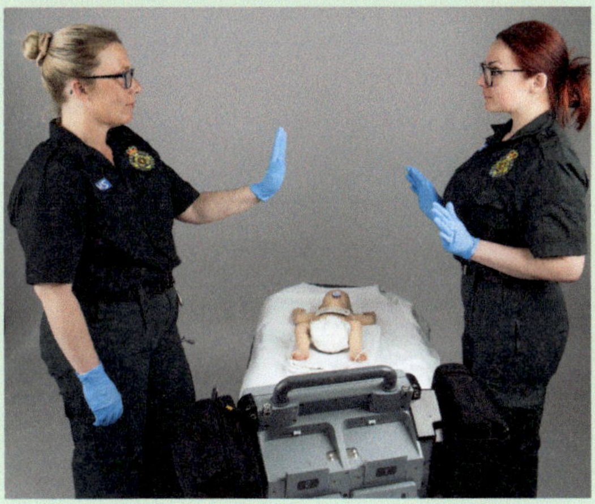	Reducing 'time off the chest' is important, but it must not compromise safety. Removing the source of oxygen, for example, reduces the risk of combustion due to an oxygen-rich environment.

Action		Rationale
19.	Immediately restart CPR at a ratio of 15:2. You should alternate chest compressions with your colleague every 2 minutes, but keep the changeover time to a minimum. 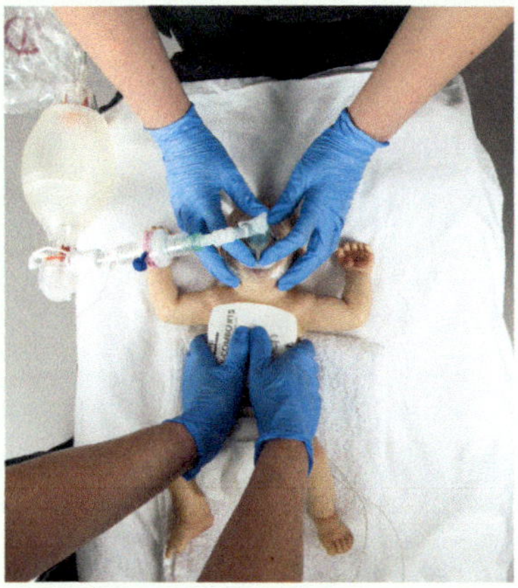	Manikin studies have demonstrated rescuer fatigue as evidenced by decreasing chest compression depth after 2 minutes (3 minutes with real-time feedback devices), so regular breaks are recommended (26).
20.	Once 2 minutes has elapsed, chest compressions should be briefly paused and the rhythm analysed. Repeat step 18 onwards.	
21.	Document the procedure.	You must keep full, clear, and accurate records for everyone you care for, treat, or provide other services to (27).

References

1. Resuscitation Council UK. *European Paediatric Advanced Life Support*. 5th edition. London: Resuscitation Council UK; 2021.
2. Joint Royal Colleges Ambulance Liaison Committee, Association of Ambulance Chief Executives. JRCALC clinical guidelines. Cited from JRCALC Plus (Version 1.2.13) [Mobile application software]. Bridgwater: Class Publishing Ltd; 2021.
3. Voorde PV de, Turner NM, Djakow J, et al. European Resuscitation Council Guidelines 2021: paediatric life support. *Resuscitation*. 2021 Apr 1;161:327–387.
4. NHS England, NHS Improvement. Standard infection control precautions: national hand hygiene and personal protective equipment policy [Internet]. 2019 [cited 2021 Nov 11]. Available from: https://www.england.nhs.uk/publication/standard-infection-control-precautions-national-hand-hygiene-and-personal-protective-equipment-policy/.
5. Kovacs G, Law JA. *Airway Management in Emergencies*. 2nd edition. Shelton: McGraw-Hill Medical; 2011.
6. Sekiguchi H, Kondo Y, Kukita I. Verification of changes in the time taken to initiate chest compressions according to modified basic life support guidelines. *American Journal of Emergency Medicine*. 2013 Aug 1;31(8):1248–1250.
7. Marsch S, Tschan F, Semmer NK, et al. ABC versus CAB for cardiopulmonary resuscitation: a prospective, randomized simulator-based trial. *Swiss Medical Weekly*. 2013 Sep 6;143:w13856.
8. Lubrano R, Cecchetti C, Bellelli E, et al. Comparison of times of intervention during pediatric CPR maneuvers using ABC and CAB sequences: a randomized trial. *Resuscitation*. 2012 Dec;83(12):1473–1477.
9. de Caen AR, Maconochie IK, Aickin R, et al. Part 6: pediatric basic life support and pediatric advanced life support. *Circulation*. 2015 Oct 20;132(16_suppl_1):S177–203.
10. Maconochie IK, Aickin R, Hazinski MF, et al. Pediatric life support: 2020 international consensus on

cardiopulmonary resuscitation and emergency cardiovascular care science with treatment recommendations. *Circulation*. 2020 Oct 20;142(16_suppl_1):S140–184.
11. Otten D, Liao MM, Wolken R, Douglas IS, Mishra R, Kao A, et al. Comparison of bag-valve-mask hand-sealing techniques in a simulated model. *Annals of Emergency Medicine*. 2014 Jan 1;63(1):6–12.e3.
12. Hart D, Reardon R, Ward C, Miner J. Face mask ventilation: a comparison of three techniques. *Journal of Emergency Medicine*. 2013 May;44(5):1028–1033.
13. Jin Y, Lee BN, Park JR, Kim YM. Comparison of two mask holding techniques for two person bag-valve-mask ventilation: a cross-over simulation study. *Resuscitation*. 2010 Dec 1;81(2):S59.
14. Del Castillo J, López-Herce J, Matamoros M, et al. Hyperoxia, hypocapnia and hypercapnia as outcome factors after cardiac arrest in children. *Resuscitation*. 2012 Dec;83(12):1456–1461.
15. Gazmuri RJ, Ayoub IM, Radhakrishnan J, et al. Clinically plausible hyperventilation does not exert adverse hemodynamic effects during CPR but markedly reduces end-tidal PCO_2. *Resuscitation*. 2012 Feb;83(2):259–264.
16. O'Neill JF, Deakin CD. Do we hyperventilate cardiac arrest patients? *Resuscitation*. 2007 Apr;73(1):82–85.
17. Wik L, Kramer-Johansen J, Myklebust H, et al. Quality of cardiopulmonary resuscitation during out-of-hospital cardiac arrest. *Journal of American Medical Association*. 2005 Jan 19;293(3):299–304.
18. Aufderheide TP, Lurie KG. Death by hyperventilation: a common and life-threatening problem during cardiopulmonary resuscitation. *Critical Care Medicine*. 2004 Sep;32(9 Suppl):S345–351.
19. Aufderheide TP, Sigurdsson G, Pirrallo RG, et al. Hyperventilation-induced hypotension during cardiopulmonary resuscitation. *Circulation*. 2004 Apr 27;109(16):1960–1965.
20. Tibballs J, Russell P. Reliability of pulse palpation by healthcare personnel to diagnose paediatric cardiac arrest. *Resuscitation*. 2009 Jan;80(1):61–64.
21. Tibballs J, Weeranatna C. The influence of time on the accuracy of healthcare personnel to diagnose paediatric cardiac arrest by pulse palpation. *Resuscitation*. 2010 Jun;81(6):671–5.
22. Topjian AA, Raymond TT, Atkins D, et al. Part 4: pediatric basic and advanced life support: 2020 American Heart Association guidelines for cardiopulmonary resuscitation and emergency cardiovascular care. *Circulation*. 2020 Oct 20;142(16):S469–523.
23. Ashoor HM, Lillie E, Zarin W, et al. Effectiveness of different compression-to-ventilation methods for cardiopulmonary resuscitation: a systematic review. *Resuscitation*. 2017 Sep;118:112–125.
24. Resuscitation Council (UK). *Advanced Life Support*. London: Resuscitation Council (UK); 2021.
25. Liddle R, Richmond W. Investigation into voltage breakdown in glyceryl trinitrate patches. *Resuscitation*. 1998 Jun;37(3):145–148.
26. Perkins GD, Handley AJ, Koster RW, et al. European Resuscitation Council Guidelines for Resuscitation 2015. Section 2. Adult basic life support and automated external defibrillation. *Resuscitation*. 2015 Oct;95:81–99.
27. Health and Care Professions Council. Standards of conduct, performance and ethics [Internet]. 2018 [cited 2019 Dec 29]. Available from: https://www.hcpc-uk.org/standards/standards-of-conduct-performance-and-ethics/.

Child Basic Life Support with Automated External Defibrillation

Indications

- Child over the age of 1 year with no apparent signs of life.

Contraindications

- Patient whose condition is unequivocally associated with death.
- Patient has a Recommended Summary Plan for Emergency Care and Treatment (ReSPECT), relevant to their current clinical presentation, indicating that cardiopulmonary resuscitation (CPR) attempts are not recommended (1).
- Patient has a valid 'do not attempt cardiopulmonary resuscitation' (DNACPR) form (2).

Advantages

- Provides blow flow to the brain and other vital organs (3).
- Good chance of a return to spontaneous circulation (ROSC) if the primary cause is cardiac (although less common in children).

Disadvantages

- Unlikely to lead to ROSC without other interventions, particularly effective ventilation and oxygenation, and treatment for reversible causes.

Procedure – Child Basic Life Support with Automated External Defibrillation

Take the following steps to perform basic life support (BLS) on an child with an automated external defibrillator (AED) (3):

Action		Rationale
1.	Ensure the scene is safe for you, your colleague, the patient and other bystanders.	Your safety and that of your colleagues is your primary concern. Some causes of cardiac arrest can present a risk to the rescuer, for example drowning and electrocution.
2.	Don appropriate personal protective equipment (PPE), and undertake appropriate hand hygiene.	This reduces the risk of cross-infection (4).

Action		Rationale
3.	Check for responsiveness by placing a hand on the child's forehead to stabilise it and tug their hair while calling their name.	Not every patient who appears to be unresponsive is in cardiac arrest.
4.	If the patient responds, assess the child's ABCDE, call for assistance and reassess regularly. If they do not respond, summon additional assistance. 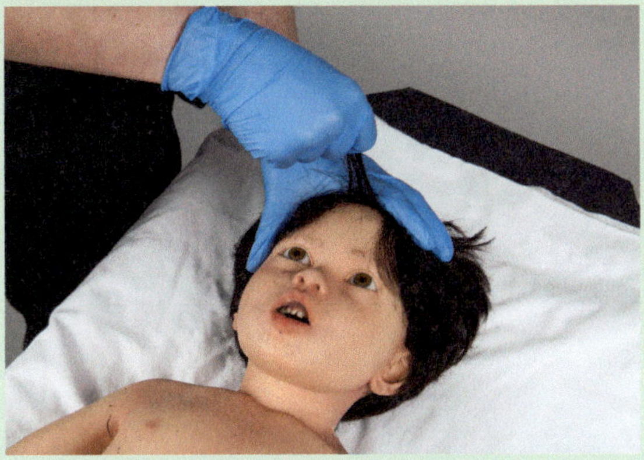	All cases where children have experienced a period of unresponsiveness or collapse should be taken seriously. The management of peri-arrest children is a team effort (1).
5.	Open the child's airway by placing one hand on their forehead and gently tilt it back until it is in a 'sniffing' position (3). Perform a chin lift by placing the fingertips of your other hand on the bony part of the lower jaw and lift upwards. Do not compress the soft tissues under the jaw, as this will occlude the airway. Younger children typically do not require any padding of the shoulders or head, but older children may benefit from a towel or pillow under the occiput (as with adults) to obtain good airway alignment (5). 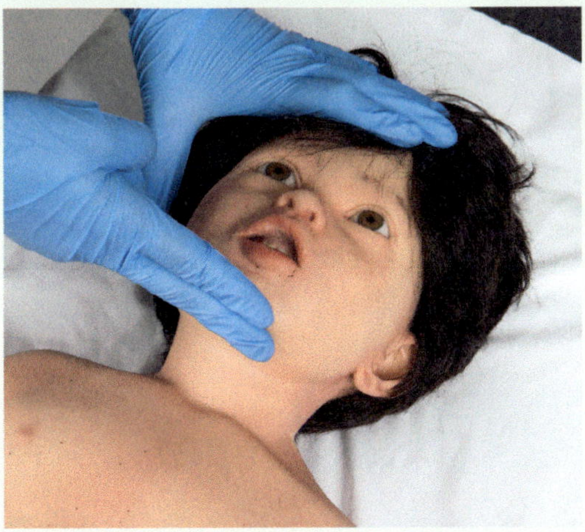	Excessive neck flexion or extension will cause obstruction of the child's airway (1).

Action		Rationale
6.	If a head tilt–chin lift does not effectively open the airway, or you suspect a cervical spinal injury, you can use a jaw thrust to open the airway: • Position yourself behind the child. • Place two fingers under both angles of the jaw. • Rest your thumbs on the child's cheeks. • Lift the jaw upwards. 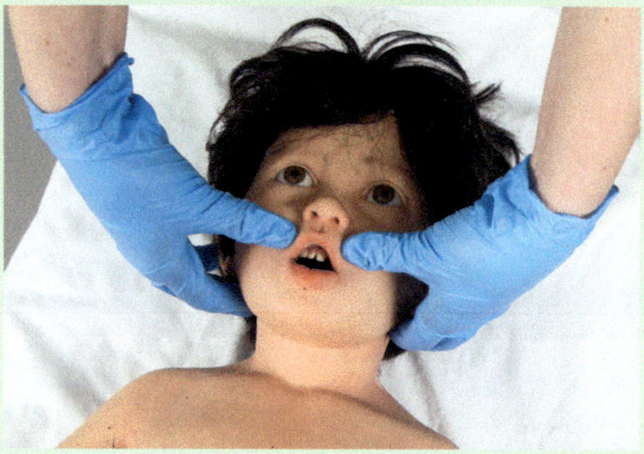	A jaw thrust results in less (but not zero) movement of the neck (1).
7.	Look, listen and feel for normal breathing and check for signs of life (swallowing, vocalising, coughing or normal breathing) for no longer than 10 seconds, by placing your face close to the child's face: • Look for chest and abdominal movements. • Listen for airflow at the mouth and nose. • Feel for airflow at the mouth and nose. 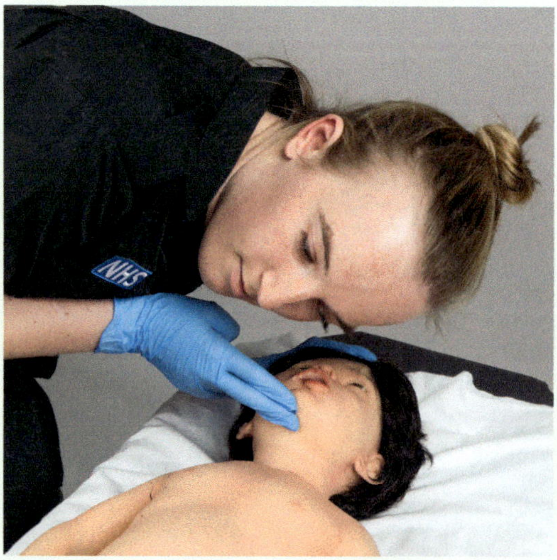	

Action		Rationale
8.	If the child is breathing normally, place them into the recovery position.	This should enable free drainage of any airway secretions or vomit (3).
9.	If the child is not breathing or there are no signs of life (no swallowing, vocalising, coughing or normal breathing), check for and carefully remove any airway obstruction, and provide five rescue breaths: • Ensure the head is in a 'sniffing' position and apply a chin lift.	There is equipoise about whether the sequence for basic life support should be chest compressions first or ventilations first. Since ventilations first has been previously advocated for paediatric patients, the current guidance is that this should remain the case (6–10).
	• Where possible, use a two-handed bag-valve-mask (BVM) technique and ensure the bag is connected to high-flow oxygen.	The two-handed technique results in a better seal and may be less fatiguing than a one-handed technique (11–13).
	• Ventilate the chest steadily for 1 second, just enough to make the chest rise. • Maintain head tilt–chin lift and watch the chest fall. 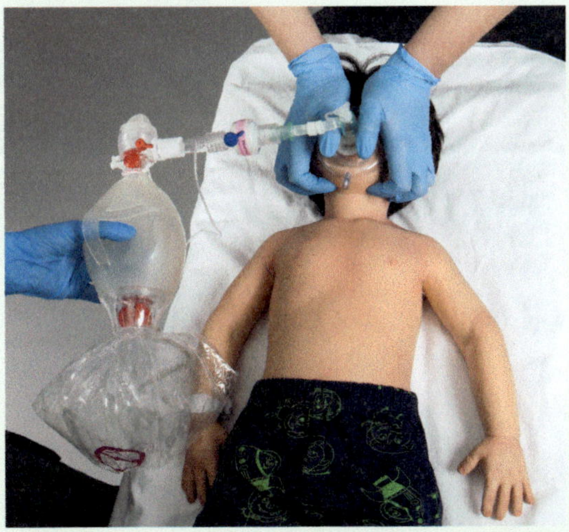	Excessive ventilation is commonly performed during CPR. Hyperventilation can lead to increased intrathoracic pressure and reduced coronary and cerebral perfusion, although the effect this has on survival is not clear (14–19).
10.	If the child's chest is not rising and falling in a similar fashion to normal breathing, open the child's mouth and check for any visible obstruction. Do not blindly sweep in the child's mouth. Reposition the head using a jaw thrust, if the head tilt–chin lift manoeuvre is not effective. The use of airway adjuncts such as an oropharyngeal airway may help too (2). Make no more than five attempts to achieve effective ventilation before moving on to chest compressions.	

Action		Rationale
11.	Check for signs of life (swallowing, vocalising, coughing or normal breathing) and if they are absent (or you are not sure), start chest compressions. If there are signs of life, continue ventilation until the child starts breathing effectively on their own.	Signs of life are prioritised over pulse checks to recognise cardiac arrest. This is because palpation of pulses to confirm cardiac arrest is unreliable in paediatric patients, even amongst healthcare professionals (20,21).
12.	If there are no signs of life (or you are unsure), start chest compressions: • Position yourself by the side of the child. • Avoid compressing the abdomen by placing your hand a finger's width above the xiphisternum. • Lock your elbow and position your body so that your shoulder is directly over the child's chest. • Compress the sternum by at least one-third of the depth of the chest (or by 5 cm) and then fully release the pressure while maintaining contact with the sternum. If this is difficult, use the two-handed technique as you would for adults. • Repeat the compressions at a rate of 100–120 per minute for 15 compressions and then give two ventilations. • Continue compressions and ventilations at a ratio of 15:2. 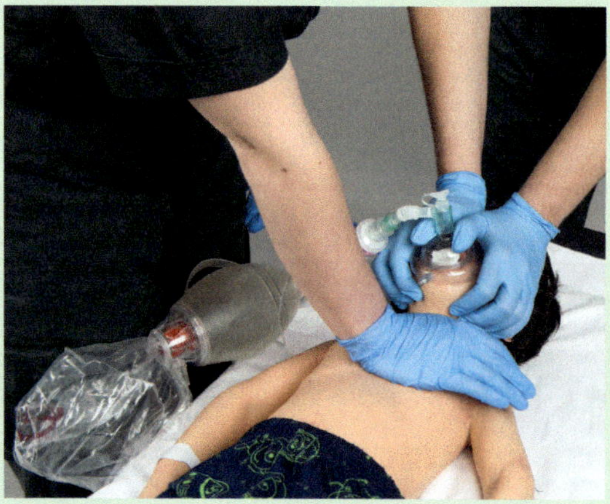	Compressing the abdomen instead of the chest will result in ineffective chest compressions and may result in abdominal injury. Allowing full chest re-expansion after a chest compression improves return of blood to the heart (22). Data from observational studies suggest that a rate of 100–120 compressions per minute results in improved blood pressures (22). Low-quality evidence suggests that alternating between chest compressions and ventilation is better than chest compressions alone (9). There is no good evidence for a ratio of 15:2 versus 30:2 in children (23), although a ratio of 15:2 results in a greater number of ventilations provided.

Action		Rationale
13.	Once BLS is established, your colleague should expose the child's chest and ensure that the pad sites are free from jewellery, piercings, medication patches, pacemakers, wounds and tumours.	There is a small theoretical risk to defibrillators and the myocardium if shocks are delivered over a pacemaker or implantable cardioverted-defibrillator (ICD). This can be minimised by placing pads more than 8 cm from such devices, where possible (24). Patches with plastic backing are unlikely to cause explosions, even with glyceryl trinitrate (GTN), but may adversely affect the defibrillator pad's contact with the skin (24,25).
14.	Switch on the AED and attach the pads to the patient, ensuring they make a good contact. Use paediatric pads if available. In smaller children, it may be more practical to place the pads in the anterior-posterior position in order to provide enough gap between the pads. 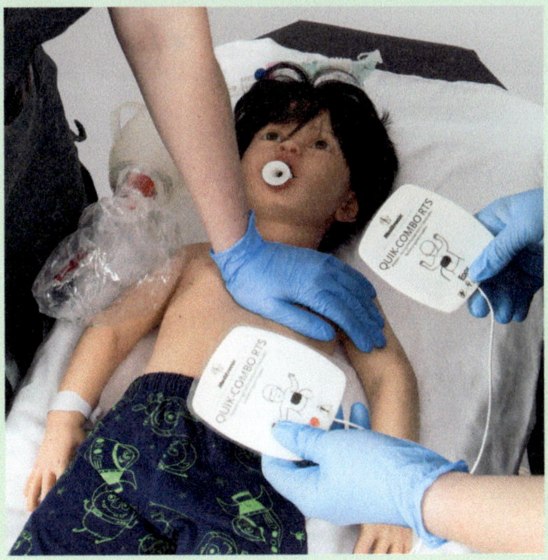	Effective defibrillation is dependent, in part, on good contact between the pads and the skin. There is some evidence that using paediatric attenuated pads in children less than 8 years old, results in higher survival rates. However, it is acceptable to use standard adult pads if that is all that is available (3).

Action		Rationale
15.	Follow visual and voice prompts, ensuring that no one touches the patient while the AED is analysing the rhythm. 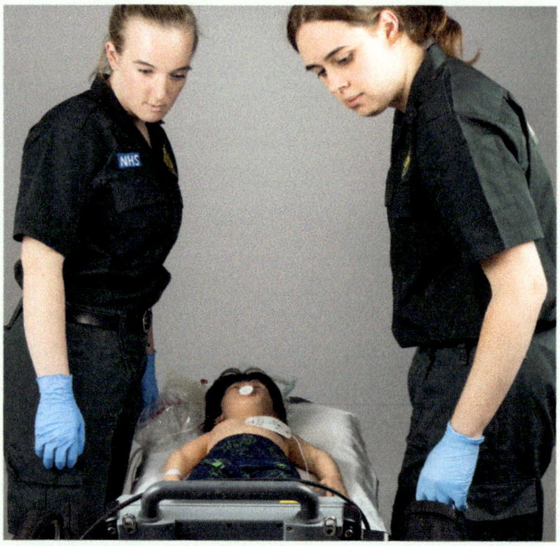	If the AED detects movement, it may result in a longer rhythm interpretation time and hence delay in defibrillation.
16.	If a shock is advised, make sure everyone is clear of the patient, oxygen is kept at least 1 metre away from the patient and push the shock button. If a shock is not advised, skip to step 17. 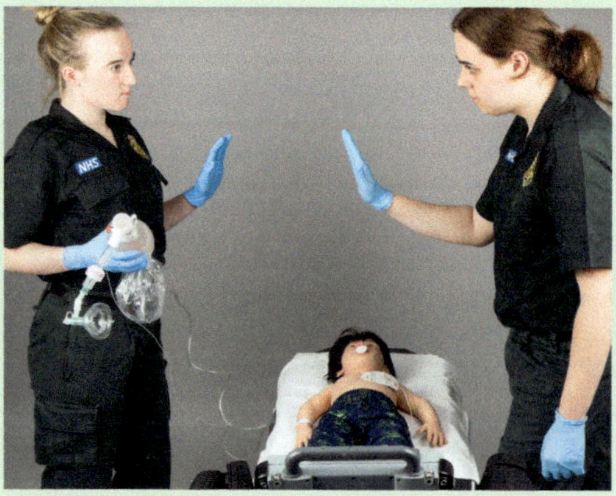	Removing the source of oxygen reduces the risk of combustion due to an oxygen-rich environment.

Action		Rationale
17.	Immediately restart CPR at a ratio of 15:2. You should alternate chest compressions with your colleague every 2 minutes, but keep the changeover time to a minimum. 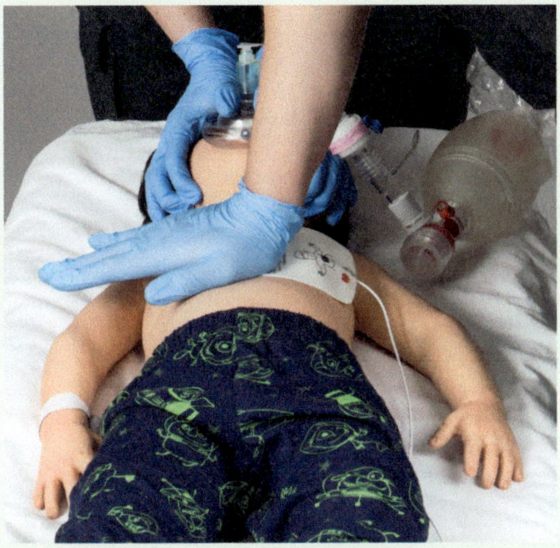	Manikin studies have demonstrated rescuer fatigue as evidenced by decreasing chest compression depth after 2 minutes (3 minutes with real-time feedback devices), so regular breaks are recommended (26).
18.	Continue to follow visual and voice prompts from the AED, ensuring that no one touches the patient while the AED is analysing the rhythm, and that oxygen is kept at least 1 metre away from the patient if defibrillation is required.	Reducing 'time of the chest' is important, but it must not compromise safety. Removing the source of oxygen, for example, reduces the risk of combustion due to an oxygen-rich environment.
19.	Document the procedure.	You must keep full, clear and accurate records for everyone you care for, treat, or provide other services to (27).

References

1. Resuscitation Council UK. *European Paediatric Advanced Life Support*. 5th edition. London: Resuscitation Council UK; 2021.
2. Joint Royal Colleges Ambulance Liaison Committee, Association of Ambulance Chief Executives. JRCALC clinical guidelines. Cited from JRCALC Plus (Version 1.2.13) [Mobile application software]. Bridgwater: Class Publishing Ltd; 2021.
3. Voorde PV de, Turner NM, Djakow J, et al. European Resuscitation Council Guidelines 2021: paediatric life support. *Resuscitation*. 2021 Apr 1;161:327–387.
4. NHS England, NHS Improvement. Standard infection control precautions: national hand hygiene and personal protective equipment policy [Internet]. 2019 [cited 2021 Nov 11]. Available from: https://www.england.nhs.uk/publication/standard-infection-control-precautions-national-hand-hygiene-and-personal-protective-equipment-policy/.
5. Kovacs G, Law JA. *Airway Management in Emergencies*. 2nd edition. Shelton: McGraw-Hill Medical; 2011.
6. Sekiguchi H, Kondo Y, Kukita I. Verification of changes in the time taken to initiate chest compressions according to modified basic life support guidelines. *American Journal of Emergency Medicine*. 2013 Aug 1;31(8):1248–1250.
7. Marsch S, Tschan F, Semmer NK, et al. ABC versus CAB for cardiopulmonary resuscitation: a prospective, randomized simulator-based trial. *Swiss Medical Weekly*. 2013 Sep 6;143:w13856.

8. Lubrano R, Cecchetti C, Bellelli E, et al. Comparison of times of intervention during pediatric CPR maneuvers using ABC and CAB sequences: a randomized trial. *Resuscitation*. 2012 Dec;83(12):1473–1477.
9. de Caen AR, Maconochie IK, Aickin R, et al. Part 6: Pediatric basic life support and pediatric advanced life support. *Circulation*. 2015 Oct 20;132(16):S177–203.
10. Maconochie IK, Aickin R, Hazinski MF, et al. Pediatric life support: 2020 international consensus on cardiopulmonary resuscitation and emergency cardiovascular care science with treatment recommendations. *Circulation*. 2020 Oct 20;142(16):S140–184.
11. Otten D, Liao MM, Wolken R, et al. Comparison of bag-valve-mask hand-sealing techniques in a simulated model. *Annals of Emergency Medicine*. 2014 Jan 1;63(1):6–12.e3.
12. Hart D, Reardon R, Ward C, Miner J. Face mask ventilation: a comparison of three techniques. *Journal of Emergency Medicine*. 2013 May;44(5):1028–1033.
13. Jin Y, Lee BN, Park JR, Kim YM. Comparison of two mask holding techniques for two person bag-valve-mask ventilation: a cross-over simulation study. *Resuscitation*. 2010 Dec 1;81(2):S59.
14. Del Castillo J, López-Herce J, Matamoros M, et al. Hyperoxia, hypocapnia and hypercapnia as outcome factors after cardiac arrest in children. *Resuscitation*. 2012 Dec;83(12):1456–1461.
15. Gazmuri RJ, Ayoub IM, Radhakrishnan J, et al. Clinically plausible hyperventilation does not exert adverse hemodynamic effects during CPR but markedly reduces end-tidal PCO_2. *Resuscitation*. 2012 Feb;83(2):259–264.
16. O'Neill JF, Deakin CD. Do we hyperventilate cardiac arrest patients? *Resuscitation*. 2007 Apr;73(1):82–85.
17. Wik L, Kramer-Johansen J, Myklebust H, et al. Quality of cardiopulmonary resuscitation during out-of-hospital cardiac arrest. *Journal of American Medical Association*. 2005 Jan 19;293(3):299–304.
18. Aufderheide TP, Lurie KG. Death by hyperventilation: a common and life-threatening problem during cardiopulmonary resuscitation. *Critical Care Medicine*. 2004 Sep;32(9 Suppl):S345-351.
19. Aufderheide TP, Sigurdsson G, Pirrallo RG, et al. Hyperventilation-induced hypotension during cardiopulmonary resuscitation. *Circulation*. 2004 Apr 27;109(16):1960–1965.
20. Tibballs J, Russell P. Reliability of pulse palpation by healthcare personnel to diagnose paediatric cardiac arrest. *Resuscitation*. 2009 Jan;80(1):61–64.
21. Tibballs J, Weeranatna C. The influence of time on the accuracy of healthcare personnel to diagnose paediatric cardiac arrest by pulse palpation. *Resuscitation*. 2010 Jun;81(6):671–675.
22. Topjian AA, Raymond TT, Atkins D, et al. Part 4: pediatric basic and advanced life support: 2020 American Heart Association guidelines for cardiopulmonary resuscitation and emergency cardiovascular care. *Circulation*. 2020 Oct 20;142(16):S469–523.
23. Ashoor HM, Lillie E, Zarin W, et al. Effectiveness of different compression-to-ventilation methods for cardiopulmonary resuscitation: a systematic review. *Resuscitation*. 2017 Sep;118:112–125.
24. Resuscitation Council (UK). *Advanced Life Support*. London: Resuscitation Council (UK); 2021.
25. Liddle R, Richmond W. Investigation into voltage breakdown in glyceryl trinitrate patches. *Resuscitation*. 1998 Jun;37(3):145–148.
26. Perkins GD, Handley AJ, Koster RW, et al. European Resuscitation Council Guidelines for Resuscitation 2015. Section 2. Adult basic life support and automated external defibrillation. *Resuscitation*. 2015 Oct;95:81–99.
27. Health and Care Professions Council. Standards of conduct, performance and ethics [Internet]. 2018 [cited 2019 Dec 29]. Available from: https://www.hcpc-uk.org/standards/standards-of-conduct-performance-and-ethics/.

Child Basic Life Support with Manual Defibrillation

Indications

- Child over the age of 1 year with no apparent signs of life.

Contraindications

- Patient whose condition is unequivocally associated with death.
- Patient has a Recommended Summary Plan for Emergency Care and Treatment (ReSPECT), relevant to their current clinical presentation, indicating that cardiopulmonary resuscitation (CPR) attempts are not recommended (1).
- Patient has a valid 'do not attempt cardiopulmonary resuscitation' (DNACPR) form (2).

Advantages

- Provides blow flow to the brain and other vital organs (3).
- Good chance of a return to spontaneous circulation (ROSC) if the primary cause is cardiac (although less common in children).
- Prompt and accurate rhythm interpretation by the clinician can result in a shorter pre-shock pause.

Disadvantages

- Unlikely to lead to ROSC without other interventions, particularly effective ventilation and oxygenation, and treatment for reversible causes.
- Relies on clinician to accurate interpret the rhythm.

Procedure – Child Basic Life Support with Manual Defibrillation

Take the following steps to perform basic life support (BLS) on an child with a manual defibrillator (3):

Action		Rationale
1.	Ensure the scene is safe for you, your colleague, the patient and other bystanders.	Your safety and that of your colleagues is your primary concern. Some causes of cardiac arrest can present a risk to the rescuer, for example drowning and electrocution.
2.	Don appropriate personal protective equipment (PPE), and undertake appropriate hand hygiene.	This reduces the risk of cross-infection (4).

Action		Rationale
3.	Check for responsiveness by placing a hand on the child's forehead to stabilise it and tug their hair while calling their name. 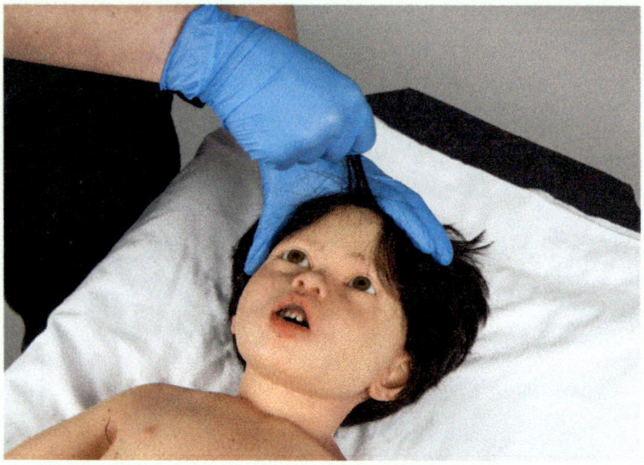	Not every patient who appears to be unresponsive is in cardiac arrest.
4.	If the patient responds, assess the child's ABCDE, call for assistance and reassess regularly. If they do not respond, summon additional assistance.	All cases where children have experienced a period of unresponsiveness or collapse should be taken seriously. The management of peri-arrest children is a team effort (1).
5.	Open the child's airway by placing one hand on their forehead and gently tilt it back until it is in a 'sniffing' position (3). Perform a chin lift by placing the fingertips of your other hand on the bony part of the lower jaw and lift upwards. Do not compress the soft tissues under the jaw as this will occlude the airway. Younger children typically do not require any padding of the shoulders or head, but older children may benefit from a towel or pillow under the occiput (as with adults) to obtain good airway alignment (5). 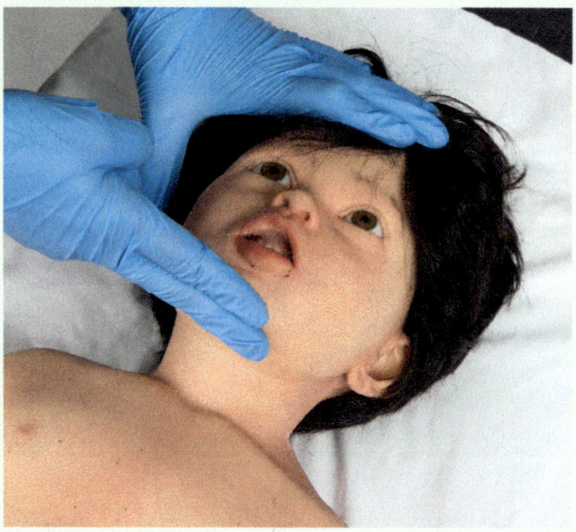	Excessive neck flexion or extension will cause obstruction of the child's airway (1).

<table>
<tr><th colspan="2">Action</th><th>Rationale</th></tr>
<tr><td>6.</td><td>If a head tilt–chin lift does not effectively open the airway, or you suspect a cervical spinal injury, you can use a jaw thrust to open the airway:
• Position yourself behind the child.
• Place two fingers under both angles of the jaw.
• Rest your thumbs on the child's cheeks.
• Lift the jaw upwards.
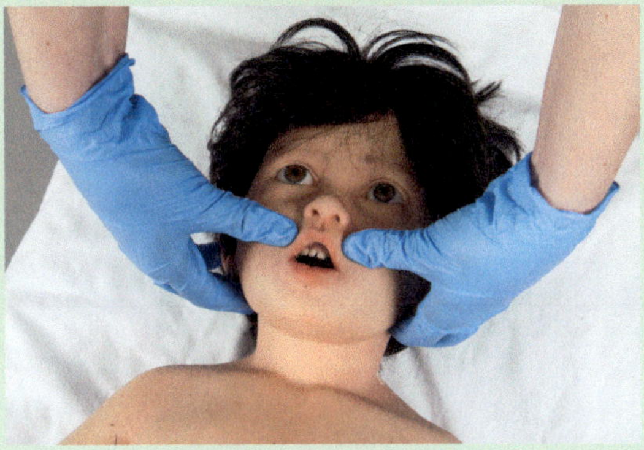</td><td>A jaw thrust results in less (but not zero) movement of the neck (1).</td></tr>
<tr><td>7.</td><td>Look, listen and feel for normal breathing and check for signs of life (swallowing, vocalising, coughing or normal breathing) for no longer than 10 seconds, by placing your face close to the child's face:
• Look for chest and abdominal movements.
• Listen for airflow at the mouth and nose.
• Feel for airflow at the mouth and nose.
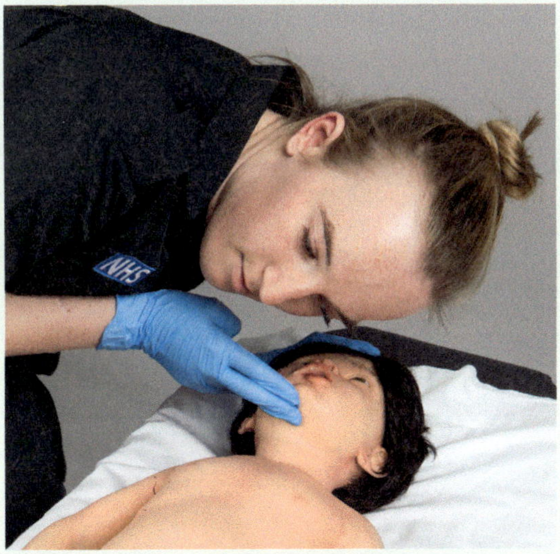
</td><td></td></tr>
<tr><td>8.</td><td>If the child is breathing normally, place them into the recovery position.</td><td>This should enable free drainage of any airway secretions or vomit (3).</td></tr>
</table>

	Action	Rationale
9.	If the child is not breathing or there are no signs of life (no swallowing, vocalising, coughing or normal breathing), check for and carefully remove any airway obstruction, and provide five rescue breaths: • Ensure the head is in a 'sniffing' position and apply a chin lift. • Where possible, use a two-handed bag-valve-mask (BVM) technique and ensure the bag is connected to high-flow oxygen. • Ventilate the chest steadily for one second, just enough to make the chest rise. • Maintain head tilt–chin lift and watch the chest fall. 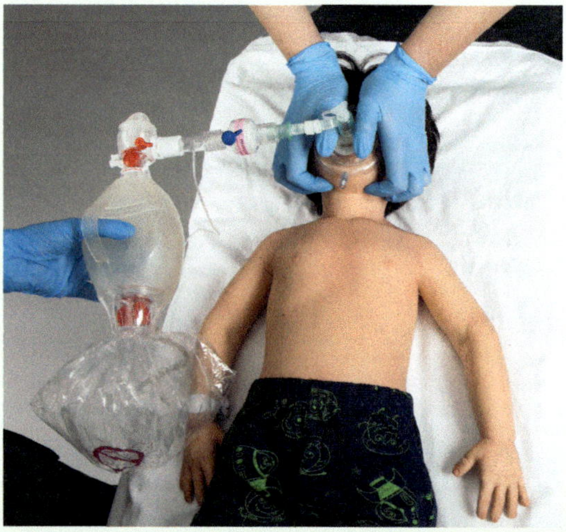	There is equipoise about whether the sequence for basic life support should be chest compressions first or ventilations first. Since ventilations first has been previously advocated for paediatric patients, the current guidance is that this should remain the case (6–10). The two-handed technique results in a better seal and may be less fatiguing than a one-handed technique (11–13). Excessive ventilation is commonly performed during CPR. Hyperventilation can lead to increased intrathoracic pressure and reduced coronary and cerebral perfusion, although the effect this has on survival is not clear (14–19).
10.	If the child's chest is not rising and falling in a similar fashion to normal breathing, open the child's mouth and check for any visible obstruction. Do not blindly sweep in the child's mouth. Reposition the head using a jaw thrust, if the head tilt–chin lift manoeuvre is not effective. The use of airway adjuncts such as an oropharyngeal airway may help too (2). Make no more than five attempts to achieve effective ventilation before moving on to chest compressions.	

Action		Rationale
11.	Check for signs of life (swallowing, vocalising, coughing or normal breathing) and if they are absent (or you are not sure), start chest compressions. If there are signs of life, continue ventilation until the child starts breathing effectively on their own.	Signs of life are prioritised over pulse checks to recognise cardiac arrest. This is because palpation of pulses to confirm cardiac arrest is unreliable in paediatric patients, even amongst healthcare professionals (20,21).
12.	If there are no signs of life (or you are unsure), start chest compressions: • Position yourself by the side of the child.	
	• Avoid compressing the abdomen by placing your hand a finger's width above the xiphisternum. • Lock your elbow and position your body so that your shoulder is directly over the child's chest.	Compressing the abdomen instead of the chest will result in ineffective chest compressions and may result in abdominal injury.
	• Compress the sternum by at least one-third of the depth of the chest (or by 5 cm) and then fully release the pressure while maintaining contact with the sternum. If this is difficult, use the two-handed technique as you would for adults.	Allowing full chest re-expansion after a chest compression improves return of blood to the heart (22).
	• Repeat the compressions at a rate of 100–120 per minute for 15 compressions and then give two ventilations.	Data from observational studies suggest that a rate of 100–120 compressions per minute results in improved blood pressures (22).
	• Continue compressions and ventilations at a ratio of 15:2. 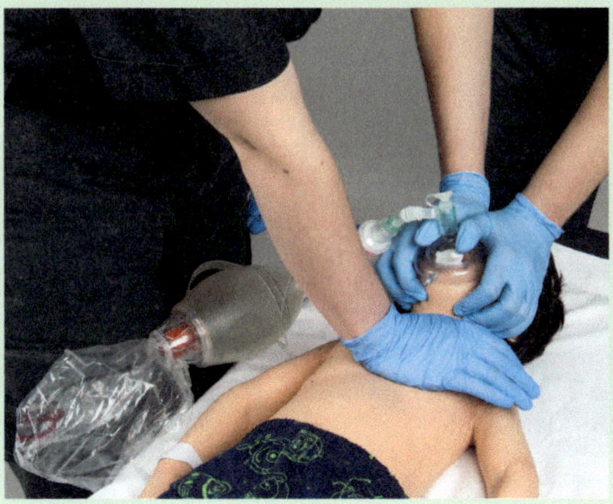	Low-quality evidence suggests that alternating between chest compressions and ventilation is better than chest compressions alone (9). There is no good evidence for a ratio of 15:2 versus 30:2 in children (23), although a ratio of 15:2 results in a greater number of ventilations provided.

	Action	Rationale
13.	Once BLS is established your colleague should expose the child's chest and ensure that the pad sites are free from jewellery, piercings, medication patches, pacemakers, wounds and tumours.	There is a small theoretical risk to defibrillators and the myocardium if shocks are delivered over a pacemaker or implantable cardioverted-defibrillator (ICD). This can be minimised by placing pads more than 8 cm from such devices, where possible (24). Patches with plastic backing are unlikely to cause explosions, even with glyceryl trinitrate (GTN), but may adversely affect the defibrillator pad's contact with the skin (24,25).
14.	Switch on the defibrillator and attach the pads to the patient, ensuring they make a good contact. Use paediatric pads if available. In smaller children, it may be more practical to place the pads in the anterior-posterior position in order to provide enough gap between the pads. 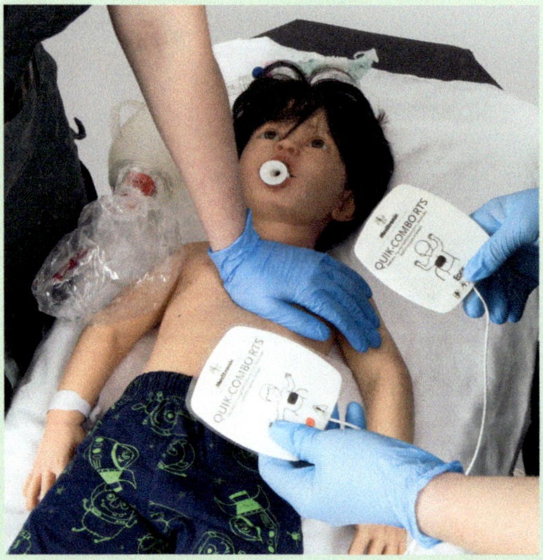	Effective defibrillation is dependent, in part, on good contact between the pads and the skin. There is some evidence that using paediatric attenuated pads in children less than 8 years old results in higher survival rates. However, it is acceptable to use standard adult pads if that is all that is available (3).
15.	Plan actions before pausing chest compressions for rhythm analysis and make sure all team members know their role and the sequence of actions.	Resuscitation guidelines suggest a target of less than 5 seconds to interpret the rhythm and decide if a shock should be delivered.

Action		Rationale
16.	A clinician not performing chest compressions, should palpate a carotid pulse to determine its location while chest compressions are being performed.	There is evidence that healthcare professionals cannot always reliably palpate pulses in cardiac arrest. This step is not in current resuscitation guidelines, but is a pragmatic step to aid in the detection of a pulse (if present), without incurring a delay, which can occur during a rhythm check and the rhythm is pulse electrical activity/ventricular tachycardia (PEA/VT).
17.	Stop chest compressions to analyse the rhythm. Confirm the presence or absence of a pulse and signs of life.	Most defibrillators do not filter chest compression interference from the electrocardiogram (ECG).
18.	If ventricular fibrillation (VF) or pulseless VT is present, follow instructions below. If the rhythm is asystole, PEA or the infant has a heart rate of less than 60 beats per minute, skip to step 19: • Immediately resume chest compressions. • The designated person should charge the defibrillator based on the child's weight (4 J/kg). If the exact energy value cannot be selected, choose the closest, higher, value (2). • While the defibrillator is charging, everyone except for the chest compressor should stand back and move oxygen 1 metre away. For safety, the clinician operating the defibrillator should keep their fingers away from the shock button. • Once the defibrillator is charged, the person defibrillating should tell the chest compressor to 'stand clear' and deliver the shock as soon as they have done so. 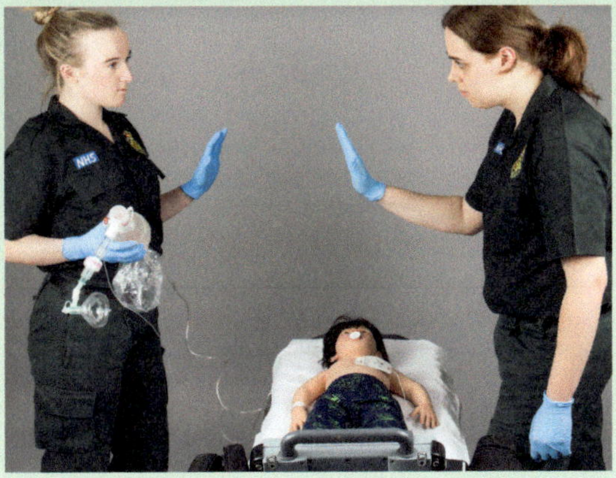	Reducing 'time off the chest' is important, but it must not compromise safety. Removing the source of oxygen, for example, reduces the risk of combustion due to an oxygen-rich environment.

Action		Rationale
19.	Immediately restart CPR at a ratio of 15:2. You should alternate chest compressions with your colleague every 2 minutes, but keep the changeover time to a minimum. 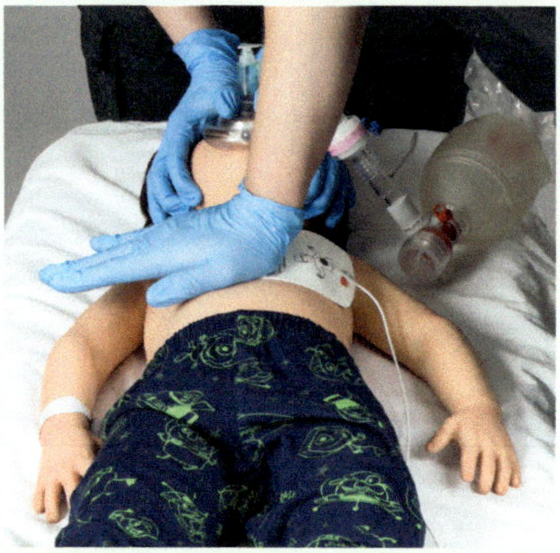	Manikin studies have demonstrated rescuer fatigue as evidenced by decreasing chest compression depth after 2 minutes (3 minutes with real-time feedback devices), so regular breaks are recommended (26).
20.	Once 2 minutes has elapsed, chest compressions should be briefly paused and the rhythm analysed. Repeat step 16 onwards.	
21.	Document the procedure.	You must keep full, clear and accurate records for everyone you care for, treat, or provide other services to (27).

References

1. Resuscitation Council UK. *European Paediatric Advanced Life Support*. 5th edition. London: Resuscitation Council UK; 2021.
2. Joint Royal Colleges Ambulance Liaison Committee, Association of Ambulance Chief Executives. JRCALC clinical guidelines. Cited from JRCALC Plus (Version 1.2.13) [Mobile application software]. Bridgwater: Class Publishing Ltd; 2021.
3. Voorde PV de, Turner NM, et al. European Resuscitation Council Guidelines 2021: paediatric life support. *Resuscitation*. 2021 Apr 1;161:327–87.
4. NHS England, NHS Improvement. Standard infection control precautions: national hand hygiene and personal protective equipment policy [Internet]. 2019 [cited 2021 Nov 11]. Available from: https://www.england.nhs.uk/publication/standard-infection-control-precautions-national-hand-hygiene-and-personal-protective-equipment-policy/.
5. Kovacs G, Law JA. *Airway Management in Emergencies*. 2nd edition. Shelton: McGraw-Hill Medical; 2011.
6. Sekiguchi H, Kondo Y, Kukita I. Verification of changes in the time taken to initiate chest compressions according to modified basic life support guidelines. *American Jounal of Emergency Medicine*. 2013 Aug 1;31(8):1248–1250.
7. Marsch S, Tschan F, Semmer NK, et al. ABC versus CAB for cardiopulmonary resuscitation: a prospective, randomized simulator-based trial. *Swiss Medical Weekly*. 2013 Sep 6;143:w13856.
8. Lubrano R, Cecchetti C, Bellelli E, et al. Comparison of times of intervention during pediatric CPR maneuvers using ABC and CAB sequences: a randomized trial. *Resuscitation*. 2012 Dec;83(12):1473–1477.
9. de Caen AR, Maconochie IK, Aickin R, et al. Part 6: pediatric basic life support and pediatric advanced life support. *Circulation*. 2015 Oct 20;132(16_suppl_1):S177–203.

10. Maconochie IK, Aickin R, Hazinski MF, et al. Pediatric life support: 2020 international consensus on cardiopulmonary resuscitation and emergency cardiovascular care science with treatment recommendations. *Circulation*. 2020 Oct 20;142(16):S140–184.
11. Otten D, Liao MM, Wolken R, et al. Comparison of bag-valve-mask hand-sealing techniques in a simulated model. *Annals of Emergency Medicine*. 2014 Jan 1;63(1):6–12.e3.
12. Hart D, Reardon R, Ward C, Miner J. Face mask ventilation: a comparison of three techniques. *Journal of Emergency Medicine*. 2013 May;44(5):1028–1033.
13. Jin Y, Lee BN, Park JR, Kim YM. Comparison of two mask holding techniques for two person bag-valve-mask ventilation: A cross-over simulation study. *Resuscitation*. 2010 Dec 1;81(2):S59.
14. Del Castillo J, López-Herce J, Matamoros M, et al. Hyperoxia, hypocapnia and hypercapnia as outcome factors after cardiac arrest in children. *Resuscitation*. 2012 Dec;83(12):1456–1461.
15. Gazmuri RJ, Ayoub IM, Radhakrishnan J, et al. Clinically plausible hyperventilation does not exert adverse hemodynamic effects during CPR but markedly reduces end-tidal PCO_2. *Resuscitation*. 2012 Feb;83(2):259–264.
16. O'Neill JF, Deakin CD. Do we hyperventilate cardiac arrest patients? *Resuscitation*. 2007 Apr;73(1):82–85.
17. Wik L, Kramer-Johansen J, Myklebust H, et al. Quality of cardiopulmonary resuscitation during out-of-hospital cardiac arrest. *Journal of American Medical Association*. 2005 Jan 19;293(3):299–304.
18. Aufderheide TP, Lurie KG. Death by hyperventilation: a common and life-threatening problem during cardiopulmonary resuscitation. *Critical Care Medicine*. 2004 Sep;32(9 Suppl):S345–351.
19. Aufderheide TP, Sigurdsson G, Pirrallo RG, et al. Hyperventilation-induced hypotension during cardiopulmonary resuscitation. *Circulation*. 2004 Apr 27;109(16):1960–1965.
20. Tibballs J, Russell P. Reliability of pulse palpation by healthcare personnel to diagnose paediatric cardiac arrest. *Resuscitation*. 2009 Jan;80(1):61–64.
21. Tibballs J, Weeranatna C. The influence of time on the accuracy of healthcare personnel to diagnose paediatric cardiac arrest by pulse palpation. *Resuscitation*. 2010 Jun;81(6):671–675.
22. Topjian AA, Raymond TT, Atkins D, et al. Part 4: Pediatric basic and advanced life support: 2020 American Heart Association guidelines for cardiopulmonary resuscitation and emergency cardiovascular care. *Circulation*. 2020 Oct 20;142(16):S469–523.
23. Ashoor HM, Lillie E, Zarin W, et al. Effectiveness of different compression-to-ventilation methods for cardiopulmonary resuscitation: a systematic review. *Resuscitation*. 2017 Sep;118:112–125.
24. Resuscitation Council (UK). *Advanced Life Support. London*: Resuscitation Council (UK); 2021.
25. Liddle R, Richmond W. Investigation into voltage breakdown in glyceryl trinitrate patches. *Resuscitation*. 1998 Jun;37(3):145–148.
26. Perkins GD, Handley AJ, Koster RW, et al. European Resuscitation Council Guidelines for Resuscitation 2015. Section 2. Adult basic life support and automated external defibrillation. *Resuscitation*. 2015 Oct;95:81–99.
27. Health and Care Professions Council. Standards of conduct, performance and ethics [Internet]. 2018 [cited 2019 Dec 29]. Available from: https://www.hcpc-uk.org/standards/standards-of-conduct-performance-and-ethics/.

Adult Basic Life Support with Automated External Defibrillation

Indications

- Adult patient with no apparent signs of life.

Contraindications

- Patient whose condition is unequivocally associated with death.
- Patient has an advance decision to refuse treatment (ADRT) or a Recommended Summary Plan for Emergency Care and Treatment (ReSPECT) that applies to their current clinical presentation (1).
- Patient has a valid 'do not attempt cardiopulmonary resuscitation' (DNACPR) form (1).

Advantages

- Provides blood flow to the heart and brain (2).
- Increases the likelihood that the heart will resume an effective rhythm and cardiac output (3).
- Most likely combination to result in return of spontaneous circulation (ROSC) in patients with a shockable rhythm.

Disadvantages

- Unlikely to lead to ROSC in a non-shockable rhythm without advanced life support.

Procedure – Adult Basic Life Support with Automated External Defibrillation

Take the following steps to perform adult basic life support (BLS) with an automated external defibrillator (AED) (1,2):

Action		Rationale
1.	Ensure the scene is safe for you, your colleague(s), the patient and other bystanders.	Your safety and that of your colleagues is your primary concern. Some causes of cardiac arrest can present a risk to the rescuer, for example drowning and electrocution.
2.	Don appropriate personal protective equipment (PPE), and undertaken appropriate hand hygiene.	This reduces the risk of cross-infection (4).

Action		Rationale
3.	Check the patient to see if they are responsive by gently shaking their shoulders and asking if they are all right. 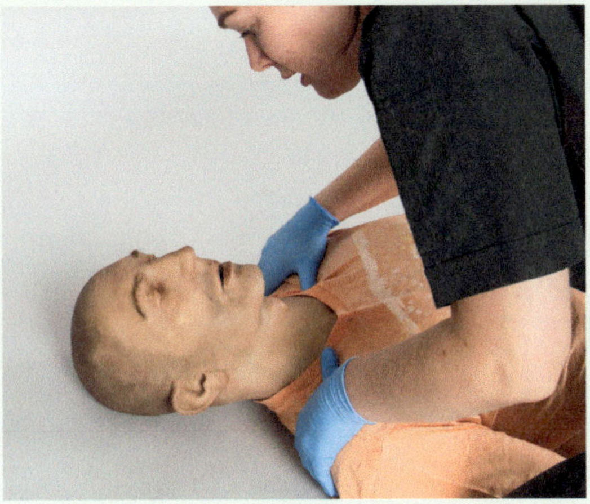	Not every patient who appears to be unresponsive is in cardiac arrest.
4.	If the patient responds, obtain a history and undertake a further patient assessment. If the patient does not respond, inform your colleague(s) so they can assist. Turn the patient onto their back.	Placing the patient on their back makes assessing breathing easier and means the patient is in an optimal position for chest compressions, if required.
5.	Open the patient's airway and look, listen and feel for breathing for no more than 10 seconds. Note that agonal breathing (occasional gasps) is common immediately following cardiac arrest, and should not be confused with normal breathing or taken as a sign of life.	It is important not to delay cardiopulmonary resuscitation (CPR) due to prolonged assessment or confusion arising as a result of agonal breathing.
	If the patient is breathing normally, place them into the recovery position. 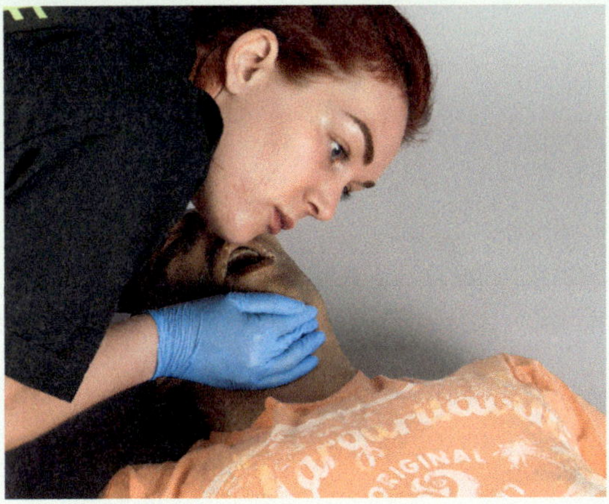	Unresponsive patients may be unable to maintain their own airway. The recovery position may decrease the risk of aspiration (5).

	Action	Rationale
6.	If the patient is not breathing normally or there are no signs of life (not moving, no normal breathing or coughing), start chest compressions: • Kneel beside the patient.	Cardiac arrest in adults is usually due to a primary cardiac cause. Since blood in the pulmonary and systemic circulation can remain oxygenated for several minutes, chest compressions are the priority (3). Manikin studies suggest that CPR starts sooner when chest compressions are commenced before ventilations (6,7).
	• Place the heel of one hand in the centre of the chest (lower half of the sternum). Place the heel of your other hand on top of the first. Interlock your fingers and ensure that pressure is not applied over the patient's ribs.	Since chest compressions are much less effective at generating blood flow than a working heart, it is important to maximise haemodynamic flow by placing the hands in the correct position and only on the sternum (8).
	• Position yourself directly over the patient's chest with your arms straight, and apply downward pressure to compress the chest to a depth of 5 cm but not more than 6 cm.	There is conflicting evidence from studies, but the consensus is that compressing to a depth of greater than 5 cm may improve survival to discharge (9), but compressing deeper than 6 cm might increase the likelihood of injury (10).
	• After each compression release the pressure on the chest, but maintain contact with the patient's skin.	Allowing complete recoil of the chest after each compression, results in better venous return to the chest and may improve the effectiveness of CPR (11,12).
	• Repeat at a rate of 100–120 compressions per minute. 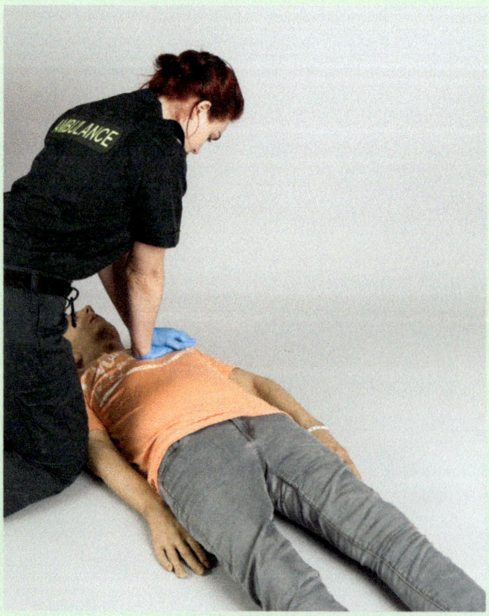	There is conflicting evidence, but some studies suggest applying 100–120 compressions per minute increases the rate of survival (9).

Action		Rationale
7.	While chest compressions are ongoing, your colleague(s) should expose the patient's chest and ensure that the pad sites are free from jewellery, piercings, medication patches, pacemakers, wounds and tumours. They should shave the chest if required. 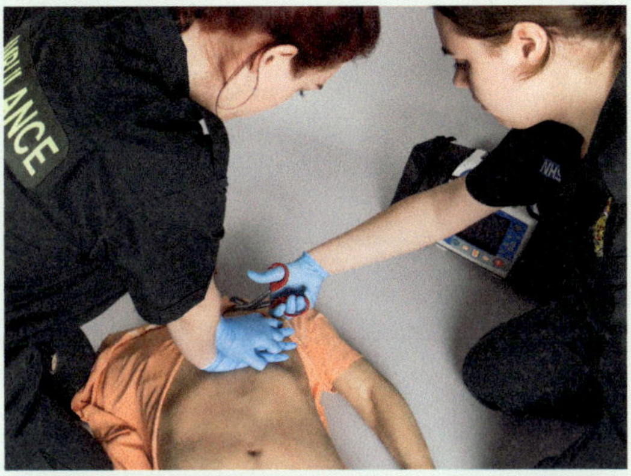	There is a small theoretical risk to defibrillators and the myocardium if shocks are delivered over a pacemaker or implantable cardioverter-defibrillator (ICD). This can be minimised by placing the pads more than 8 cm from such devices, where possible (13). Patches with plastic backing are unlikely to cause explosions, even those with glyceryl trinitrate (GTN), but may adversely affect the defibrillator pad's contact with the skin (13,14).
8.	Switch on the AED and attach the pads to the patient, ensuring they make good contact. Do not interrupt chest compressions while applying the self-adhesive pads. 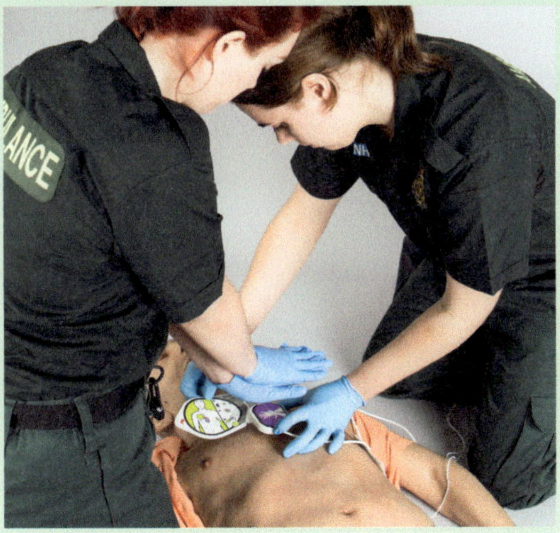	Effective defibrillation is dependent, in part, on good contact between the pads and the skin.

	Action	Rationale
9.	Follow visual and voice prompts, ensuring that no one touches the patient while the AED is analysing the rhythm. 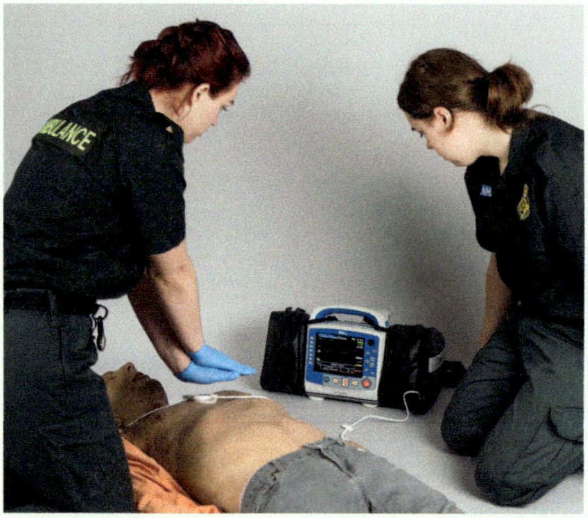	If the AED detects movement, it may result in a longer rhythm interpretation time and hence delay in defibrillation.
10.	If a shock is advised, make sure everyone is clear of the patient and push the shock button. If a shock is not advised, skip to step 11. 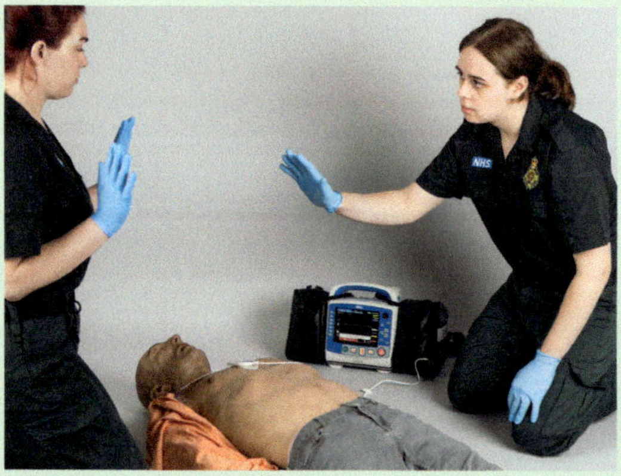	It is preferable if you do not shock your colleague(s).
11.	Immediately restart CPR at a ratio of 30:2.	

	Action	Rationale
12.	After 30 compressions, open the airway (you can insert an oropharyngeal airway (OPA) if available) and provide two rescue breaths with a bag-valve-mask (BVM). If your colleague(s) is available, they may well have already assembled the equipment and be prepared to ventilate.	There is some low-quality evidence that suggests compression-only CPR is as good as CPR with ventilations, but this has not been of sufficient quality to change guidelines (3).
	Each ventilation should cause the chest to rise and take about 1 second to deliver.	A ventilation of around 500–600 ml should be sufficient to make the chest rise and provide adequate oxygenation while minimising the risk of gastric inflation (3).
	Do not attempt to compress the chest while ventilations are being provided, but keep your hands in the correct position so that chest compressions can immediately resume once the ventilations have been administered. 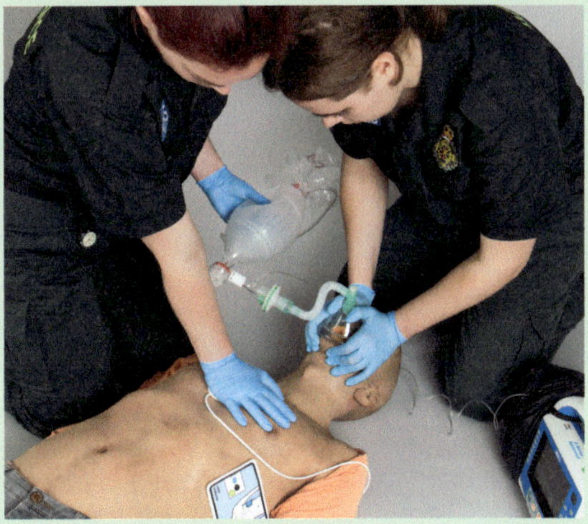	This will help minimise any delay with restarting chest compressions (15–17).

Action		Rationale
13.	Continue with chest compressions and ventilations at a ratio of 30:2. You should alternate chest compressions with your colleague every 2 minutes, but keep the changeover time to a minimum. 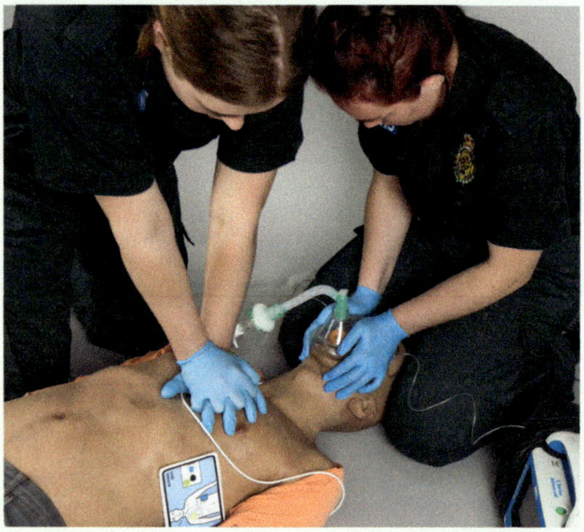	There is some evidence from observational studies of marginally improved outcomes after the change from 15:2 to 30:2 (18–20). Manikin studies have demonstrated rescuer fatigue as evidenced by decreasing chest compression depth after 2 minutes (3 minutes with real-time feedback devices), so regular breaks are recommended (3).
14.	Follow visual and voice prompts from the AED, ensuring that no one touches the patient while the AED is analysing the rhythm and that oxygen is kept at least 1 metre away from the patient if defibrillation is required.	
15.	Document the procedure.	You must keep full, clear and accurate records for everyone you care for, treat, or provide other services to (21).

References

1. Joint Royal Colleges Ambulance Liaison Committee, Association of Ambulance Chief Executives. JRCALC clinical guidelines. Cited from JRCALC Plus (Version 1.2.13) [Mobile application software]. Bridgwater: Class Publishing Ltd; 2021.
2. Olasveengen TM, Semeraro F, Ristagno G, et al. European Resuscitation Council Guidelines 2021: basic life support. *Resuscitation*. 2021 Apr 1;161:98–114.
3. Perkins GD, Handley AJ, Koster RW, et al. European Resuscitation Council Guidelines for Resuscitation 2015. Section 2. Adult basic life support and automated external defibrillation. *Resuscitation*. 2015 Oct;95:81–99.
4. NHS England, NHS Improvement. Standard infection control precautions: national hand hygiene and personal protective equipment policy [Internet]. 2019 [cited 2021 Nov 11]. Available from: https://www.england.nhs.uk/publication/standard-infection-control-precautions-national-hand-hygiene-and-personal-protective-equipment-policy/.
5. Zideman DA, Singletary EM, Borra V, et al. European Resuscitation Council Guidelines 2021: first aid. *Resuscitation*. 2021 Apr;161:270–290.
6. Sekiguchi H, Kondo Y, Kukita I. Verification of changes in the time taken to initiate chest compressions according to modified basic life support guidelines. *American Journal of Emergency Medicine*. 2013 Aug 1;31(8):1248–1250.
7. Marsch S, Tschan F, Semmer NK, et al. ABC versus CAB for cardiopulmonary resuscitation: a prospective, randomized simulator-based trial. *Swiss Medical Weekly*. 2013 Sep 6;143:w13856.
8. Cha KC, Kim HJ, Shin HJ, et al. Hemodynamic effect of external chest compressions at the lower end of the sternum in cardiac arrest patients. *Journal of Emergency Medicine*. 2013 Mar 1;44(3):691–697.
9. Considine J, Gazmuri RJ, Perkins GD, et al. Chest compression components (rate, depth, chest wall recoil and leaning): a scoping review. *Resuscitation*. 2020 Jan;146:188–202.
10. Hellevuo H, Sainio M, Nevalainen R, et al. Deeper chest compression – more complications for cardiac arrest patients? *Resuscitation*. 2013 Jun;84(6):760–765.
11. Zuercher M, Hilwig RW, Ranger-Moore J, et al. Leaning during chest compressions impairs cardiac output and left ventricular myocardial blood flow in piglet cardiac arrest. *Critical Care Medicine*. 2010 Apr;38(4):1141–1146.
12. Niles DE, Sutton RM, Nadkarni VM, et al. Prevalence and hemodynamic effects of leaning during CPR. *Resuscitation*. 2011 Dec;82 Suppl 2:S23–26.
13. Resuscitation Council (UK). *Advanced Life Support*. London: Resuscitation Council (UK); 2021.
14. Liddle R, Richmond W. Investigation into voltage breakdown in glyceryl trinitrate patches. *Resuscitation*. 1998 Jun;37(3):145–148.
15. Cheskes S, Turner L, Foggett R, et al. Paramedic contact to balloon in less than 90 minutes: a successful strategy for st-segment elevation myocardial infarction bypass to primary percutaneous coronary intervention in a Canadian emergency medical system. *Prehospital Emergency*. 2011 Dec;15(4):490–498.
16. Vaillancourt C, Everson-Stewart S, Christenson J, et al. The impact of increased chest compression fraction on return of spontaneous circulation for out-of-hospital cardiac arrest patients not in ventricular fibrillation. *Resuscitation*. 2011 Dec;82(12):1501–1507.
17. Cheskes S, Schmicker RH, Verbeek PR, et al. The impact of peri-shock pause on survival from out-of-hospital shockable cardiac arrest during the Resuscitation Outcomes Consortium PRIMED trial. *Resuscitation*. 2014 Mar;85(3):336–342.
18. Steinmetz J, Barnung S, Nielsen SL, et al. Improved survival after an out-of-hospital cardiac arrest using new guidelines. *Acta Anaesthesiologica Scandinavica*. 2008;52(7):908–913.
19. Olasveengen TM, Vik E, Kuzovlev A, et al. Effect of implementation of new resuscitation guidelines on quality of cardiopulmonary resuscitation and survival. *Resuscitation*. 2009 Apr 1;80(4):407–411.
20. Sayre MR, Cantrell SA, White LJ, et al. Impact of the 2005 American Heart Association Cardiopulmonary Resuscitation and Emergency Cardiovascular Care guidelines on out-of-hospital cardiac arrest survival. *Prehospital Emergency Care*. 2009 Jan 1;13(4):469–477.
21. Health and Care Professions Council. Standards of conduct, performance and ethics [Internet]. 2018 [cited 2019 Dec 29]. Available from: https://www.hcpc-uk.org/standards/standards-of-conduct-performance-and-ethics/.

Adult Basic Life Support with Manual Defibrillation

Indications

- Adult patient with no apparent signs of life.

Contraindications

- Patient whose condition is unequivocally associated with death.
- Patient has an advance decision to refuse treatment (ADRT) or a Recommended Summary Plan for Emergency Care and Treatment (ReSPECT) that applies to their current clinical presentation (1).
- Patient has a valid 'do not attempt cardiopulmonary resuscitation' (DNACPR) form (1).

Advantages

- Provides blood flow to the heart and brain (2).
- Increases the likelihood that the heart will resume an effective rhythm and cardiac output (3).
- Most likely combination to result in return of spontaneous circulation (ROSC) in patients with a shockable rhythm.
- Prompt and accurate rhythm interpretation by the clinician can result in a shorter pre-shock pause.

Disadvantages

- Unlikely to lead to ROSC in non-shockable rhythm without advanced life support.
- Relies on clinician to accurately interpret the rhythm.

Procedure – Adult Basic Life Support on an Adult with Manual Defibrillation

Take the following steps to perform adult basic life support (BLS) with a manual defibrillator (1,2):

Action		Rationale
1.	Ensure the scene is safe for you, your colleague(s), the patient and other bystanders.	Your safety and that of your colleague(s) is your primary concern. Some causes of cardiac arrest can present a risk to the rescuer, for example drowning and electrocution.
2.	Don appropriate personal protective equipment (PPE), and undertaken appropirate hand hygiene.	This reduces the risk of cross-infection (4).
3.	Check the patient to see if they are responsive by gently shaking their shoulders and asking if they are all right. 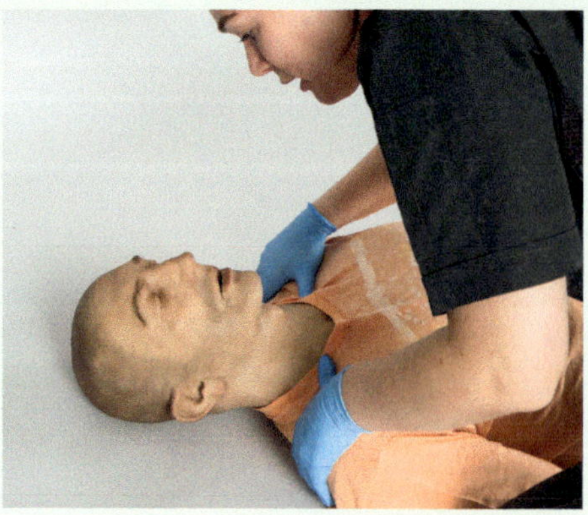	Not every patient who appears to be unresponsive is in cardiac arrest.

Action		Rationale
4.	If the patient responds, obtain a history and undertake a further patient assessment. If the patient does not respond, inform your colleague(s) so they can assist. Turn the patient onto their back.	Placing the patient on their back makes assessing breathing easier and means the patient is in an optimal position for chest compressions, if required.
5.	Open the patient's airway and look, listen and feel for breathing for no more than 10 seconds. Note that agonal breathing (occasional gasps) is common immediately following cardiac arrest, and should not be confused with normal breathing or taken as a sign of life. If the patient is breathing normally, place them into the recovery position. 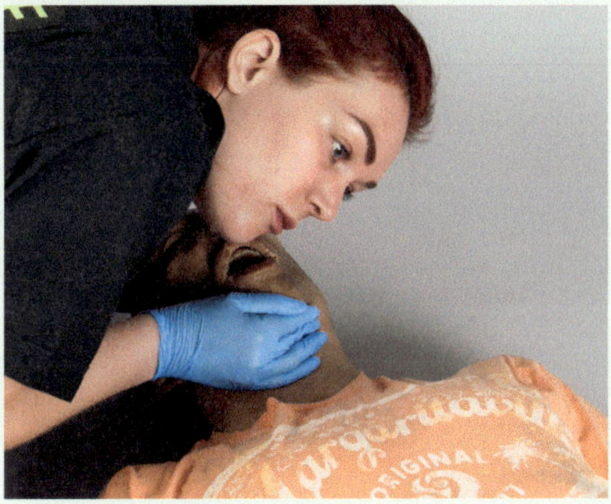	It is important not to delay cardiopulmonary resuscitation (CPR) due to prolonged assessment or confusion arising as a result of agonal breathing. Unresponsive patients may be unable to maintain their own airway. The recovery position may decrease the risk of aspiration (5).
6.	If the patient is not breathing normally or there are no signs of life (not moving, no normal breathing or coughing), start chest compressions: • Kneel beside the patient.	Cardiac arrest in adults is usually due to a primary cardiac cause. Since blood in the pulmonary and systemic circulation can remain oxygenated for several minutes, chest compressions are the priority (3). Manikin studies suggest that CPR starts sooner when chest compressions are commenced before ventilations (6,7).
	• Place the heel of one hand in the centre of the chest (lower half of the sternum). Place the heel of your other hand on top of the first. Interlock your fingers and ensure that pressure is not applied over the patient's ribs.	Since chest compressions are much less effective at generating blood flow than a working heart, it is important to maximise haemodynamic flow by placing the hands in the correct position and only on the sternum (8).
	• Position yourself directly over the patient's chest with your arms straight, and apply downward pressure to compress the chest to a depth of 5 cm but not more than 6 cm.	There is conflicting evidence from studies, but consensus is that compressing to a depth of greater than 5 cm may improve survival to discharge (9), but compressing deeper than 6 cm might increase the likelihood of injury (10).

	Action	Rationale
	• After each compression release the pressure on the chest, but maintain contact with the patient's skin. • Repeat at a rate of 100–120 compressions per minute. 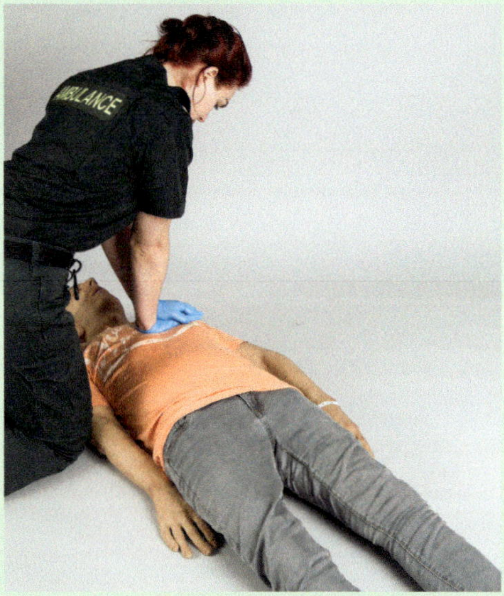	Allowing complete recoil of the chest after each compression results in better venous return to the chest and may improve the effectiveness of CPR (11,12). There is conflicting evidence, but some studies suggest applying 100–120 compressions per minute increases the rate of survival (9).
7.	While chest compressions are ongoing, your colleague(s) should expose the patient's chest and ensure that the pad sites are free from jewellery, piercings, medication patches, pacemakers, wounds and tumours. They should shave the chest if required. 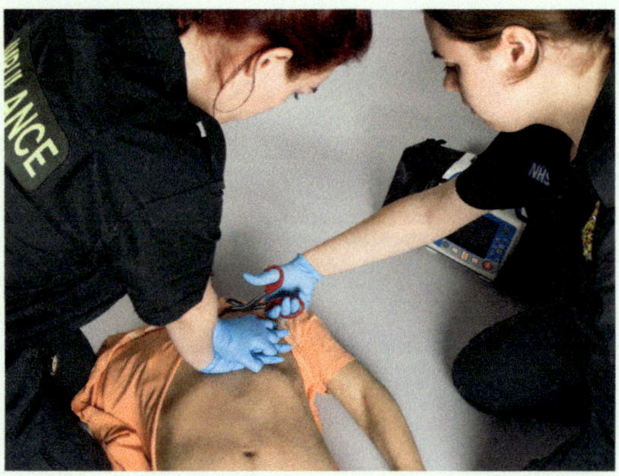	There is a small theoretical risk to the device and the myocardium if shocks are delivered over a pacemaker or implantable cardioverter-defibrillator (ICD). This can be minimised by placing the pads more than 8 cm from such devices, where possible (13). Patches with plastic backing are unlikely to cause explosions, even those with glyceryl trinitrate (GTN), but may adversely affect the defibrillator pad's contact with the skin (13,14). Pads placed directly over metal jewellery and piercings may cause burns.

Action		Rationale
8.	Switch on the defibrillator and attach the pads to the patient, ensuring they make good contact. Do not interrupt chest compressions while applying the self-adhesive pads. 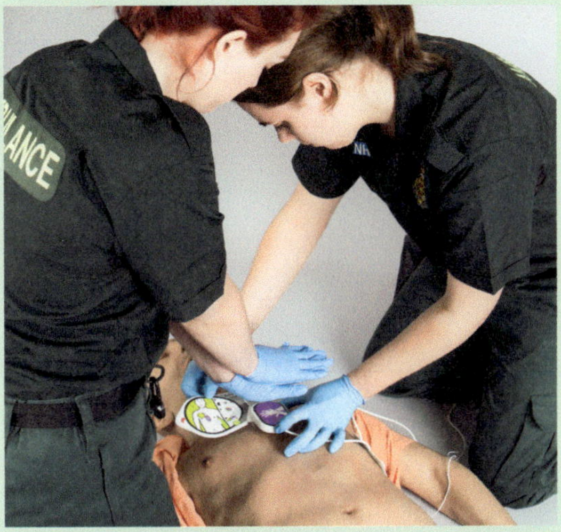	Effective defibrillation is dependent, in part, on good contact between the pads and the skin.
9.	Plan actions before pausing chest compressions for rhythm analysis and make sure all team members know their role and the sequence of actions.	Resuscitation guidelines suggest a target of less than 5 seconds to interpret the rhythm and decide whether a shock should be delivered.
10.	A clinician not performing chest compressions should palpate a carotid pulse to determine its location while chest compressions are being performed. 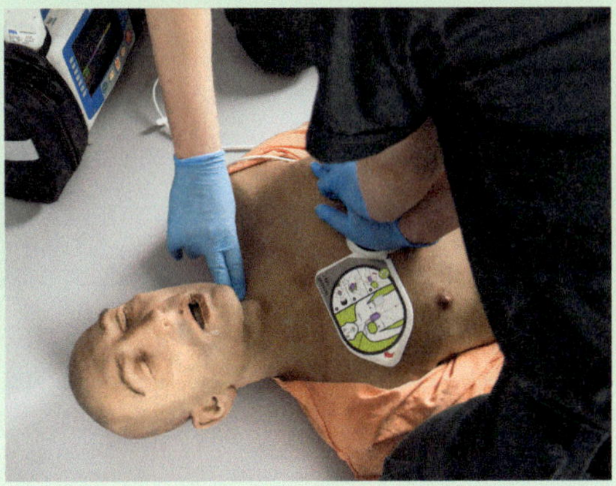	There is evidence that healthcare professionals cannot always reliably palpate pulses in cardiac arrest. This step is not in current resuscitation guidelines but is a pragmatic step to aid in the detection of a pulse (if present), without incurring a delay, which can occur during a rhythm check and the rhythm is pulse electrical activity/ventricular tachycardia (PEA/VT).

	Action	Rationale
11.	Stop chest compressions to analyse the rhythm. Confirm the presence or absence of a pulse and signs of life. 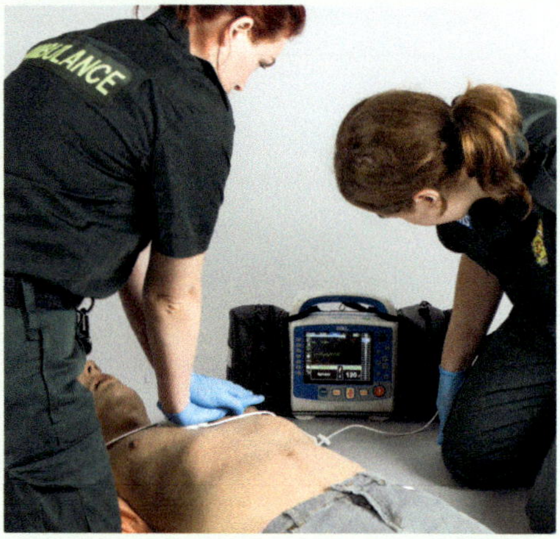	Most defibrillators do not filter chest compression interference from the electrocardiogram (ECG).
12.	If the rhythm is identified as ventricular fibrillation (VF) or pulseless VT, follow instructions below, otherwise skip to step 13: • Immediately resume chest compressions. • The designated person should charge the defibrillator according to the manufacturer's recommendation. • While the defibrillator is charging, everyone except for the chest compressor should stand back and move oxygen 1 metre away. For safety, the clinician operating the defibrillator should keep their fingers away from the shock button. • Once the defibrillator is charged, the person defibrillating should tell the chest compressor to 'stand clear' and deliver the shock as soon as they have done so. 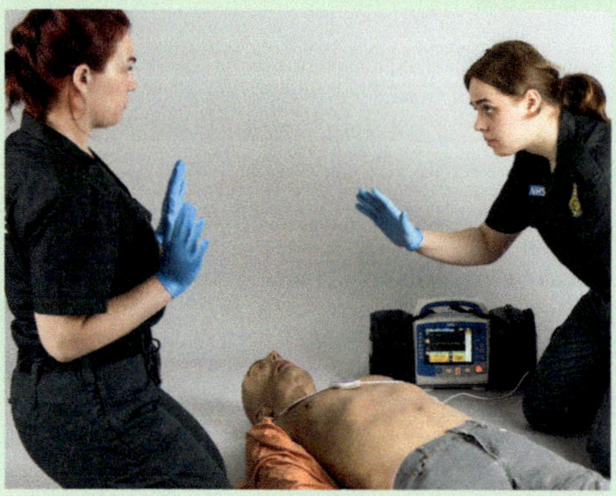	This reduces the risk of combustion due to an oxygen-rich environment.

Action		Rationale
13.	Restart CPR immediately at a ratio of 30:2 without checking for a pulse or assessing the rhythm.	This minimises interruptions in chest compressions.
14.	After 30 compressions, open the airway (you can insert an oropharyngeal airway (OPA) if available) and provide two rescue breaths with a bag-valve-mask. If your colleague(s) is available, they may well have already assembled the equipment and be prepared to ventilate.	There is some low-quality evidence that suggests compression-only CPR is as good as CPR with ventilations, but this has not been of sufficient quality to change guidelines (3).
	Each ventilation should cause the chest to rise and take about 1 second to deliver.	A ventilation of around 500–600 ml should be sufficient to make the chest rise and provide adequate oxygenation while minimising the risk of gastric inflation (3).
	Do not attempt to compress the chest while ventilation is being provided, but keep your hands in the correct position so that chest compressions can immediately resume once the ventilations have been administered.	This will help minimise any delay with restarting chest compressions (15–17).
	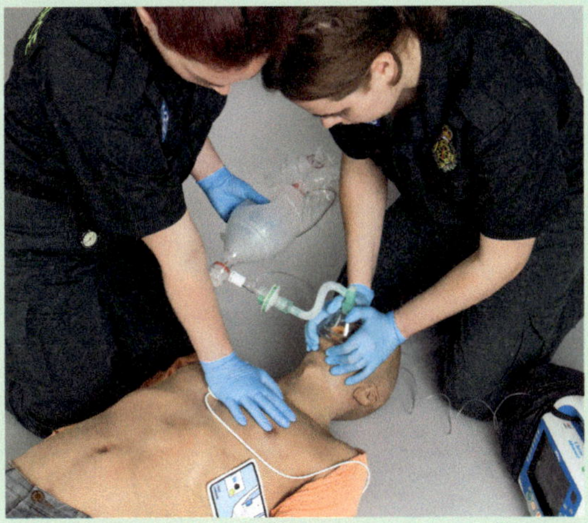	

Action		Rationale
15.	Continue with chest compressions and ventilations at a ratio of 30:2. You should alternate chest compressions with your colleague every 2 minutes, but keep the changeover time to a minimum. 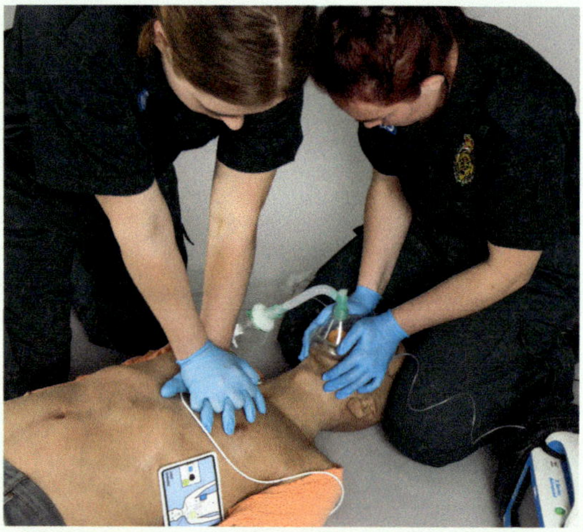	There is some evidence from observational studies of marginally improved outcomes after the change from 15:2 to 30:2 (18–20). Manikin studies have demonstrated rescuer fatigue as evidenced by decreasing chest compression depth after 2 minutes (3 minutes with real-time feedback devices), so regular breaks are recommended (3).
16.	Once 2 minutes have elapsed, chest compressions should be briefly paused and the rhythm analysed. Repeat from step 12 onwards.	
17.	Document the procedure.	You must keep full, clear and accurate records for everyone you care for, treat, or provide other services to (21).

References

1. Joint Royal Colleges Ambulance Liaison Committee, Association of Ambulance Chief Executives. JRCALC clinical guidelines. Cited from JRCALC Plus (Version 1.2.13) [Mobile application software]. Bridgwater: Class Publishing Ltd; 2021.
2. Olasveengen TM, Semeraro F, Ristagno G, et al. European Resuscitation Council Guidelines 2021: basic life support. *Resuscitation*. 2021 Apr 1;161:98–114.
3. Perkins GD, Handley AJ, Koster RW, et al. European Resuscitation Council Guidelines for Resuscitation 2015. Section 2. Adult basic life support and automated external defibrillation. *Resuscitation*. 2015 Oct;95:81–99.
4. NHS England, NHS Improvement. Standard infection control precautions: national hand hygiene and personal protective equipment policy [Internet]. 2019 [cited 2021 Nov 11]. Available from: https://www.england.nhs.uk/publication/standard-infection-control-precautions-national-hand-hygiene-and-personal-protective-equipment-policy/.
5. Zideman DA, Singletary EM, Borra V, et al. European Resuscitation Council Guidelines 2021: first aid. *Resuscitation*. 2021 Apr;161:270–290.
6. Sekiguchi H, Kondo Y, Kukita I. Verification of changes in the time taken to initiate chest compressions according to modified basic life support guidelines. *American Journal of Emergency Medicine*. 2013 Aug 1;31(8):1248–1250.
7. Marsch S, Tschan F, Semmer NK, et al. ABC versus CAB for cardiopulmonary resuscitation: a prospective, randomized simulator-based trial. *Swiss Medical Weekly*. 2013 Sep 6;143:w13856.

8. Cha KC, Kim HJ, Shin HJ, et al. Hemodynamic effect of external chest compressions at the lower end of the sternum in cardiac arrest patients. *Journal of Emergency Medicine*. 2013 Mar 1;44(3):691–697.
9. Considine J, Gazmuri RJ, Perkins GD, et al. Chest compression components (rate, depth, chest wall recoil and leaning): a scoping review. *Resuscitation*. 2020 Jan;146:188–202.
10. Hellevuo H, Sainio M, Nevalainen R, et al. Deeper chest compression – more complications for cardiac arrest patients? *Resuscitation*. 2013 Jun;84(6):760–765.
11. Zuercher M, Hilwig RW, Ranger-Moore J, et al. Leaning during chest compressions impairs cardiac output and left ventricular myocardial blood flow in piglet cardiac arrest. *Critical Care Medicine*. 2010 Apr;38(4):1141–1146.
12. Niles DE, Sutton RM, Nadkarni VM, et al. Prevalence and hemodynamic effects of leaning during CPR. *Resuscitation*. 2011 Dec;82 Suppl 2:S23–26.
13. Resuscitation Council (UK). *Advanced Life Support*. London: Resuscitation Council (UK); 2021.
14. Liddle R, Richmond W. Investigation into voltage breakdown in glyceryl trinitrate patches. *Resuscitation*. 1998 Jun;37(3):145–148.
15. Cheskes S, Turner L, Foggett R, et al. Paramedic contact to balloon in less than 90 minutes: a successful strategy for ST-segment elevation myocardial infarction bypass to primary percutaneous coronary intervention in a Canadian emergency medical system. *Prehospital Emergency Care*. 2011 Dec;15(4):490–498.
16. Vaillancourt C, Everson-Stewart S, Christenson J, et al. The impact of increased chest compression fraction on return of spontaneous circulation for out-of-hospital cardiac arrest patients not in ventricular fibrillation. *Resuscitation*. 2011 Dec;82(12):1501–1507.
17. Cheskes S, Schmicker RH, Verbeek PR, et al. The impact of peri-shock pause on survival from out-of-hospital shockable cardiac arrest during the Resuscitation Outcomes Consortium PRIMED trial. *Resuscitation*. 2014 Mar;85(3):336–342.
18. Steinmetz J, Barnung S, Nielsen SL, et al. Improved survival after an out-of-hospital cardiac arrest using new guidelines. *Acta Anaesthesiologica Scandinavica*. 2008;52(7):908–913.
19. Olasveengen TM, Vik E, Kuzovlev A, et al. Effect of implementation of new resuscitation guidelines on quality of cardiopulmonary resuscitation and survival. *Resuscitation*. 2009 Apr 1;80(4):407–411.
20. Sayre MR, Cantrell SA, White LJ, et al. Impact of the 2005 American Heart Association Cardiopulmonary Resuscitation and Emergency Cardiovascular Care guidelines on out-of-hospital cardiac arrest survival. *Prehospital Emergency Care*. 2009 Jan 1;13(4):469–477.
21. Health and Care Professions Council. Standards of conduct, performance and ethics [Internet]. 2018 [cited 2019 Dec 29]. Available from: https://www.hcpc-uk.org/standards/standards-of-conduct-performance-and-ethics/.

LUCAS Chest Compression System

Indications

- Adult patient in cardiac arrest who requires prolonged resuscitation at the scene or transport to hospital.

Contraindications

- Patient whose condition is unequivocally associated with death.
- Oxygen-rich environments.
- Flammable agents (for example, petrol) nearby.
- Patient too small or large for the device to be fitted or function correctly.

Advantages

- Enables safe chest compressions during transport.
- Does not fatigue during prolonged resuscitation attempts.
- Can be connected to external power supply during use.

Disadvantages

- Not superior to manual chest compressions in improving rates of favourable neurological outcome following cardiac arrest (1).
- High centre of gravity can adversely affect quality of chest compressions when travelling in an ambulance.

Procedure – LUCAS Chest compression System

Take the following steps to undertake mechanical chest compressions (MCC) with the LUCAS chest compression system (2,3):

Action		Rationale
1.	During an ongoing resuscitation attempt identify the need for a MCC device.	A LUCAS device should not be used on every cardiac arrest (1).
2.	Open the carrying case and power on the device by pressing the ON/OFF button for 1 second. 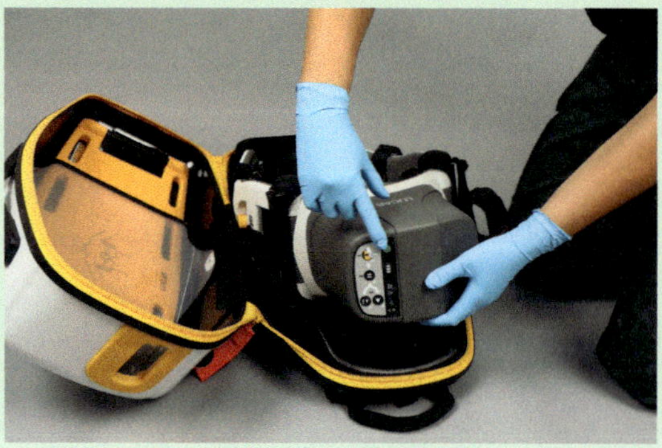	Powering on the device will enable the self-test process to be completed before the device is required for used.

Action		**Rationale**
3.	Remove the back plate from the bag. At a suitable time during the arrest (for example, during a pulse check or instead of one cycle of ventilation) and in a smooth co-ordinated fashion, lift the patient's torso so the device can be slid in behind. Ensure that the tops of the handles are immediately below the armpits. 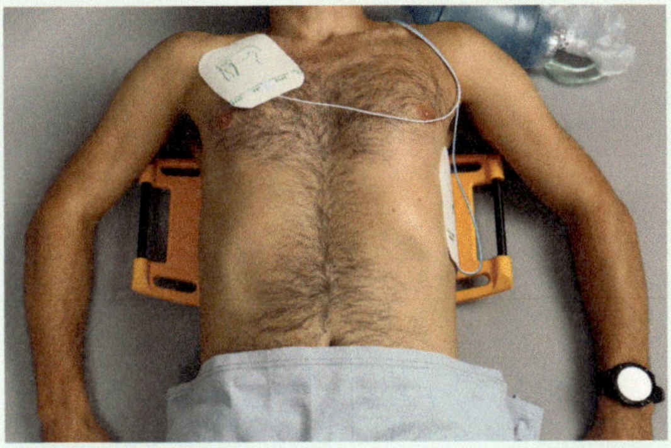	Placing the back board in the correct position will make it easier and faster to position the suction cup accurately.
4.	Recommence manual CPR.	Minimising interruptions in chest compressions is important for good patient outcomes from cardiac arrest (4).
5.	Using the handles on the support legs, remove the upper part of the LUCAS device from the bag. Pull the release rings once and ensure that the claw locks open. 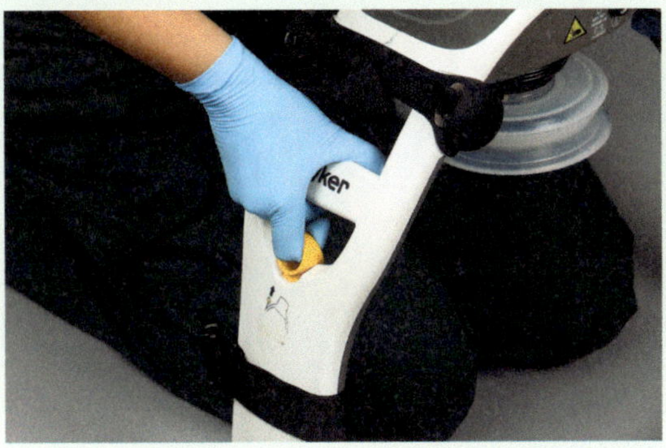	Check that the locking mechanism for the upper part of the device is functioning correctly.

Action		Rationale
6.	Without interrupting manual CPR, the clinician should attach the support leg closest to them. Present the support leg at an angle of about 45° and push it onto the backboard pin. Listen for a click to indicate correct attachment. 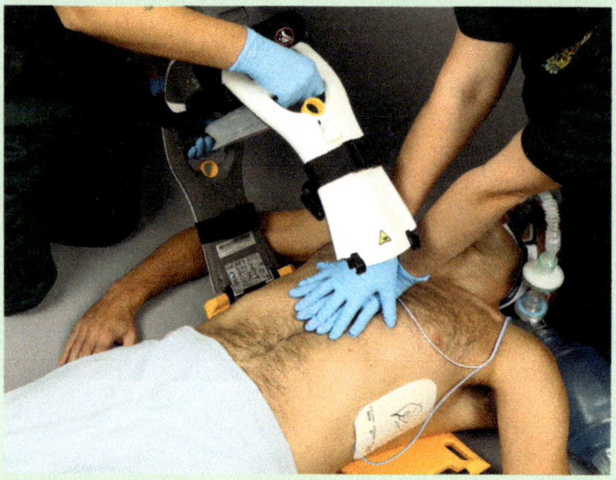	Minimising interruptions in chest compressions is important for good patient outcomes from cardiac arrest (4).
7.	Stop manual CPR and attach the other support leg to the backboard. Again, listen for the click and then pull up once on both support legs to ensure they are locked to the backboard correctly. 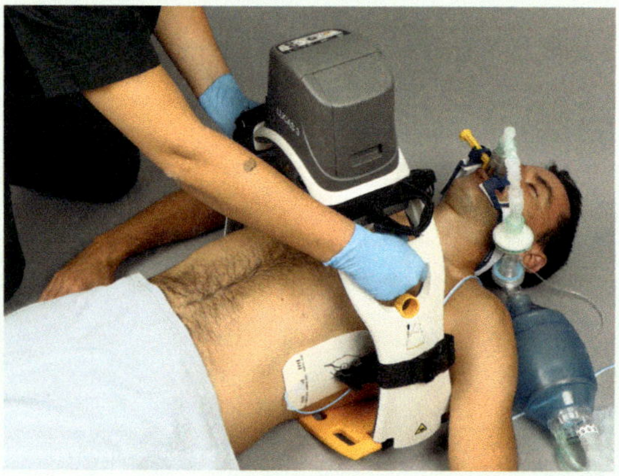	

Action		Rationale
8.	Check that the suction cup is in the correct position by using a finger to confirm that the edge of the suction cup furthest from the head, is just above where the body of the sternum meets the xiphoid process. If necessary, use the support legs to move the device into the correct position. 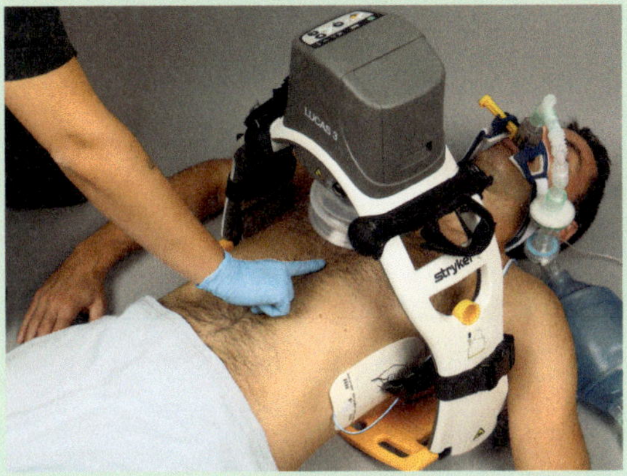	
9.	Confirm the LUCAS device is in ADJUST mode (the LED next to the number-1 button should be illuminated), then use two fingers to push the suction cup down until the pressure pad makes contact with the patient's chest, but does not compress it. 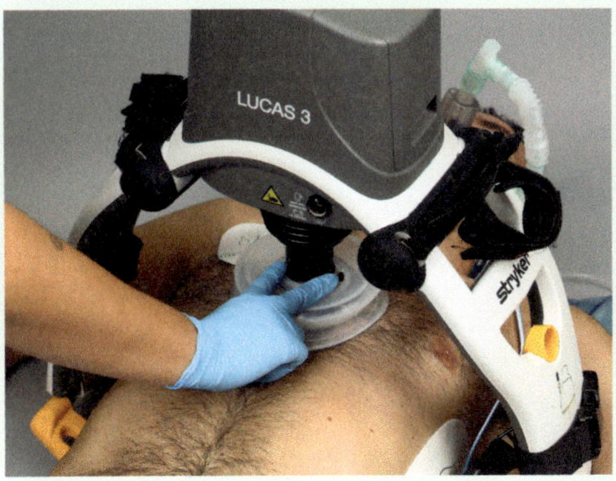	

Action		Rationale
10.	Push the PAUSE button to lock the start position. 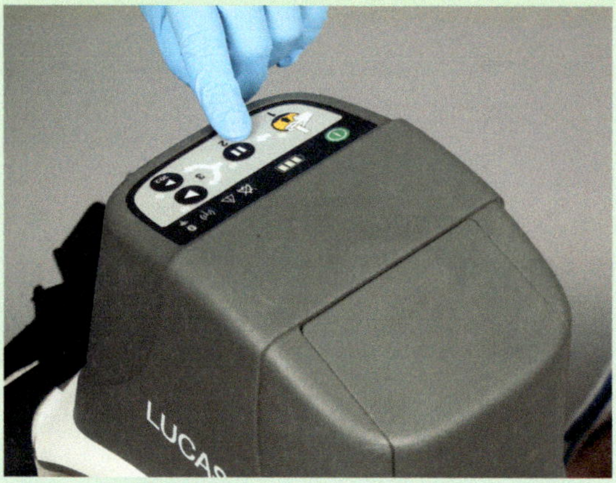	
11.	Push the ACTIVE or ACTIVE (30:2) button to start chest compressions. 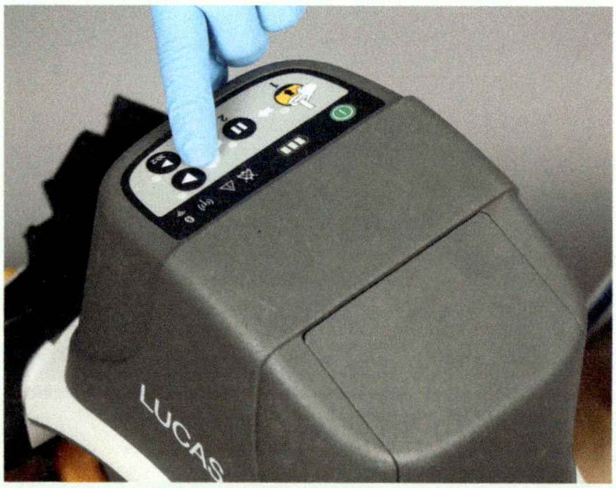	
12.	Pass the stabilising strap under the head and click into clips mounted on the upright arms of the device. Once in place pull the strap so it is firm. 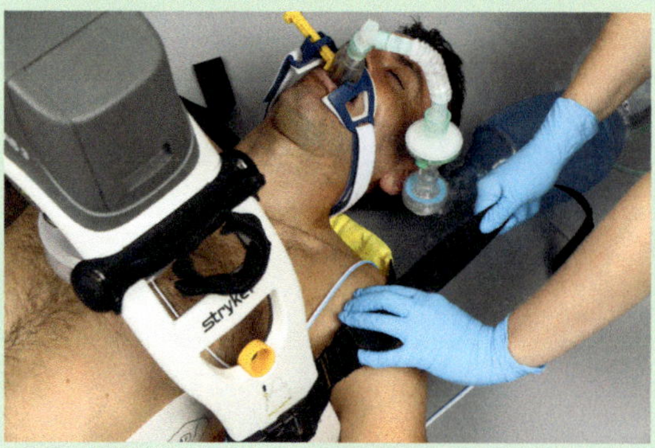	The strap helps to keep the LUCAS device in place whilst it is providing CPR.

Action		Rationale
13.	When ready to move the patient, secure their arms to the upper part of the LUCAS device using the patient straps. 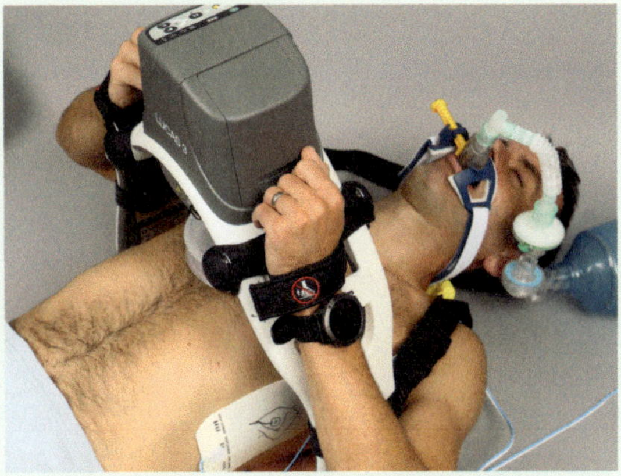	
14.	Remember to pause the device when performing rhythm analysis. 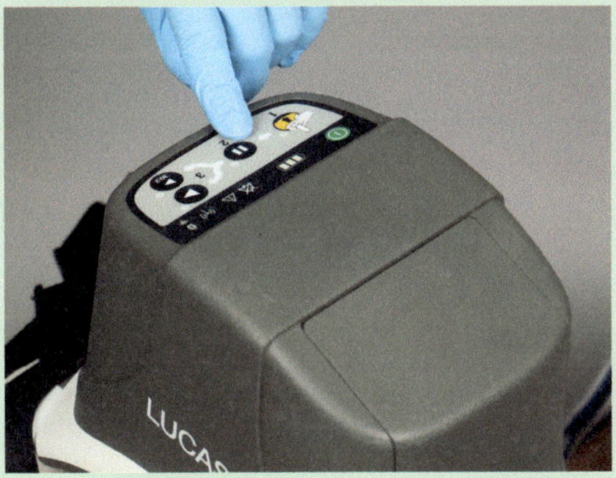	As with chest compression, chest wall movement by the device will make rhythm analysis difficult or impossible.
15.	Document the procedure.	You must keep full, clear and accurate records for everyone you care for, treat, or provide other services to (5).

References

1. Soar J, Böttiger BW, Carli P, et al. European Resuscitation Council Guidelines 2021: adult advanced life support. *Resuscitation*. 2021 Apr;161:115–151.
2. Physio-Control. LUCAS 2 chest compression system Hemsley Grant Instructor Guidebook. Redmond: Physio Control, Inc.; 2016.
3. Physio-Control. LUCAS 3 chest compression system Instructions for Use. Sweden: Jolife AB; 2017.
4. Olasveengen TM, Semeraro F, Ristagno G, et al. European Resuscitation Council Guidelines 2021: basic life support. *Resuscitation*. 2021 Apr 1;161:98–114.
5. Health and Care Professions Council. Standards of conduct, performance and ethics [Internet]. 2018 [cited 2019 Dec 29]. Available from: https://www.hcpc-uk.org/standards/standards-of-conduct-performance-and-ethics/.

AutoPulse®

Indications

- Adult patient in cardiac arrest who requires prolonged resuscitation at the scene or transport to hospital.

Contraindications

- Cause of cardiac arrest is traumatic in origin.
- Patient whose condition is unequivocally associated with death.
- Oxygen-rich (more than 25% oxygen) atmosphere.
- Flammable anaesthetic gases or other flammable agents (for example, petrol) nearby.
- Patient weighing in excess of 136 kg (21 st 6 lbs).
- Patient too small or large for the device to be fitted or function correctly.

Advantages

- Enables safe chest compressions during transport.
- Does not fatigue during prolonged resuscitation attempts.

Disadvantages

- Limited battery life of 30 minutes.
- Not superior to manual chest compressions in improving rates of favourable neurological outcome following cardiac arrest (1).
- Inadvertent covering of the cooling vents can lead to device shutdown.

Procedure – AutoPulse®

Take the following steps to undertake mechanical chest compressions (MCC) with an AutoPulse® (2):

Action		Rationale
1.	During an ongoing resuscitation attempt identify the need for an MCC device. 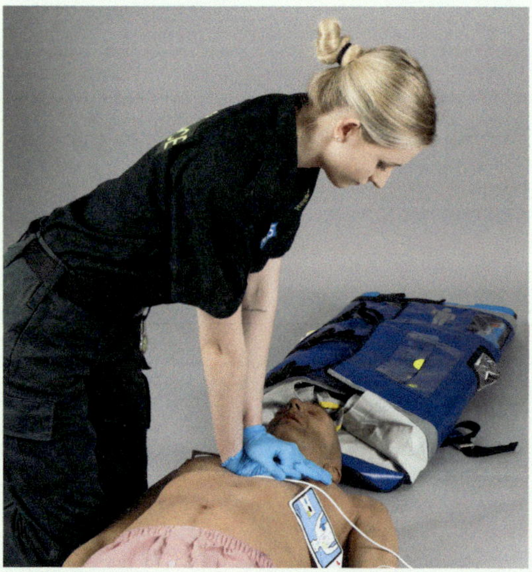	The AutoPulse® should not be used on every cardiac arrest (1).

Action		Rationale
2.	Place the AutoPulse® at the head of the patient, power the device on and unpack. 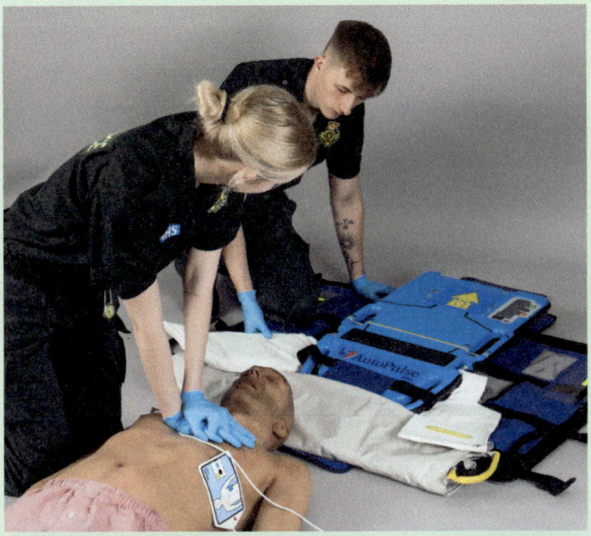 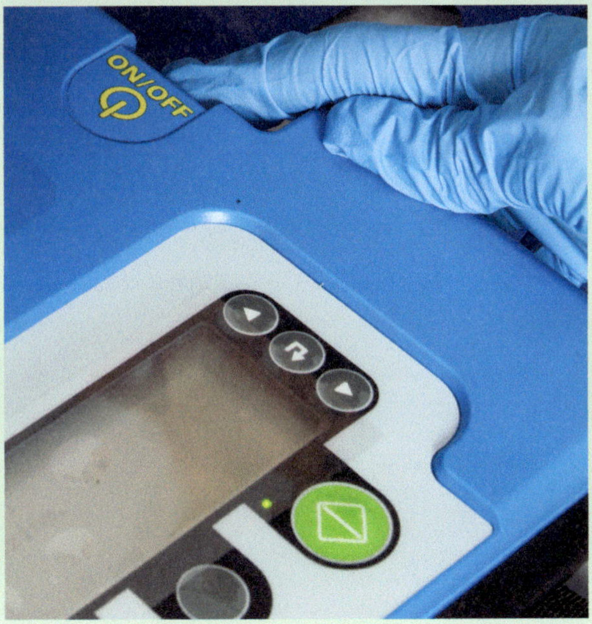 	Powering on the device will enable the initialisation process to be completed before the device is required for use. The device will usually be slid in from the patient's head, although can be slid in from the side, if required.

	Action	Rationale
3.	In a smooth co-ordinated fashion, lift the patient's torso so the device can be slid in behind. If not already undertaken, any clothing covering the patient's torso should be removed. 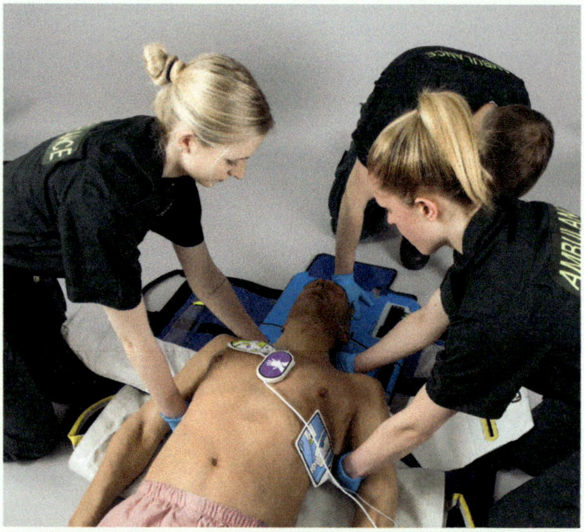	Interruptions to chest compressions should be minimised.
4.	Ensure the patient is positioned centrally on the board and the yellow line is visible below the axilla. 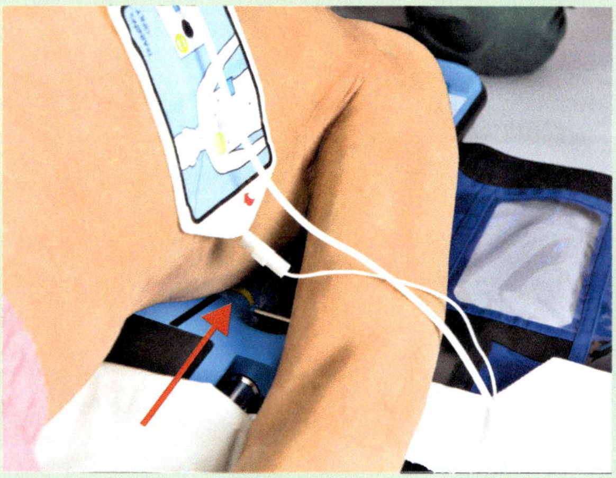	Correct positioning of the patient on the board will ensure chest compressions are administered correctly.

	Action	Rationale
5.	Close the LifeBand around the patient's chest and over the defibrillation pads. Band 1 should rest on top of the patient's chest and band 2 should be placed over band 1, ensuring that the alignment tab on band 1 inserts through the alignment slot of band 2. Press the Velcro of the bands together. 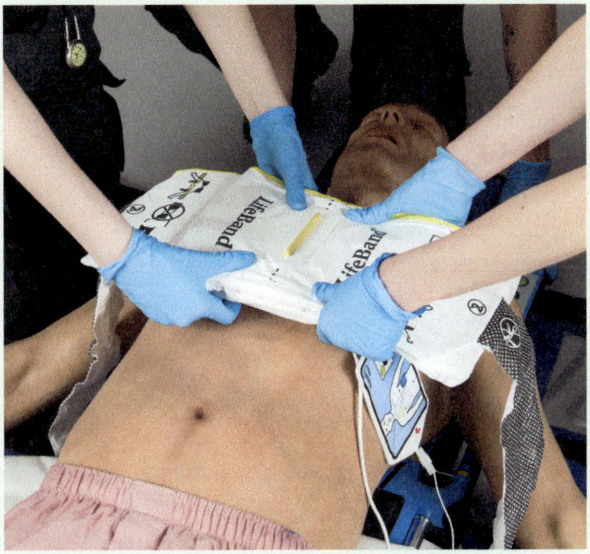	
6.	Lift up the LifeBand to full extension, checking that the side bands are at 90° to the board and are not twisted or obstructed. 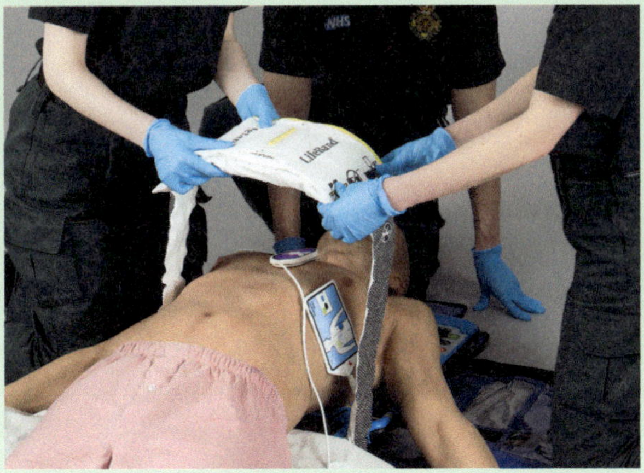	This helps ensure the device performs correctly.

Action		Rationale
7.	Place the LifeBand onto the patient's chest, ensuring it is centred over the location where manual chest compressions have been performed. 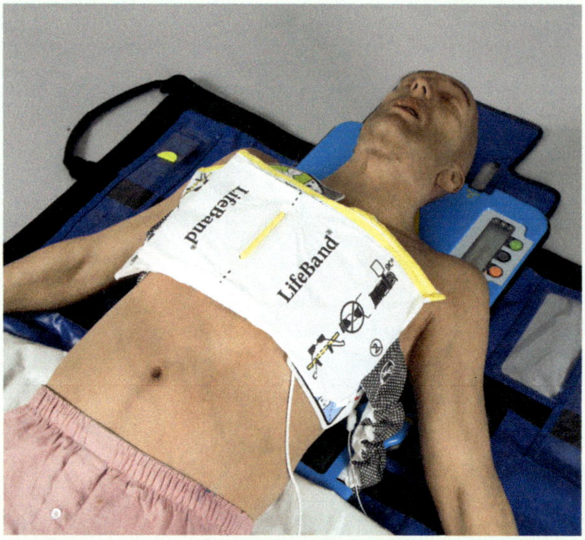	Failure to properly position a patient, both vertically and laterally with respect to the AutoPulse® board, may cause injury to the patient.
8.	Press and release the START/CONTINUE button (green button) once. The AutoPulse® will adjust the band to the patient's chest and then pause for 3 seconds before commencing chest compressions. 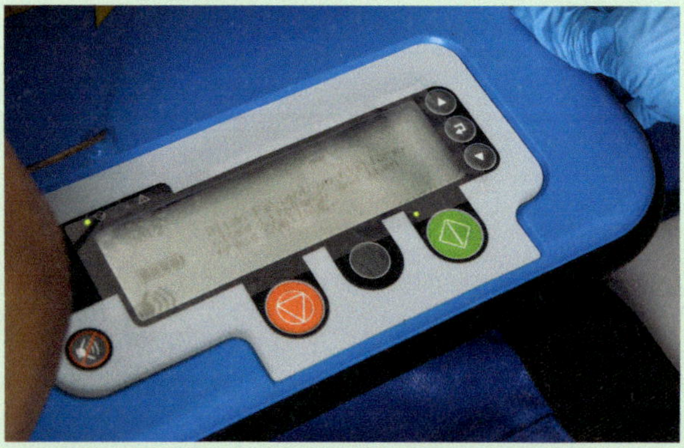	The pause allows time for the clinicians to verify correct alignment between the patient and the LifeBand.
9.	Prior to extricating the patient, the shoulder strap should be applied. Connect the black straps to the loops near the patient's head and the yellow strap to the pin close to the patient's armpits. Make sure you do not interfere with the LifeBand or over-tighten the straps.	This will help minimise displacement of the AutoPulse from the correct position.

Action		Rationale
10.	Pull down on the yellow straps of the carry sheet until it is fully unfolded. 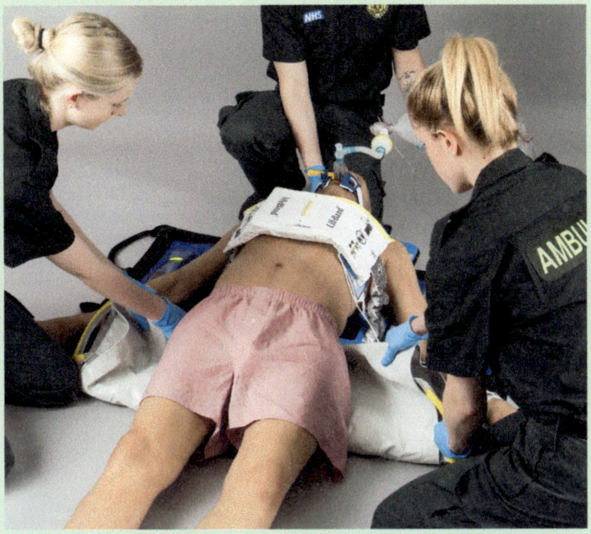 	
11.	Fasten the waist belt and prepare to move the patient. 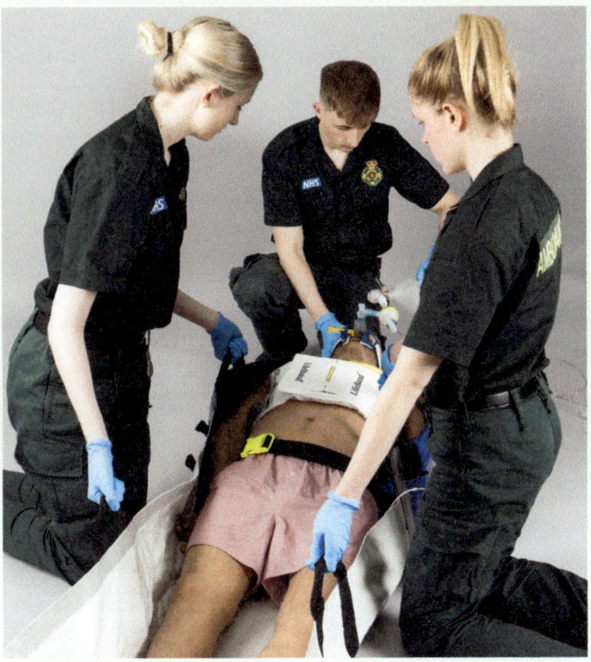 	

Action		Rationale
12.	Document the procedure.	You must keep full, clear and accurate records for everyone you care for, treat, or provide other services to (3).

References

1. Soar J, Böttiger BW, Carli P, et al. European Resuscitation Council Guidelines 2021: adult advanced life support. *Resuscitation*. 2021 Apr;161:115–151.
2. Zoll. *AutoPulse Resuscitation System Model 100 User Guide*. 7th edition. San Jose, CA: Zoll Circulation, Inc.; 2018.
3. Health and Care Professions Council. Standards of conduct, performance and ethics [Internet]. 2018 [cited 2019 Dec 29]. Available from: https://www.hcpc-uk.org/standards/standards-of-conduct-performance-and-ethics/.

Chapter 8

Infection Prevention and Control

The COVID-19 pandemic has brought infection prevention and control (IPC) into sharp focus for everyone, not just healthcare staff. However, for healthcare professionals IPC extends beyond the impact that COVID-19 has had. In 2020 it was estimated that healthcare-associated infections (HCAIs) were responsible for nearly 23,000 deaths and cost the NHS a staggering £2.1 billion annually (1).

Poor IPC practice increases the risk to both you as a clinician and to your patients. Simple things done well, such as regular hand hygiene, can substantially contribute to improving IPC and reducing HCAIs. The prehospital environment is well recognised as being a 'dirty environment', but this does not excuse poor standards of IPC. You should ensure that you practise to a high standard of IPC to protect yourself, your friends and family, your colleagues and also your patients.

Reference

1. Guest JF, Keating T, Gould D, et al. Modelling the annual NHS costs and outcomes attributable to healthcare-associated infections in England. *BMJ Open*. 2020;10(1): e033367.

Hand Hygiene with Soap and Running Water

Indications (1)

- Before touching a patient.
- Before clean or aseptic procedures.
- After body fluid exposure risk.
- After touching a patient.
- After touching patient surroundings.
- Before putting on and after removing gloves.

Contraindications

- None.

Caution

- Alcohol-based hand rubs should be used for routine hand hygiene during care to reduce the skin damage that can occur with repeated soap-based hand-washing, unless (2):
  - hands are visibly soiled or dirty
  - you are caring for patients with vomiting or diarrhoeal illnesses
  - you are caring for a patient with a suspected or known gastrointestinal infection, for example norovirus or a spore-forming organism such as *Clostridium difficile*.

Disadvantages

- Repeated hand hygiene can result in dermatitis developing (3). Use emollient hand cream regularly during breaks and when off duty.

Procedure – Hand Hygiene with Soap and Running Water

Take the following steps to wash your hands (4):

Note: This procedure assumes that you have adopted a 'bare below the elbows' dress code. The entire process should take around 40–60 seconds (5).

Action		Rationale
1.	Wet hands with water. 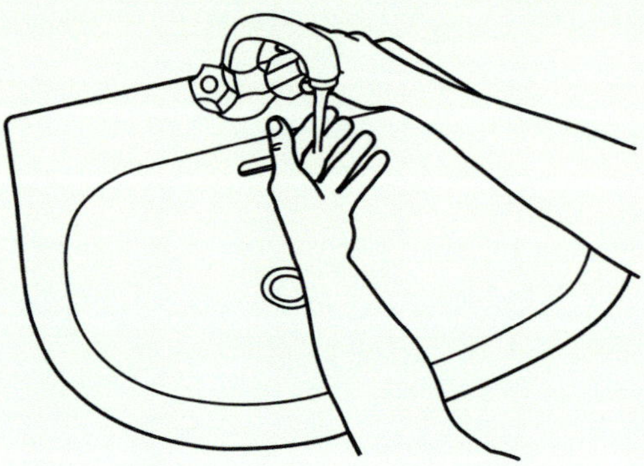	This will help the soap to lather when you rub your hands together from step 3 onwards.

	Action	Rationale
2.	Apply enough soap to cover all hand surfaces. 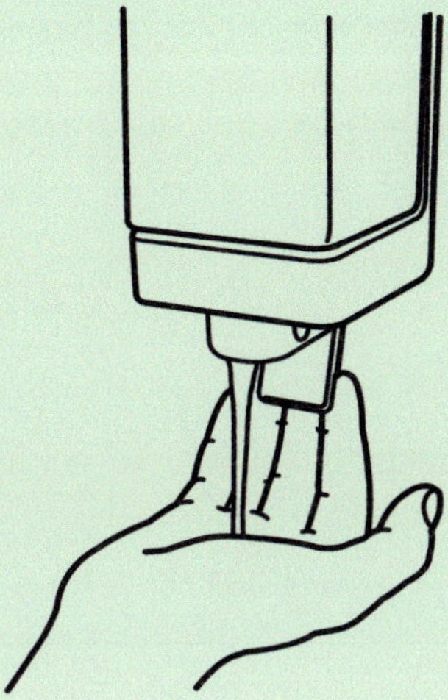	You should thoroughly cover your hands with soap prior to the process of physically cleaning for best results.
3.	Rub hands palm to palm. 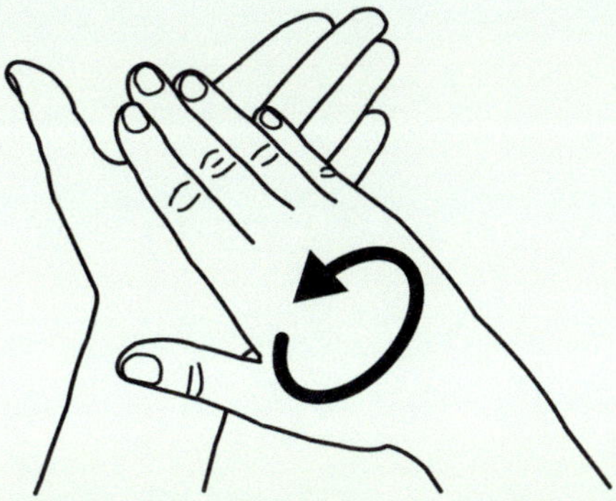	Steps 3–8 are to ensure the hands are thoroughly cleaned and areas that are commonly missed or difficult to clean, are thoroughly decontaminated.
4.	Rub your right palm over the back of the left hand with interlaced fingers and vice versa. 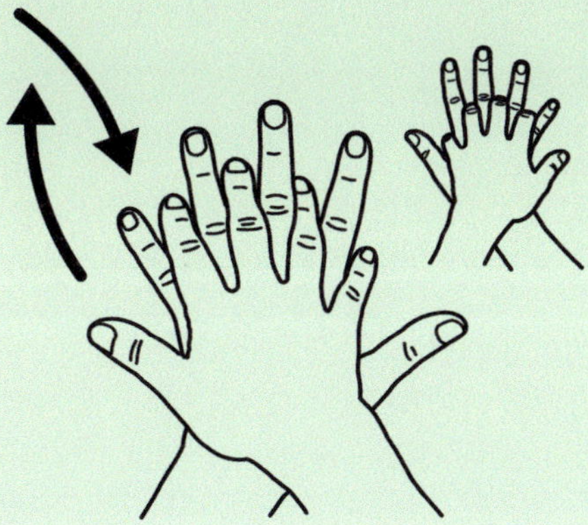	

Action		Rationale
5.	Rub palm to palm with fingers interlaced. 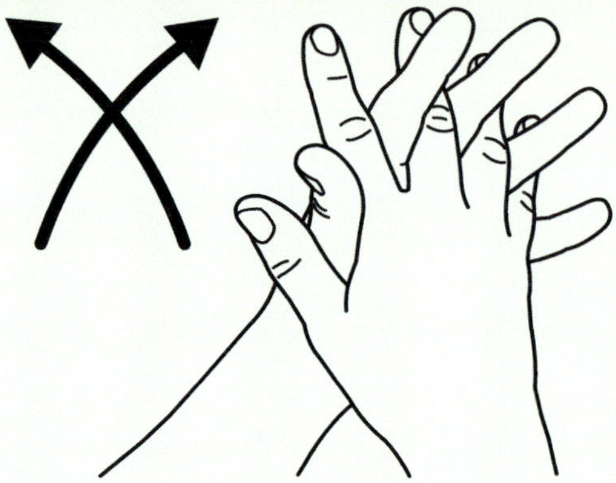	
6.	Rub the backs of your fingers to opposing palms with fingers interlocked. 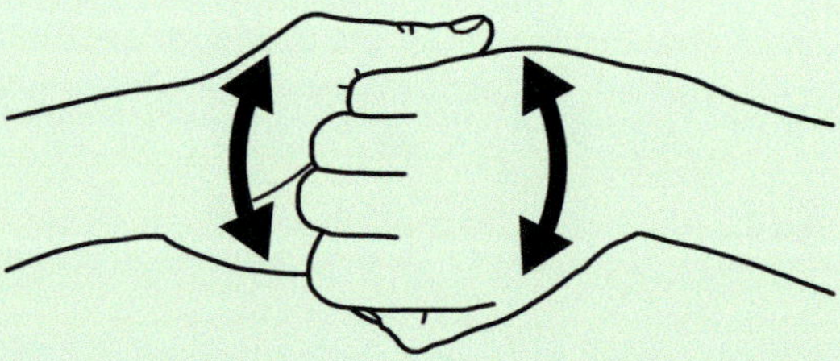	
7.	Rub the left thumb in your right palm in a rotational motion and vice versa. 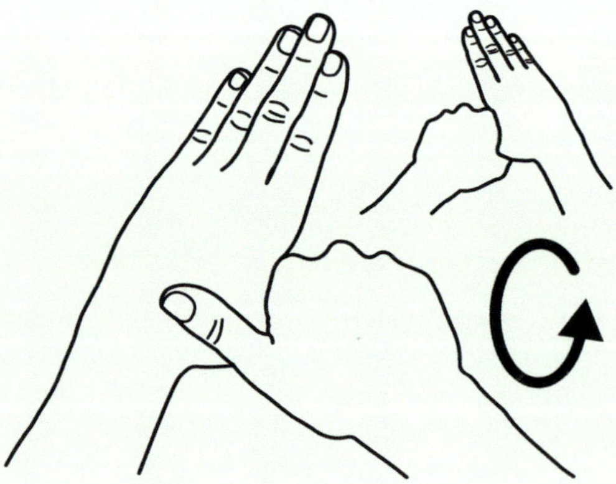	

Action		Rationale
8.	Clasp the fingers of your right hand in your left palm and rub in a rotational motion, backwards and forwards, and vice versa. 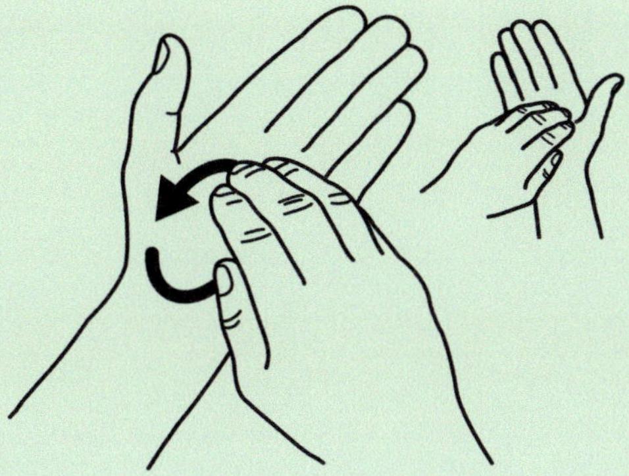	
9.	Rinse hands with water. 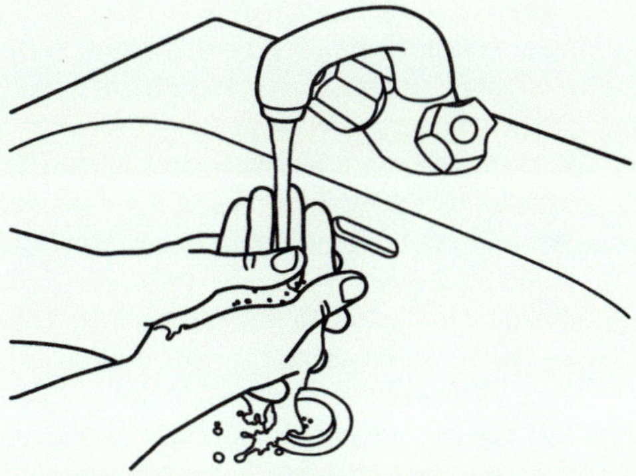	
10.	Dry thoroughly with a disposable towel. 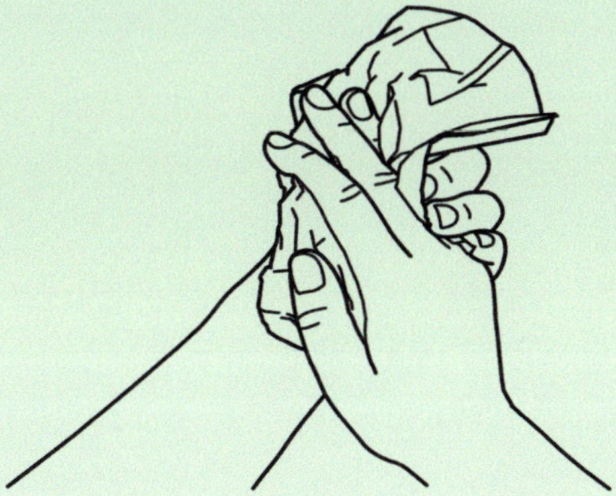	Air dryers are more likely to spread microbiological contamination than paper towels, so are no longer allowed in healthcare settings (6).

	Action	Rationale
11.	Where possible, use your elbows to turn off taps. However, if this is not possible, use a towel to turn off taps. 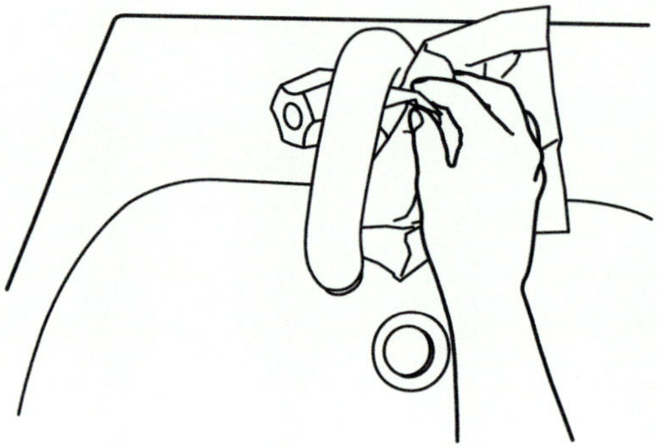	Use your elbows or a hand towel to turn off the tap to avoid touching a contaminated surface with your clean hand.

References

1. World Health Organization. Your 5 moments of hand hygiene [Internet]. 2009 [cited 2022 Aug 30]. Available from: https://cdn.who.int/media/docs/default-source/integrated-health-services-(ihs)/infection-prevention-and-control/your-5-moments-for-hand-hygiene-poster.pdf?sfvrsn=83e2fb0e_16.
2. NHS England. Hand hygiene [Internet]. 2022 [cited 2022 Jul 25]. Available from: www.england.nhs.uk/standard-infection-control-precautions-sicps/hand-hygiene/.
3. Health and Safety Executive. Dermatitis [Internet]. 2022 [cited 2022 Aug 30]. Available from: www.hse.gov.uk/skin/employ/dermatitis.htm.
4. NHS. National infection prevention and control manual for England [Internet]. 2022 [cited 2022 Aug 30]. Available from: www.england.nhs.uk/wp-content/uploads/2022/04/C1676_National-Infection-Prevention-and-Control-IPC-Manual-for-England-V-2.3.pdf.
5. World Health Organization. How to handwash? 2009 Jul [cited 2022 Aug 30]. Available from: www.who.int/docs/default-source/patient-safety/how-to-handwash-poster.pdf?sfvrsn=7004a09d_2.
6. Best EL, Parnell P, Wilcox MH. Microbiological comparison of hand-drying methods: The potential for contamination of the environment, user, and bystander. *Journal of Hospital Infection*. 2014;88(4):199–206.

Hand Hygiene with Alcohol-Based Hand Rub

Indications (1)

- Before touching a patient.
- Before cleaning or aseptic procedures.
- After body fluid exposure risk.
- After touching a patient.
- After touching patient surroundings.
- Before putting on and after removing gloves.

Contraindications

Alcohol hand rub should not be used when (2):

- hands are visibly soiled or dirty
- caring for patients with vomiting or diarrhoeal illnesses
- caring for a patient with a suspected or known gastrointestinal infection, for example norovirus or a spore-forming organism such as *Clostridium difficile*.

Disadvantages

- Repeated hand hygiene can result in dermatitis developing (3). Use emollient hand cream regularly during breaks and when off duty.

Procedure – Hand Hygiene with Alcohol-Based Hand Rub

Take the following steps to clean your hands with an alcohol-based hand rub (4):

Note: This procedure assumes that you have adopted a 'bare below the elbows' dress code. The entire process should take around 40–60 seconds (5).

Action		Rationale
1.	Apply a palmful of the product into a cupped hand and cover all surfaces. 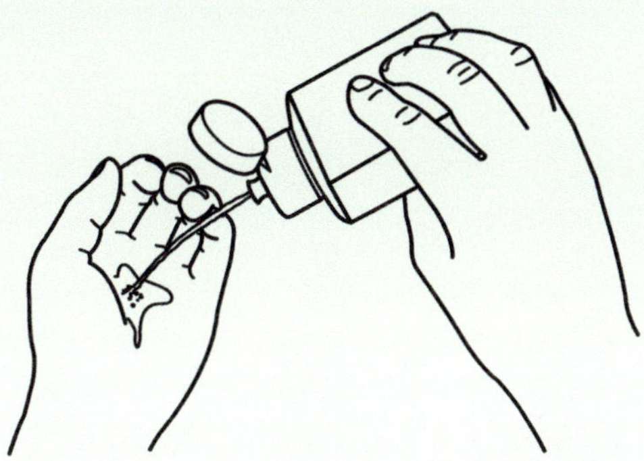	You should thoroughly cover your hands with hand rub prior to the process below to ensure effective decontamination.

<table>
<tr><th colspan="2">Action</th><th>Rationale</th></tr>
<tr><td>2.</td><td>Rub hands palm to palm.
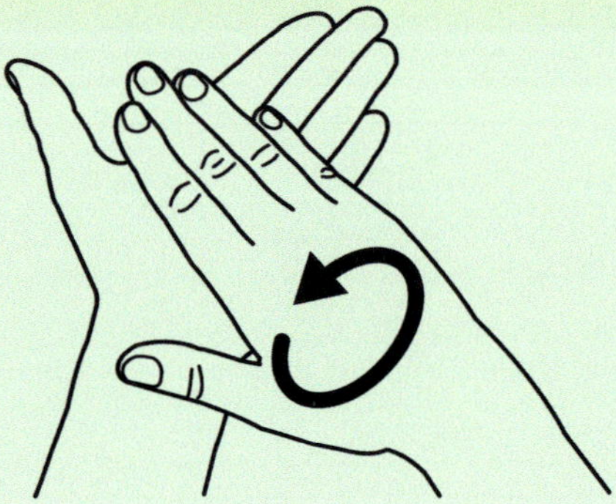</td><td>Steps 2–7 are to ensure the hands are thoroughly cleaned and areas that are commonly missed or difficult to clean are thoroughly decontaminated.</td></tr>
<tr><td>3.</td><td>Rub your right palm over the back of the left hand with interlaced fingers and vice versa.
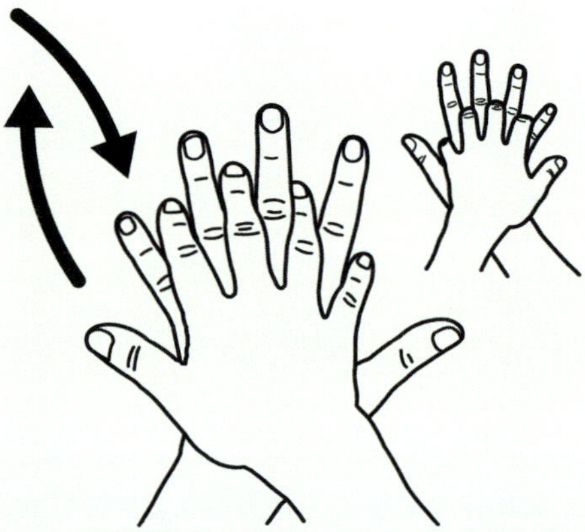</td><td></td></tr>
<tr><td>4.</td><td>Rub palm to palm with fingers interlaced.
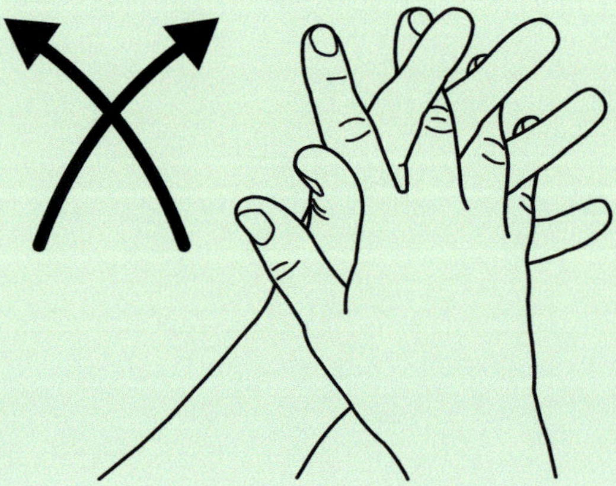</td><td></td></tr>
</table>

Action		Rationale
5.	Rub the backs of your fingers to opposing palms with fingers interlocked. 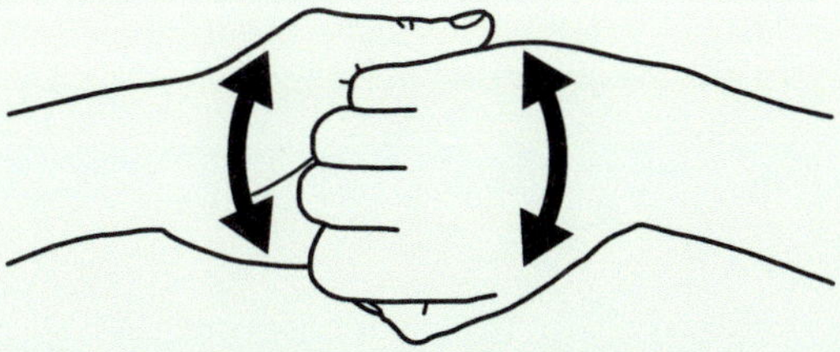	
6.	Rub the left thumb in your right palm in a rotational motion and vice versa. 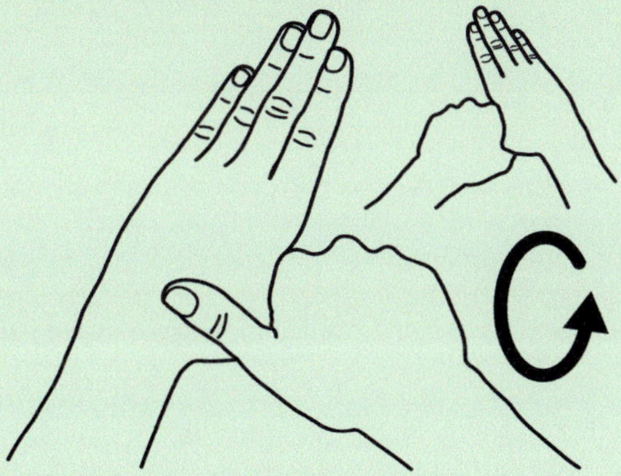	
7.	Clasp the fingers of your right hand in your left palm and rub in a rotational motion, backwards and forwards, and vice versa. 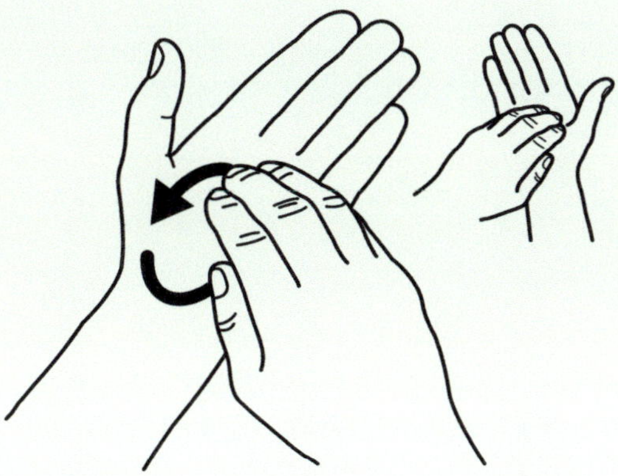	

Action		Rationale
8.	Once dry, your hands are safe. 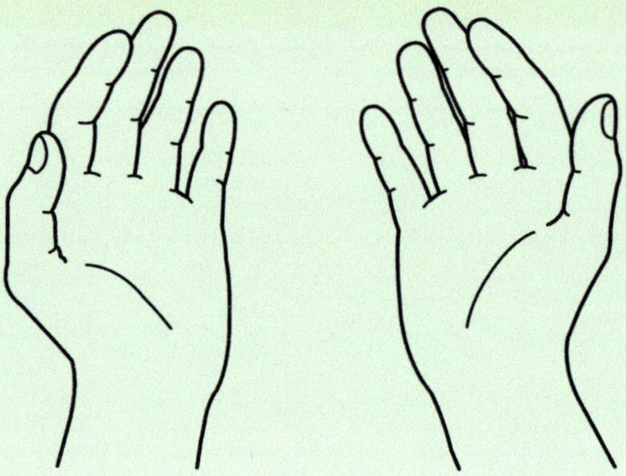	

References

1. World Health Organization. Your 5 moments of hand hygiene [Internet]. 2009 [cited 2022 Aug 30]. Available from: https://cdn.who.int/media/docs/default-source/integrated-health-services-(ihs)/infection-prevention-and-control/your-5-moments-for-hand-hygiene-poster.pdf?sfvrsn=83e2fb0e_16.
2. NHS England. Hand hygiene [Internet]. 2022 [cited 2022 Jul 25]. Available from: www.england.nhs.uk/standard-infection-control-precautions-sicps/hand-hygiene/.
3. Health and Safety Executive. Dermatitis [Internet]. 2022 [cited 2022 Aug 30]. Available from: www.hse.gov.uk/skin/employ/dermatitis.htm.
4. NHS. National infection prevention and control manual for England [Internet]. 2022 [cited 2022 Aug 30]. Available from: www.england.nhs.uk/wp-content/uploads/2022/04/C1676_National-Infection-Prevention-and-Control-IPC-Manual-for-England-version-21_July-2022.pdf.
5. World Health Organization. How to handwash? 2009 Jul [cited 2022 Aug 30]. Available from: www.who.int/docs/default-source/patient-safety/how-to-handwash-poster.pdf?sfvrsn=7004a09d_2.

Donning PPE for Standard Infection Prevention Control

Indications

- The risk of transmission of infection requires clinicians to wear personal protective equipment (PPE).

Contraindications

- Situations where PPE is not required.

Advantages

- Helps protect clinicians and patients from infection.

Disadvantages

- Can delay patient care as donning takes time.

Procedure – Donning PPE for Standard Infection Prevention Control

Take the following steps to don PPE for Standard Infection Prevention Control (1):

Action		Rationale
1.	Ensure you have the required PPE in the correct sizes. This should include: • Disposable apron • Surgical face mask • Disposable gloves • Eye protection (goggles or visor, if required) • Alcohol-based hand rub.	Prepare your PPE in sizes you know are comfortable for you before commencing donning.
2.	Remove any items from the pockets of your clothing, tie back hair and remove jewellery. Where possible, ensure you are adequately hydrated prior to donning PPE.	Items should be removed from pockets to ensure nothing is uncomfortable, as once you are in PPE, you will not be able to access your pockets. Wearing PPE can cause heavy perspiration, especially over prolonged periods.
3.	Perform hand hygiene using an alcohol-based hand rub.	This decontaminates your hands from any accidental exposure during removal of the gloves.

Action		Rationale
4.	Place your head through the neck loop of the apron and fasten the apron to your body by tying the ties behind your back. Try to cover as much of the front of your uniform as you can. 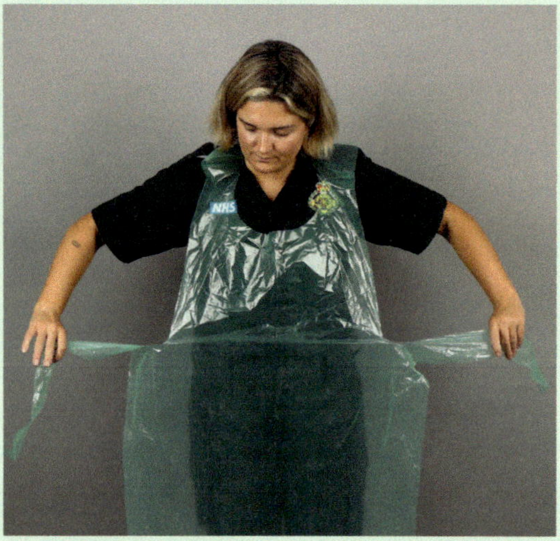	
5.	Put on the face mask: 1. Place the mask over your nose, mouth and chin. 2. If you have elastic ear loops, hook these over your ears. 3. If you have ties, tie the upper straps on the crown of your head and the lower straps at the nape of the neck. 4. Mould the nose piece over the bridge of your nose. 5. Ensure the mask extends under the chin. 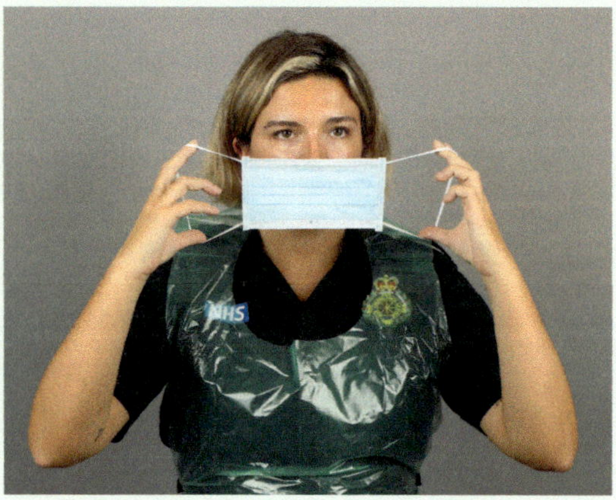	

	Action	Rationale
	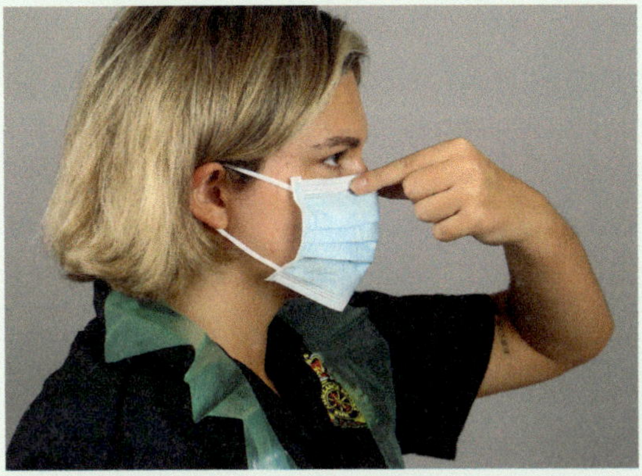	
6.	Apply eye protection and adjust as required to ensure a secure fit. 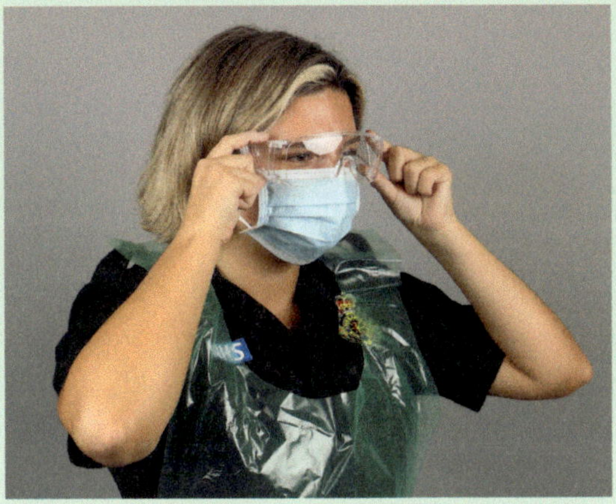	This helps protect against splashes of contaminated liquid entering the eyes. Note that prescription glasses are not considered to be eye protection.

Action		Rationale
7.	Put on disposable gloves. 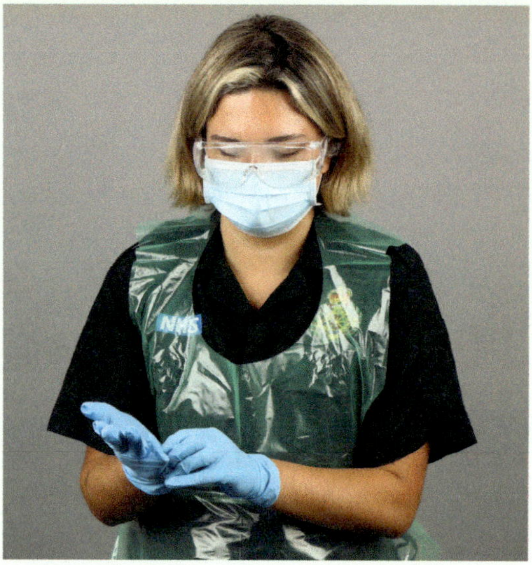 	

References

1. UK Health Security Agency. COVID-19: Personal protective equipment use for non-aerosol generating procedures [Internet]. 2022 [cited 2022 Oct 2]. Available from: https://www.gov.uk/government/publications/covid-19-personal-protective-equipment-use-for-non-aerosol-generating-procedures.

Donning PPE for Aerosol-Generating Procedures

Indications

- Performing a recognised aerosol-generating procedure (AGP).

Contraindications

- Situations where a lower level of personal protective equipment (PPE) would be appropriate.

Advantages

- Provides enhanced respiratory protection for the clinician.

Disadvantages

- Takes considerable time to don.

Procedure – Donning PPE for AGPs

Take the following steps to don PPE for AGP environments (1):

Action		Rationale
1.	Ensure you have the required PPE in the correct sizes. This should include: • Disposable coveralls • Respiratory protection • Disposable gloves • Eye protection (goggles or visor).	Prepare your PPE in sizes you know are comfortable for you before commencing donning.
2.	Remove any items from the pockets of your clothing, tie back hair and remove jewellery. Where possible, ensure you are adequately hydrated prior to donning PPE.	Items should be removed from pockets to ensure nothing is uncomfortable, as once you are in PPE you will not be able to access your pockets. Wearing PPE can cause heavy perspiration, especially over prolonged periods.
3.	Don coveralls: 1. Step into them. 2. Pull them up to your waist. 3. Insert your arms into the sleeves – if thumb holes exist in the end of the sleeves, insert your thumbs into them. 4. Pull the coveralls over your shoulder. 5. Fasten the zip all the way to the top.	Depending on availability, you may find gowns are provided instead of disposable coveralls. These can also be used for AGP protection.

Action		Rationale
	Current national recommendations suggest there is no requirement to use the hood. 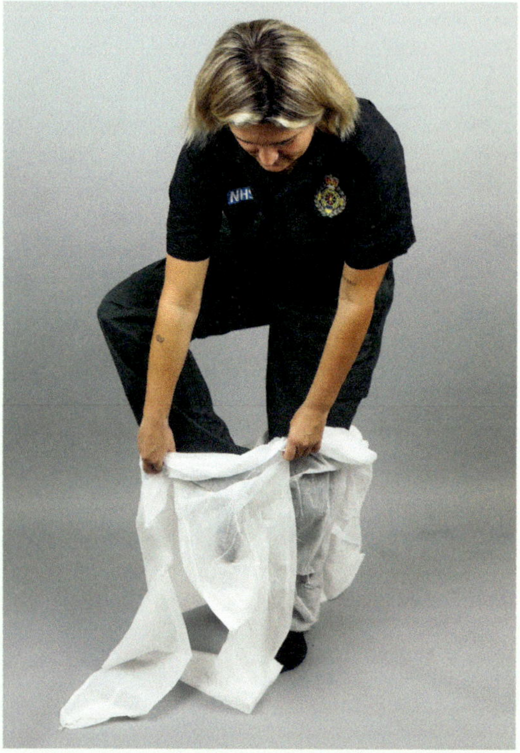 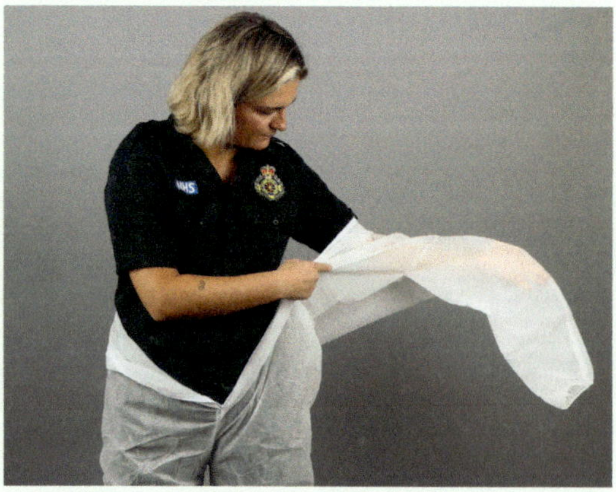	

Action		Rationale
	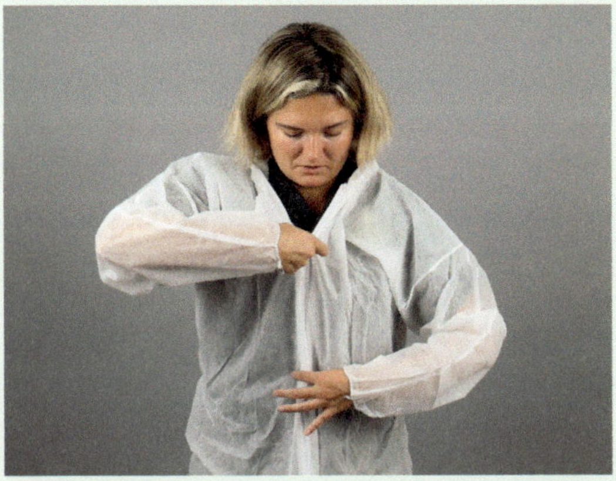	
4.	Apply an appropriate respirator, either a mask or powered hood. Ensure a secure fit by adjusting the respirator according to the manufacturer's recommendation. 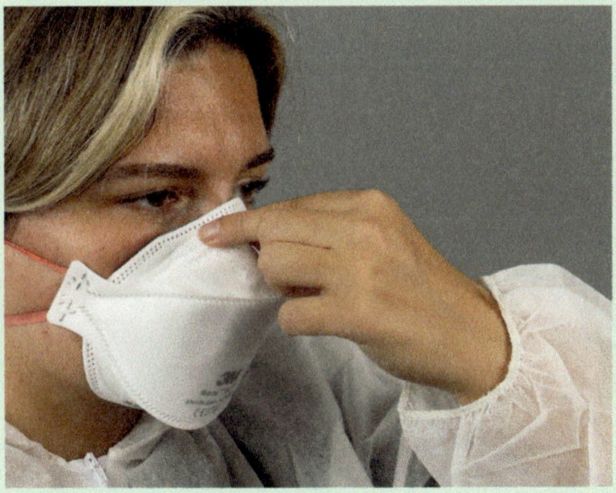	Many different masks are available, and it is not possible to describe the differences in application for them all here. You should have been fit-tested for the masks in use in your work setting, and as part of that process you should have been shown how to adjust the masks appropriately. The mask is the most important aspect of PPE against aerosolised transmission, so take time to ensure a good fit and appropriate seal.

Action		Rationale
5.	Apply eye protection and adjust as required to ensure a secure fit. 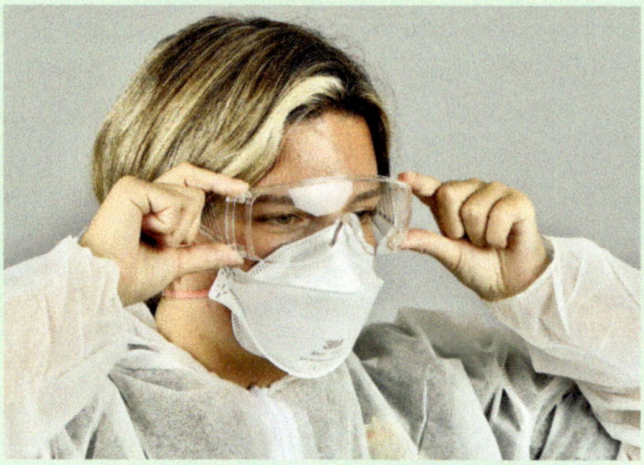	
6.	Put on disposable gloves, ensuring that the cuff of the glove covers the cuff of the coveralls. 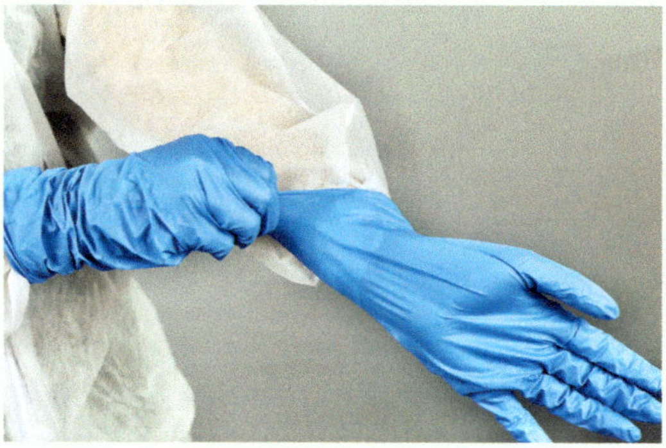	Ensuring the cuffs overlap will prevent your wrists from becoming exposed and contaminated while caring for the patient.

References

1. UK Health Security Agency. Putting on (donning) personal protective equipment (PPE) including coveralls for aerosol generating procedures (AGPs) [Internet]. 2020 [cited 2022 Aug 31]. Available from: https://assets.publishing.service.gov.uk/government/uploads/system/uploads/attachment_data/file/1020016/20200821_COVID-19_Airborne_precautions_Putting_on_PPE_coveralls.pdf.

Doffing PPE for Standard Infection Prevention Control

Indications

- Once patient care episode or procedure requiring PPE for standard infection prevention control purposes is completed.

Contraindications

- None.

Advantages

- Reduces the risk of inadvertent contamination of the clinician or other persons nearby.

Disadvantages

- Must be completed in a systematic method to ensure minimising risk of contamination.

Procedure – Doffing PPE for Standard Infection Prevention Control

Take the following steps to doff personal protective equipment (PPE) for standard Infection Prevention Control (IPC) purposes (1):

Action		Rationale
1.	Plan your movements: gloves, aprons and eye protection should be removed prior to leaving the ambulance or the patient's immediate environment. Face masks should be removed after you have left the environment.	Reduce risk of spreading contaminants to other areas or personnel.
2.	Grasp the outside of a glove with the opposite gloved hand and peel off. Hold the removed glove in the hand that is still wearing a glove. 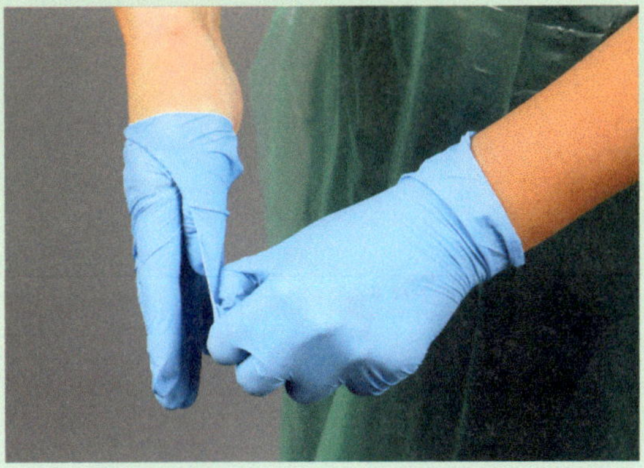	

	Action	Rationale
3.	Slide a finger from the ungloved hand under the wrist of the gloved hand, hook the glove and peel it off over the glove being held in the hand. 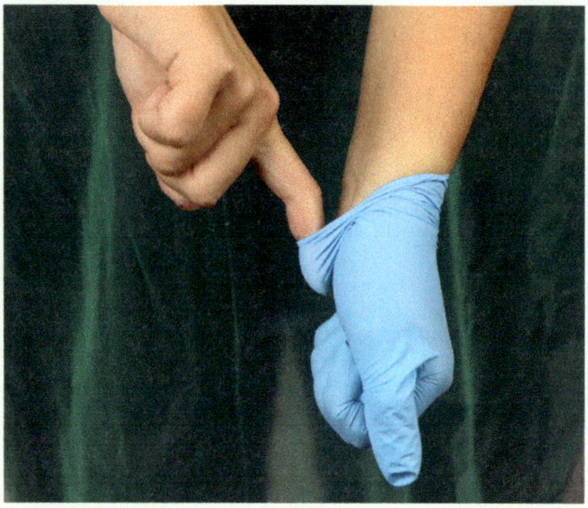 Discard both gloves into a clinical waste bag.	This process minimises the risk of touching the contaminated surface of the gloves.
4.	Perform hand hygiene using an alcohol-based hand rub.	This decontaminates your hands from any accidental exposure during removal of the gloves.
5.	Remove the disposable apron: 1. Unfasten or break apron ties at the neck. 2. Let the apron fall forwards to fold onto itself. 3. Break the ties at the waist. 4. Fold the apron in on itself. 5. Roll up apron sufficiently so that it can be discarded easily. 6. Dispose of apron into clinical waste. 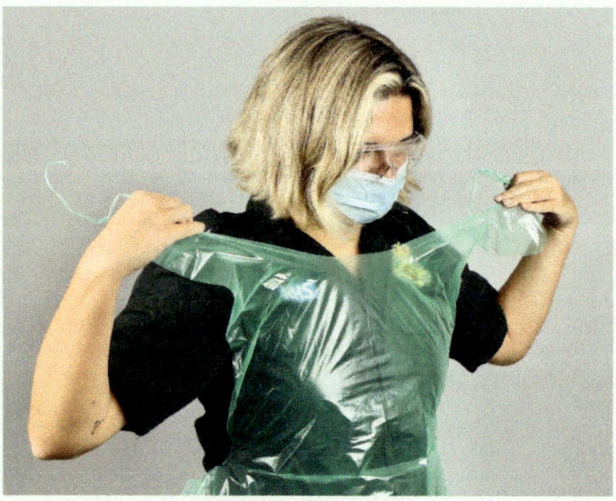	This method should ensure you do not touch the outside of the apron and contaminate yourself.

Action		Rationale
	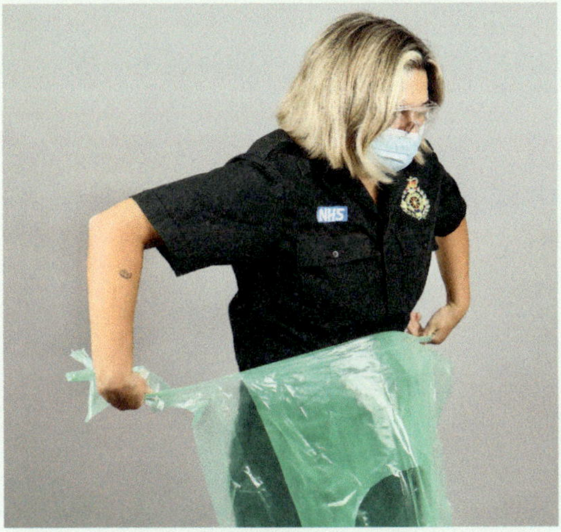 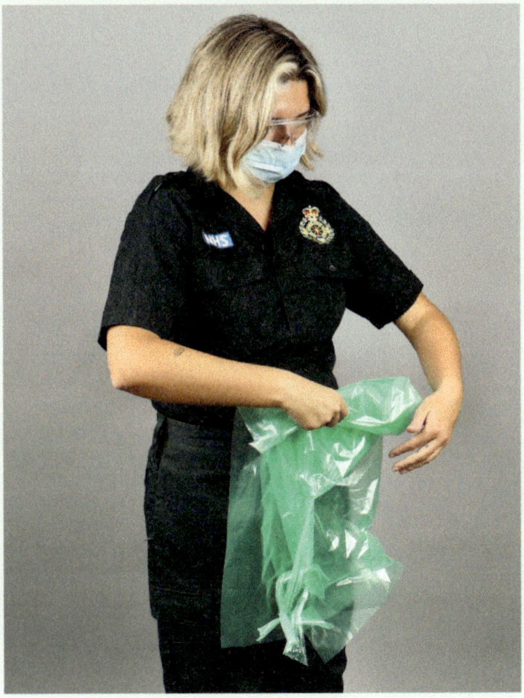	

	Action	Rationale
6.	Remove eye protection by holding both arms of the eye protection, then lift and pull it away from your face. 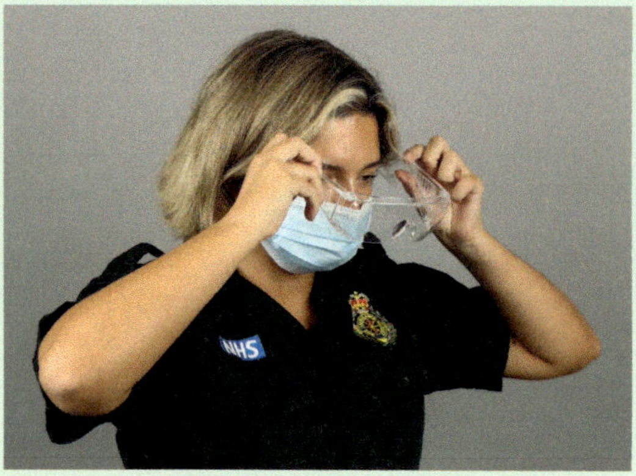	
7.	Dispose of eye protection into clinical waste.	
8.	Perform hand hygiene using an alcohol-based hand rub.	This decontaminates your hands from any accidental exposure during removal of the eye protection.
9.	Once outside of the ambulance or the patient's immediate environment, remove the surgical face mask: 1. Untie or break bottom ties. 2. Untie or break top ties. 3. Handling the mask by the ties only, lean forward and pull mask away from your face. 4. Dispose of the mask into clinical waste. 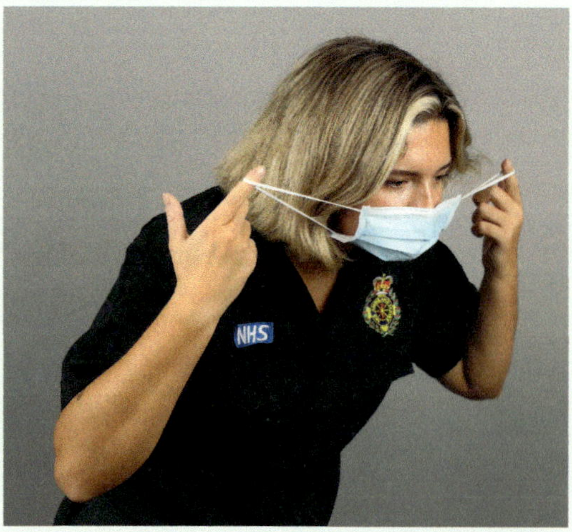	This process allows careful removal of the mask without contaminating your face. Note that if your mask has elastic loops, you can hook your fingers under the elastic and stretch the loops instead of breaking them.

Action		Rationale
10.	Perform hand hygiene with soap and water if available; if not, use an alcohol-based hand rub.	This decontaminates your hands from any accidental exposure.

References

1. UK Health Security Agency. COVID-19: Personal protective equipment use for non-aerosol generating procedures [Internet]. 2022 [cited 2022 Oct 2]. Available from: https://www.gov.uk/government/publications/covid-19-personal-protective-equipment-use-for-non-aerosol-generating-procedures.

Doffing PPE for Aerosol-Generating Procedures

Indications

- When leaving an environment where aerosol-generating procedures (AGPs) have been performed.

Contraindications

- Do not remove the respirator while still in proximity to the patient.

Advantages

- Reduces the risk of inadvertent contamination of the clinician or other persons nearby.

Disadvantages

- Must be completed in a systematic method to ensure risk of contamination is minimised.
- Takes time to undertake properly.

Procedure – Doffing PPE for AGPs

Take the following steps to doff personal protective equipment (PPE) for AGP environments (1):

Action		Rationale
1.	Move away from the patient. In the community this may mean outside a property (though not the back of the ambulance as this may contaminate it). In hospital there is likely to be a dedicated doffing area.	You must be in a safe environment when you remove your PPE, but also consider the risk of contaminating areas during your doffing. Outside in a well-ventilated space is ideal, but you should not doff in a rainy environment.
2.	Grasp the outside of a glove with the opposite gloved hand and peel off. Hold the removed glove in the hand that still wears a glove. 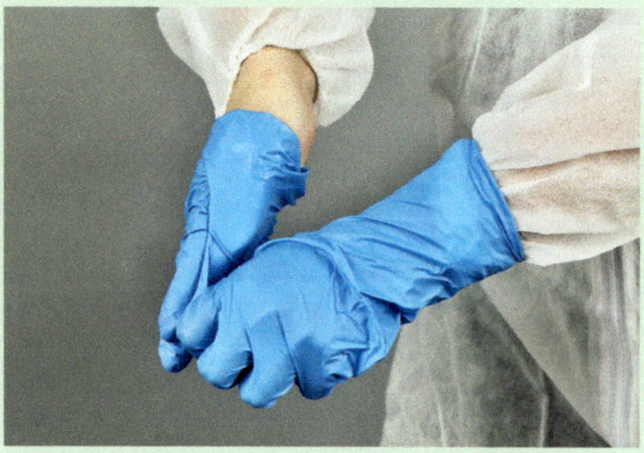	

	Action	Rationale
3.	Slide a finger from the ungloved hand under the wrist of the gloved hand, hook the glove and peel it off over the glove being held in the hand. 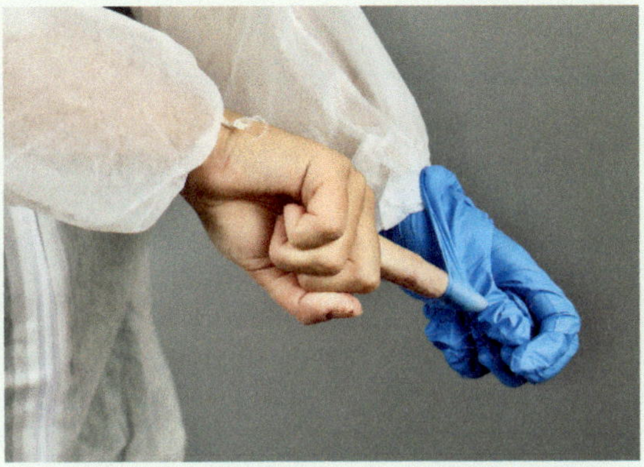 Dispose of both gloves into a clinical waste bag.	This process minimises the risk of touching the contaminated surface of the gloves.
4.	Perform hand hygiene using an alcohol-based hand rub.	This decontaminates your hands from any accidental exposure during removal of the gloves.
5.	Remove the coveralls from top to bottom: 1. Tilt your head back and pull the coveralls away from your body. 2. Unzip the coveralls without touching any skin, clothes or uniform. 3. Free your shoulders and pull your arms out. 4. Roll the coveralls from the waist down and from the inside of the coveralls all the way to the shoes, taking care to only touch the inside of the coveralls. 5. Use one shoe-covered foot to pull off the coveralls from the other leg and repeat for the second leg. 6. Step away from the coveralls and dispose of them into clinical waste.	This process of only touching the inside of the coveralls and rolling them so that the exposed surface is continually covered reduces the risk of transmission and contamination.

	Action	Rationale
	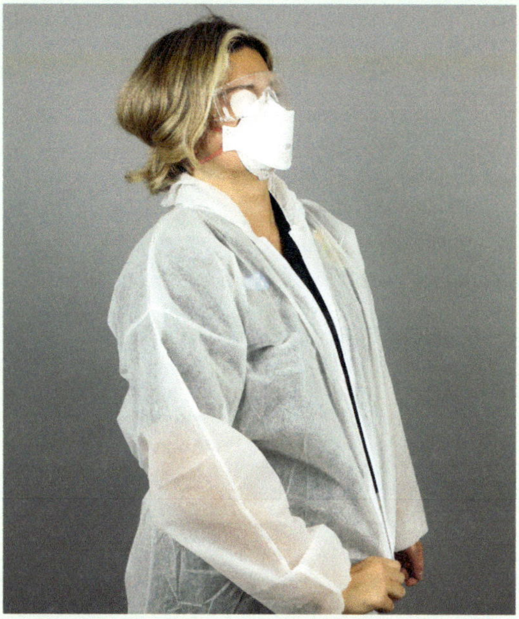 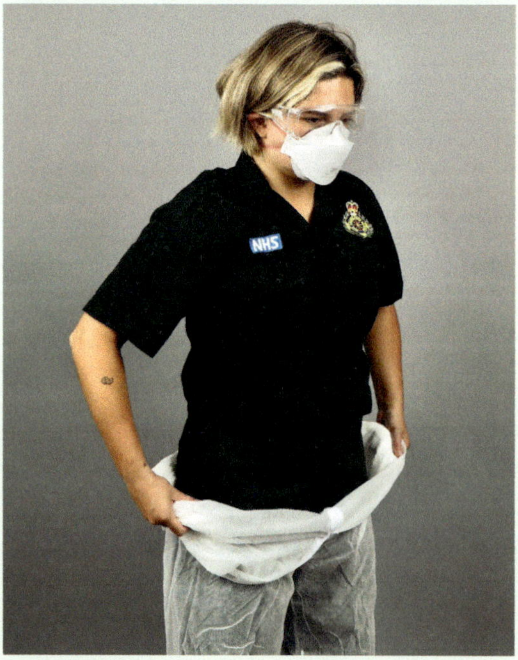	
6.	Perform hand hygiene using an alcohol-based hand rub.	This decontaminates your hands from any accidental exposure during removal of the coveralls.

<table>
<tr><th colspan="2">Action</th><th>Rationale</th></tr>
<tr><td>7.</td><td>Remove eye protection and dispose of it into a clinical waste bin.
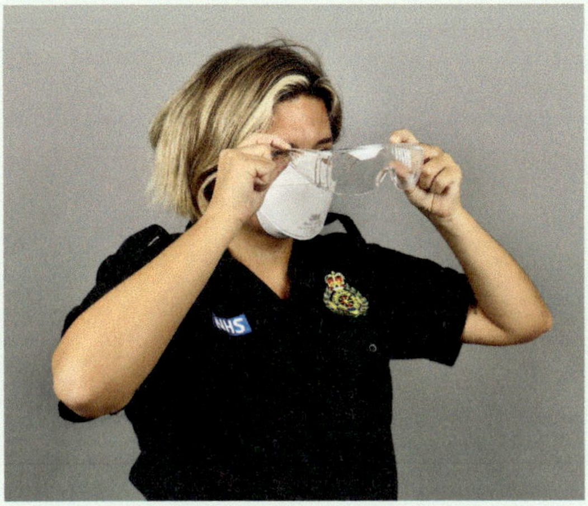</td><td></td></tr>
<tr><td>8.</td><td>Perform hand hygiene using an alcohol-based hand rub.</td><td>This decontaminates your hands from any accidental exposure during removal of the eye protection.</td></tr>
<tr><td>9.</td><td>Remove the respirator.
Different devices will have different requirements, but in general for a mask:
1. Lean slightly forwards.
2. Reach to the back of the head with both hands, feel for the bottom strap and bring it up to the top strap.
3. Lift both straps over your head.
4. Allow the respirator to fall away from your face and dispose of it into a clinical waste bin.
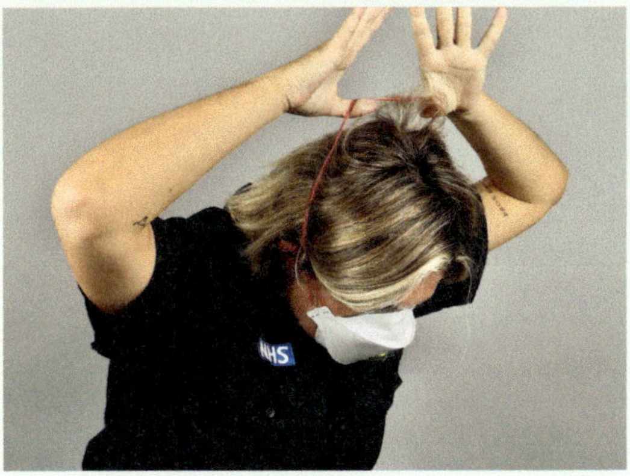</td><td>This process allows careful removal of the respirator without contaminating your face.</td></tr>
</table>

Action		Rationale
	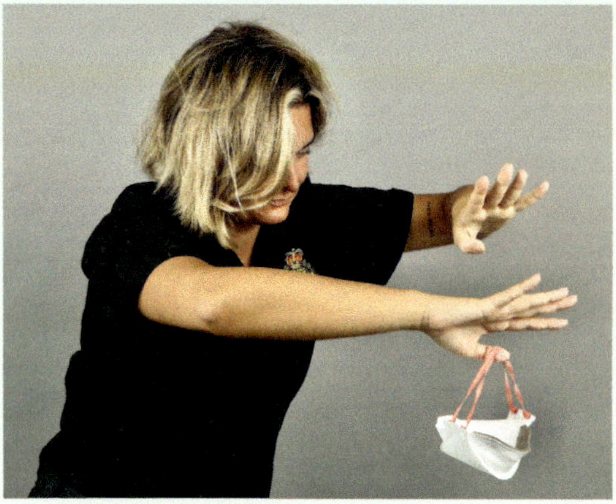	
10.	Perform hand hygiene with soap and water if available; if not, use an alcohol-based hand rub.	This decontaminates your hands from any accidental exposure.

References

1. UK Health Security Agency. Removing (doffing) personal protective equipment (PPE) including coveralls for aerosol generating procedures (AGPs) [Internet]. 2020 [cited 2022 Aug 31]. Available from: https://assets.publishing.service.gov.uk/government/uploads/system/uploads/attachment_data/file/1020078/20200821_COVID-19_Airborne_precautions_Removing_PPE_coveralls.pdf.

Index

NOTE: Page numbers followed by *f* denote figures.